D1718669

Personalized Nutrition for the Diverse Needs of Infants and Children

Nestlé Nutrition Workshop Series
Pediatric Program, Vol. 62

Personalized Nutrition for the Diverse Needs of Infants and Children

Editors

Dennis M. Bier, Houston, TX, USA
J. Bruce German, Davis, CA, USA
Bo Lönnerdal, Davis, CA, USA

KARGER

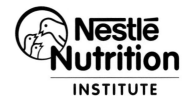

Nestec Ltd., 55 Avenue Nestlé, CH–1800 Vevey (Switzerland)
S. Karger AG, P.O. Box, CH–4009 Basel (Switzerland)   www.karger.com

Printed in Switzerland on acid-free and non-aging paper (ISO 9706) by Reinhardt Druck, Basel
ISBN 978–3–8055–8553–8
ISSN 1661–6677

Library of Congress Cataloging-in-Publication Data

Nestlé Nutrition Workshop (62nd : 2007 : Helsinki, Finland)
    Personalized nutrition for the diverse needs of infants and children / editors, Dennis M. Bier, J. Bruce German, Bo Lönnerdal.
       p. ; cm. – (Nutrition workshop series pediatric program, ISSN 1661–6677 ; v. 62)
    Includes bibliographical references and index.
    ISBN 978–3–8055–8553–8 (hard cover : alk. paper)
1.   Infants–Nutrition–Genetic aspects–Congresses.   2. Children–Nutrition–Genetic aspects–Congresses.   3. Infants–Nutrition–Requirements–Congresses.   4. Children–Nutrition–Requirements–Congresses.   5. Human genetics–Variation–Congresses.   I. Bier, Dennis M.   II. German, J. Bruce. III.   Lönnerdal, Bo, 1938–   IV. Nestlé Nutrition Institute.   V. Title.   VI. Series: Nestlé Nutrition workshop series. Paediatric programme ; v.   62.
    [DNLM: 1.   Child Nutrition Physiology–genetics–Congresses.   2.   Infant Nutrition Physiology–genetics–Congresses.   3. Nutritional Requirements–Congresses. 4.   Variation (Genetics)–physiology–Congresses. W1 NE228D v.62 2008 / WS 115 N468p 2008]
    RJ216.N473 2008
    618.92′39–dc22

                                    2008021123

Basel · Freiburg · Paris · London · New York · Bangalore · Bangkok · Shanghai · Singapore · Tokyo · Sydney

Contents

Contents

Preface

The field of nutrition is building the basic science necessary to produce a revolutionary shift in agriculture and public health, moving from dietary guidelines for populations to foods and diets for individuals. Considerable epidemiologic and mechanistic research has documented that humans respond differently to diets and display varying predispositions to many diet-dependent metabolic and degenerative diseases. The field of *nutrigenomics* is emerging with the goal of assigning this human diversity in nutritional response to diet and the subsequent consequences to human health to specific genetic elements. At the same time, breakthroughs in our understanding of developmental biology and the importance of diet to early human maturation and lifelong health have emphasized that diet is itself a critical determinant of human diversity. These two major emerging trends in nutrition converge on one life stage and one issue: how different are humans as infants and children with respect to nutritional needs and responses to diet? International experts in various fields whose research work interfaces with the nutrition of infants and children came together in Helsinki, Finland, for a workshop to address this critical subject to human health. The workshop focused on 4 clear questions.

How do children differ?
The first scientific issue addressed by the workshop was the most fundamental and yet the most bold: how do children differ? Just how much diversity is there in the human population as infants and what is the nature of important differences with respect to dietary needs? This question was separated into various determinants of biological variation: genetic diversity; environmental inputs; prior imprinting, and resident microflora. Unquestionably there are important genetic variations among humans that lead to unique nutritional requirements. The issue is how many children in the population experience deleterious consequences in their immediate and long-term health due to diets unmatched to their genetic makeup? Surprisingly with the tools of modern genomics it can be seen that many infants and children are distinguishable as genetically at risk for particular diets. From the well-known disease phenylketonuria to inborn errors of metabolism and genetic predispositions for allergies, although the absolute proportion of the population is small, the numbers of children affected are significant.

Preface

The environments into which infants arrive and within which infants grow and develop are improving throughout the world, yet discouragingly in much of the world environmental conditions are threatening the optimal health of young children. Pathogen and allergen exposure, nutrient quality of indigenous diets and the presence and timing of vaccination are now recognized to be environmental variables that can translate into diverse outcomes in children's health. The implications of these environmental variables are profound. The tools of genomics are enabling scientists to understand the regulation of developmental patterning in biology and with this understanding has come the means to document the mechanisms by which early environments imprint individual organisms. From a nutritional perspective, it is becoming increasingly clear that early dietary effects prior to and immediately after birth can persist throughout the lives of individual humans.

The largest reservoir of genes in humans are not their own genome but the genomes of the thousands of bacteria that co-habit the human intestine and body surfaces. For the infant, birth is the emergence from a sterile environment into this cacophony of microbial colonizers. During the first few hours and days, the infant must become reconciled to peaceful coexistence with an ecological population of microorganisms numbering ten times its own cell numbers. Science still does not understand how this process takes place, nor all of the consequences of the varying success that different infants achieve. Remarkably, for each of us, these bacterial ecosystems once established in infancy remain relatively constant throughout life. In a strictly cellular sense, our environment is largely defined by these bacteria.

What are the consequences of these differences?

The workshop then addressed the critical pragmatic question: what are the immediate and long-term consequences of these various sources of individual difference? Are some children faced with important negative consequences of diets that are designed for the average or population mean and further, are some children limited in their future potential by diets that are considered appropriate for the average? Perhaps the most important and yet least understood of the bodily processes is the successful development of *immunity*. The rapid establishment of innate immunity is more variable than previously thought, with clear differences in the ability of different individuals to mount an immediate protective response to pathogens. Further, the timing and diversity of acquired immunity is not solely the consequence of diversity of exposure, but varies with genotypic determinants and with critical environmental cues, not the least of which are the colonizing bacteria in and on the developing infant. In addition to varying susceptibilities to pathogen invasion, intestinal disease and the success of its resolution, many infants are now recognized to carry genetic predispositions to the immunological failures that lead to *allergy*. Genetics, however, cannot account for the astonishing rise in allergic and autoimmune diseases throughout the world during the past 50 years. These increases must be assigned to changes in environmental factors acting upon a background of genetic susceptibilities. Varying outcomes in immune protection and autoimmune diseases are not the only aspects of health that are being documented to be on the rise in the world's infants and children. Metabolic dysregulation and its most visible signpost *obesity* has been frustrating health researchers around the world as it is seen to be moving inexorably into younger and younger children. Scientific mechanisms and epidemiological data together point to the conclusion that early diets in some infants are both promoting excess weight gain as children, but establishing a phenotype that persists throughout adult life. The most recent research has even more disturbing implications. Obesity in this generation's children carries greater risk of other metabolic consequences than the same apparent 'level' of obesity in previous generations. The progression in children and adolescents towards a broad range of metabolic disturbances is unprecedented in recorded human history. If these trends continue, a substantial number of adults will transition to type-2 *diabetes* as young adults. The potential for early diets to alter the basic mechanisms of infant and childhood development through several mechanisms ranging from methylation of chromosomal DNA to alteration of endogenous microflora has many other implications than metabolic regulation. Many cellular processes of immunity, protection, tissue proliferation and cellular elimination are known in simpler biological systems to be modified during development. If these basic processes are acting similarly in humans, early infant diets and their effects on these persistent developmental mechanisms could alter many diseases of late adulthood including heart disease, neurodegeneration and cancer. Interestingly, the implications of these developmental changes would even extend to altering the responses of individuals to standard therapeutic approaches for these diseases once established.

Can we accurately assess differences?

Participants at the workshop explored the next logical steps in bringing scientific knowledge to effective practice and intervention. Is it possible with currently available diagnostic and measurement technologies to assess the differences between infants and children that are the basis of these health outcomes prior to the deterioration of their health? The possibilities for measuring human diversity are quite broad ranging from cellular, tissue and whole body imaging to detailed analysis of constituent molecules in biofluids even to genotyping. The technologies of medical imaging have reached remarkable capabilities in providing spatial information on biological structures and processes. The attendees at the workshop were treated to a literal view of the visual future that imaging of humans will provide medical sciences for the treatment of disease. The workshop participants then considered the question: can these imaging approaches, so successful in delivering diagnostic accuracy to disease management, provide equally valuable insights into the personal variations that anticipate disease? The key issues that must be resolved include not only spatial precision but chemical accuracy. The variations among healthy infants and children are subtle and it is still not known which of the differences that are measurable are indeed associated with important variations in subsequent health. The tools necessary for genotyping individuals are moving forward rapidly and only time stands in the way of being able to genotype every individual. However, knowing an individual's genome does not translate immediately into the knowledge of what the variations mean for the multiple interactions between diet and health. The field of nutrigenomics is building this knowledge and there is much knowledge to build but relatively few scientists engaged. The difficulties posed by sequencing of entire genomes unfortunately do not end there. With the new knowledge that during development each individual's DNA is specifically methylated and that the pattern of methylation is both sensitive to diet and influences subsequent response to diet poses a dilemma for human assessment. If the pattern of methylation of an individual's DNA is important to their diet and health, can these methylation patterns be measured? The workshop explored the technologies that have emerged that are capable of such analyses and, indeed, it is possible to accurately measure DNA methylation at a research level. Only time will be required to translate these techniques into routine tools of human measurement. However, once again, interpreting patterns into accurate predictions of future health is a massive research challenge. The more direct evaluations of genetic variation include gene expression profiling or transcriptomics, protein expression, proteomics or metabolite distributions, metabolomics. Transcriptomic analyses are capable of becoming a routine component of disease management and the example of stratifying cancer patients for therapeutics based on straightforward expression patterns provides a vivid proof of principle. Proteomic technologies are not as well developed, nonetheless their application to disease is equally appropriate. It is not yet clear whether either technology is capable of providing the accuracy and precision necessary to resolve the subtle differences between healthy infants. This basic question has indeed been answered for metabolic profiling, albeit for a small proportion of children and a small number of metabolites. The principle of measuring concentrations of metabolites in infant blood as a means of distinguishing those with diet-dependent metabolic dysregulation is already a worldwide system of blood spot analyses. Currently used for genetically based inborn errors of metabolism whose phenotype makes certain diets toxic such as phenylketonuria, the potential of this simple technology to revolutionize the management of infant and childhood diet management is apparent.

Can we act on these differences?

The workshop finally addressed the most central and defining question for nutrition as a science: knowing that infants and children differ in their responses to diet and that these differences imply that diets delivered during infancy and childhood could improve the lives of these individuals, do we know what diets they should be guided to? The participants took the various nutrient classes in turn to examine where we stand, what we know and what we still need to know. The simple abundance of protein in the early diets of infants has emerged as a focus of considerable attention in the search for factors that could explain imprinting to predisposition of obesity. With the massive variations in protein sequence and the ability of proteins to interact biologically with different intestinal targets, with the tendency of this same sequence variation to lead to diversity of subsequent peptide fragments released during digestion and with the capability of proteins and peptides to conjugate with and bind virtually all other nutrient classes, it is clear that we have just begun to explore proteins as components capable of influencing development. Lipids have been the subject of intensive research due to the potential of polyunsaturated fatty acids to influence the development of infant neurological tissues and the obvious implications for long-term cognitive functions. While the simple presence of the different families of polyunsaturated fatty acids was long thought to be sufficient, breakthrough research on variations in humans are suggesting that differences in requirements can be traced to infant genetics, maternal phenotype during pregnancy and even infant microflora. Nutrition scientists have invested in decades of research to establish quantitative recommendations for the various micronutrients required by infants and children. Underpinning this global mandate was the assumption that all infants have the same quantitative requirements for all of these micronutrients. Groundbreaking research is beginning to cast doubt on this basic assumption. In fact, iron supplements in particular at the same dose may be highly beneficial to some children in one circumstance and yet deleterious to other children in other circumstances. Examining the consequences of evolution on the components of human milk produced by mammary biosynthesis during lactation has revealed a remarkable class of biologically active compounds, oligosaccharides. What is remarkable about this class of molecules is that they are apparently most biologically active not to the human infant that cannot digest them but to the bacteria inhabiting the intestine of the infant for whom they are astonishingly selective as a fermentation source. With the realization that human milk is highly concentrated in a class of molecules whose principle purpose is to nourish the endogenous microflora of infants, the implications of the bacteria themselves is becoming inescapable. Should all children be inoculated with the same bacteria, with different bacteria at different life stages, or should each individual's microflora be considered a personal choice?

Recommendations for future research

After 3 days of intensive discussion, the workshop participants arrived at the obvious point of decision: what recommendations should be made for scientists and for the industries whose products feed infants and children? Research and epidemiological data are quite convincing, waiting until adulthood to attempt to resolve metabolic and immunologic problems of disease progression is not appropriate. It is critical to act as early as possible to improve the health in each individual. Scientists studying the nutritional implications of diets for infants need to be brought together with all the tools of modern life sciences. Also, nutrition scientists need to guide and validate the technologies of human assessment for *infants and children*. These technologies can then be brought to clinical trials to build accurate databases of infant and childhood health. Within those trials, scientists should include the perspective that differences between children, not just their common biological processes, are critical to the ability to discriminate endpoints. Finally, the ongoing issue of the nutrition field needs to be reconciled for studies on children every bit as much as for all ages. Nutrition desperately needs to gain control of its independent variable: food. Studies need to measure and report in detail the ingredients used as input variables.

For the Industries that are actively involved in developing foods for infants and children, the recommendations are equally compelling. Their ability to provide standardized and compositionally defined diets for multiple clinical trials should be advanced as one of the most immediate and yet powerful and unifying principles for nutrition research. For the near future, however, as assessment technologies provide the means to distinguish differences among infants and children, industries must be able to provide parallel technologies capable of metering distinct diets to each individual with compositions and concentrations appropriate to their metabolic, physiological or nutritional needs.

D.M. Bier
J.B. German
B. Lönnerdal

Foreword

With the completion of the human genome sequence just a few years ago, it is most interesting to note that 99.9% of the genetic information is similar in all humans; it is the remaining 0.1% that varies and which makes each of us individual. Epigenetic studies have demonstrated that variation in nutrient requirements depends upon individual variations in genes which can affect nutrient metabolism. It was in this context, that the 62nd Nestlé Nutrition Workshop was dedicated to 'Personalized Nutrition for the Diverse Needs of Infants and Children' and took place in Helsinki, Finland, on September 2–6, 2007.

This was the first workshop within the 27-year history of the Nestlé Nutrition Workshops – Pediatric Program that addressed personalized nutrition in infants and young children. Individuality was discussed at the genetic, biochemical, environmental, metabolic and nutritional levels. The first food in life, breast milk, has been reported to dynamically vary between mothers, between feeds and during the lactation period. This natural individualized nutritional concept can explain in part the differences of growth pattern between breastfed and formula-fed infants. By gradually changing the composition of infant formula in a manner similar to that of breast milk, it may be possible to come closer to the goal of achieving similar growth and development of formula-fed infants relative to those which are breastfed. Bioactive factors, such as prebiotics and probiotics were discussed in the context of mimicking nature's example, breast milk. Additionally, factors that distort 'healthy' development, such as gene defects leading to inherited diseases, or epigenetic factors that can influence individual susceptibility to obesity and type-2 diabetes/insulin resistance were emphasized. Key questions during the workshop were during which time window modification of the effects can be possible, and to which extent nutrition and its personalization can contribute to optimal growth and development.

We wish to warmly thank the three chairpersons of this workshop, *Dennis M. Bier, J. Bruce German* and *Bo Lönnerdal* for establishing an exciting scientific workshop program. Many thanks also to *Annette Järvi* and her team from Nestlé Nutrition Nordics for the excellent logistic support and for enabling the workshop participants to enjoy the charm of Finnish culture.

Foreword

Our special thanks go to *Denis Barclay* who has coordinated the last five Nestlé Nutrition Workshops. He will move as scientific advisor for adult nutrition and enrich the Nestlé Nutrition Institute activities.

Prof. Ferdinand Haschke, MD, PhD
Chairman
Nestlé Nutrition Institute
Vevey, Switzerland

Dr. Petra Klassen, PhD
Scientific Advisor
Nestlé Nutrition Institute
Vevey, Switzerland

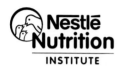

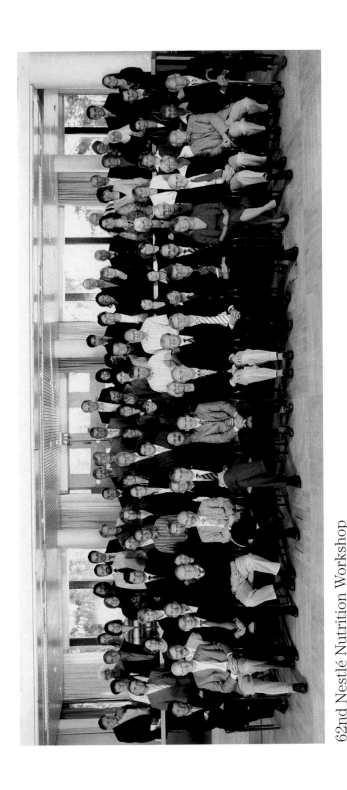

62nd Nestlé Nutrition Workshop
Pediatric Program
Helsinki, Finland, September 2–6, 2007

Contributors

Chairpersons & Speakers

Dr. Ingegerd Adlerberth

Department of Clinical Bacteriology
Göteborg University
Gudhedsgatan 10
SE–413 46 Göteborg
Sweden
E-Mail ia@microbio.gu.se

Prof. Gerard Berry

Children's Hospital
Division of Genetics and
Program in Genomics
Harvard Medical School
300 Longwood Avenue
Boston, MA 02115
USA
E-Mail gerard.berry@
childrens.harvard.edu

Prof. Dennis M. Bier

Children's Nutrition Research Center
Baylor College of Medicine
1100 Bates Street
Houston, TX 77030
USA
E-Mail dbier@bcm.tmc.edu

Dr. Jason Chou Chieh

Nutrition and Health Department
Nestlé Research Center
PO Box 44
CH–1000 Lausanne 26
Switzerland
E-Mail chieh-jason.chou@
rdls.nestle.com

Prof. Bruce German

Department of Nutrition
University of California
One Shields Ave
Davis, CA 95616
USA
E-Mail jbgerman@ucdavis.edu

Prof. Peter Gluckman

Liggins Institute
University of Auckland
Private Bag 92019
1023 Auckland
New Zealand
E-Mail pd.gluckman@auckland.ac.nz

Prof. Olle Hernell

Department of Clinical Sciences,
Pediatrics
Umeå University
SE–901 85 Umeå
Sweden
E-Mail olle.hernell@pediatri.umu.se

Prof. Dr. J.W. (Hans) Hofstraat

Healthcare Strategic Partnerships
Philips Research Laboratories/CTMM
High Tech Campus 11 (HTC 11 P 2.41)
NL–5656 AE Eindhoven
The Netherlands
E-Mail hans.Hofstraat@philips.com

Contributors

Prof. Berthold Koletzko

Division of Metabolic Diseases and
Nutritional Medicine
Dr. von Hauner Children's Hospital
Ludwig Maximilians University of
Munich
Lindwurmstrasse 4
D–80337 Munich
Germany
E-Mail berthold.koletzko@
med.uni-muenchen.de

Prof. Ching Lau

Baylor College of Medicine
Texas Children's Cancer Center
6621 Fannin Stret, MC 3-3320
Houston, TX 77030
USA
E-Mail cclau@txccc.org

Prof. Bo Lönnerdal

Department of Nutrition
University of California
One Shields Ave
Davis, CA 95616
USA
E-Mail bllonnerdal@ucdavis.edu

Prof. Piero Rinaldo

Biochemical Genetics Laboratory –
Hilton 360C
Department of Laboratory Medicine
and Pathology
Mayo Clinic College of Medicine
200 First Street SW
Rochester, MN 55905
USA
E-Mail rinaldo@mayo.edu

Prof. Seppo Salminen

Functional Foods Forum
University of Turku
FI–20100 Turku
Finland
E-Mail seppo.salminen@utu.fi

Prof. Erkki Savilahti

Pediatric Gastroenterology and
Immunology Department
Helsinki University Central Hospital
Hospital for Children and
Adolescents
POB 281
FI–00029 Hus
Finland
E-Mail erkki.savilahti@hus.fi

Prof. W. Allan Walker

Developmental Gastroenterology
Laboratory
Massachusetts General Hospital for
Children
Department of Pediatrics
Harvard Medical School
114 16th Street (114–35 03)
Charleston, MA 02129–4404
USA
E-Mail wwalker@partners.org

Prof. Robert A. Waterland

Department of Pediatrics and
Molecular and Human Genetics
Baylor College of Medicine
USDA Children's Nutrition Research
Center
1100 Bates Street
Houston, TX 77030
USA
E-Mail waterland@bcm.edu

Moderators

Prof. Bengt Björkstén

Allergy Prevention and Pediatrics
Institute of Environmental Medicine
Karolinska Institute
SE–17177 Stockholm
Sweden
E-Mail bengt.bjorksten@ki.se

Prof. Mikko Hallman

Department of Pediatrics
Faculty of Medicine
Kajanintie 50
Oulu University Hospital
FI–902 20 Oulu
Finland
E-Mail mikko.hallman@oulu.fi

Prof. Erika Isolauri

Department of Pediatrics
Turku University Central Hospital
Kiinamyllankatu 4–8
FI–205 20 Turku
Finland
E-Mail eriiso@utu.fi

Prof. Olli Simell

Department of Pediatrics
Turku University Central Hospital
Kiinamyllynkatu 4–8
FI–205 20 Turku
Finland
E-Mail olli.simell@utu.fi

Prof. Outi Vaarala

Laboratory for Immunobiology
Department of Viral Diseases and
Immunology
National Public Health Institute
Mannerheimintie 166
FI–003 00 Helsinki
Finland
E-Mail outi.vaarala@ktl.fi

Invited Attendees

Susan Prescott/Australia
Nadja Haiden/Austria
Karl Zwiauer/Austria
Bosco Paes/Canada
Simon Lam/China
Rosanna Ming Sum Wong/China
Kim Fleischer Michaelsen/Denmark
Rafael Aulestia/Ecuador
May Nassar/Egypt
Anne Ormission/Estonia
Merle Paluste/Estonia
Heli Kuusipalo/Finland
Kirsi Laitinen/Finland
Harri Niinikoski/Finland
Anneli Pouta/Finland
Tuula Simell/Finland
Suvi Virtanen/Finland

Agnés Guiseppi/France
Clemens Kunz/Germany
Axel Von der Wense/Germany
Iraklis Salvanos/Greece
Maria Trigka/Greece
Diane Devy Sondakh/Indonesia
Dr. Wistiani/Indonesia
Luca Bernardo/Italy
Giovanni Corsello/Italy
Mario De Curtis/Italy
Ieve Eglite/Latvia
Ruta Kuciskiene/Lithuania
Vaidotas Urbanos/Lithuania
Sigita Zindziuviene/Lithuania
Yael Enricas Bravo/Mexico
Ulises Leal/Mexico
Victoria Lima/Mexico

Contributors

Ignacio Ortiz/Mexico
Francis H. Bloomfield/New Zealand
Steve Hodgkinson/New Zealand
Per Brandtzaeg/Norway
Per H. Finne/Norway
Janusz Ksiazyk/Poland
Hania Szajewska/Poland
Abdurrachid Nurmamodo/Portugal
Susanna M. Saraiva Pissarra da
Silva/Portugal
Tatiana Loskucherjavaja/Russia

Bengt Björkstén/Sweden
Hugo Lagercrantz/Sweden
Inger Öhlund/Sweden
Staffan Polberger/Sweden
Niels Räihä/Sweden
Birgitta Strandvik/Sweden
Anan Alhaffar/Syria
Pimol Srisuparp/Thailand
Deniz Ertrem/Turkey
Ayşe Mukkadder Selimoglu/Turkey
Carina Venter/UK

Nestlé Participants

Mr. Xavier Payrard/Australia
Ms. Lisa Beausoleil/Canada
Dr. Louis-Dominque Van Egroo/France
Mr. Mike Possner/Germany
Mr. Panagotis Bagkas/Greece
Dr. Inguna Berzina/Latvia
Dr. Darius Praninskas /Lithuania
Dr. Fernando Carvalho/Portugal
Prof. Olga Netrebenko/Russia
Dr. Sergey Ukraintsev/Russia
Mr. Robert Aderbauer/Sweden
Dr. Anette Järvi/Sweden
Dr. Denis Barclay/Switzerland

Mrs. Elisabeth Chappuis/Switzerland
Dr. Irene Corthésy/Switzerland
Mrs. Ulrike Deland/Switzerland
Dr. Marie-Claire Fichot/Switzerland
Prof. Ferdinand Haschke/Switzerland
Dr. Petra Klassen/Switzerland
Dr. Françoise Maynard/Switzerland
Dr. Bruce McConnell/Switzerland
Mr. Giovanni Pascalicchio/Switzerland
Dr. Evelyn Spivey-Krobath/Switzerland
Dr. Thierry Von der Weid/Switzerland
Mrs. Zelda Wilson/UK
Prof. Jose Saavedra/USA

Bier DM, German JB, Lönnerdal B (eds): Personalized Nutrition for the Diverse Needs of Infants and Children.
Nestlé Nutr Workshop Ser Pediatr Program, vol 62, pp 1–12,
Nestec Ltd., Vevey/S. Karger AG, Basel, © 2008.

Developmental Perspectives on Individual Variation: Implications for Understanding Nutritional Needs

Peter D. Gluckman[a], *Alan S. Beedle*[a], *Mark A. Hanson*[b], *Eric P. Yap*[c]

[a]Liggins Institute, University of Auckland, Auckland, New Zealand; [b]Developmental Origins
of Health and Disease Centre, Institute of Developmental Sciences, University of
Southampton, Southampton, UK; and [c]Defence Research and Technology Office, Ministry of
Defence, Singapore

Abstract

Genetic research has focused on identifying linkages between polymorphisms and
phenotypic traits to explain variations in complex biologies. However, the magnitude of
these linkages has not been particularly high. Conversely, the ability of developmental
plasticity to generate biological variation from one genotype is well understood, while
interest has emerged in the clinical significance of epigenetic processes, particularly
those influenced by the external environment. Environmental cues in early development may induce responses that provide adaptive advantage later in life. The benefit of
such responses depends on the fidelity of the prediction of the future environment. Life
history and physiological changes mediated through epigenetic processes then follow,
determining the later phenotype. Developmental mismatch, leading to disease, can arise
from discordance between the fetal environment, which is relatively constant across
generations, and the postnatal nutritional environment, which can change drastically
within and between generations. Metabolic disorders represent the outcome of an individual living in an energetically inappropriate environment. Experimental and clinical
evidence suggests that individual capacity to live in a given energetic environment is
influenced by developmental factors acting through epigenetic mechanisms. Epigenetic
biomarkers may be able to identify a risk of developmental mismatch and thus offer the
opportunity for nutritional or other intervention.

Introduction

The genetics and genomic revolutions focused attention on genes as the
basis of individual variation. As has been reviewed elsewhere [1], this led to a

reduced appreciation of the role of developmental factors in such diversity. Recent progress in our understanding of developmental plasticity, particularly in comparative biology, has led to the recognition that developmental processes act through epigenetic mechanisms to have a major influence on phenotypic variation. This article reviews the extent to which these processes contribute to variation in body composition and insulin sensitivity.

An individual's phenotype and capacity to live healthily in a given nutritional environment are influenced by developmental, epigenomic and genomic profiles. In all populations the incidence of obesity and its associated disorders such as type-2 diabetes and cardiovascular disease represents a growing concern. Simplistically, this has been attributed to the changing patterns of nutrition and exercise (the nutritional transition), but there has been little consideration of individual variation in the propensity to develop obesity in a given environment. There is growing evidence that there are important developmental elements in, and several developmental pathways to, obesity. But adipose tissue is not homogeneous, there are functional differences between visceral and subcutaneous fat, and there is increasing consideration of the role of muscular and intramuscular fat. However, the relationship between different patterns of obesity and disease risk is poorly understood – for example, Singaporeans have a high rate of diabetes relative to the rate of overt obesity [2]. These considerations are critical for population and individual strategies for prevention and intervention.

A further complexity is provided by the growing recognition that different fat depots have very different properties in terms of both metabolic lability and cytokine/adipokine profile. Visceral fat is considered to be that most associated with metabolic disease [3], although new imaging techniques now raise the question of the role of intramuscular fat as a source of peripheral insulin resistance [4]. The use of magnetic resonance imaging allows accurate in-life assessment of visceral fat, and it is now apparent that smaller children already have visceral obesity at birth [5] and that some individuals can have visceral obesity without obvious subcutaneous obesity (the thin outside/fat inside (TOFI) syndrome). This appears to be more common in some populations [3]. A major defect in virtually all current population studies is the reliance on simple measures of obesity without any attempt to understand it in terms of the different fat masses.

Genetic Variation

The initial thrifty genotype model of Neel proposed that humans had been selected in Pleistocene environments for genes that would promote energy (fat) storage, conferring a fitness benefit in the supposed environment of 'feast and famine' and a high protein/low glycemic index diet. Neel proposed that in recent decades, as humans lived longer and were now exposed to higher nutrient burdens and lower energy expenditure, this formerly adaptive trait had become maladaptive in the form of an increased burden of disease in middle age. However, this model had significant weaknesses [6], including the failure to find genes to explain the very high incidence of type-2 diabetes in some populations (e.g. Pima Indians), the extremely rapid appearance of type-2 diabetes in some populations and at a declining age, and population differences – for example, in India type-2 diabetes is appearing at nutritional levels and body compositions well within the normal range.

There has been a large international effort seeking genetic linkages to explain variations in body composition and the propensity to diabetes. A number of polymorphisms have been identified which confer added risk [7], but even for those with the greatest linkage the attributable risk is not great, for example, the risk allele of *FTO* confers an added risk of obesity of 1.67-fold [7]. Only rare forms of obesity (for example, leptin receptor deficiency) and type-2 diabetes (for example, glucokinase deficiency) have been linked to monogenic disease.

Developmental Factors

In the late 1980s, epidemiological studies [for review see 8] started to show linkages between birth size and later risks of cardiovascular disease and type-2 diabetes and, more recently, with body composition. A critical feature which was not initially understood was that the relationship is continuous across the full range of body sizes – this led to the recognition that later disease was not a result of a disruption of development, as initially suggested, but was the adverse outcome of the normative processes of developmental plasticity [9].

Developmental plasticity can be defined as the processes by which one genotype can lead to a range of phenotypes as a result of environmental influences acting during development. There has been an enormous surge of comparative research in developmental plasticity in recent years (particularly in the field of ecological developmental biology [1]) and only in the last 5 years have the implications for human medicine become truly apparent [10]. A major mechanism underpinning developmental plasticity is that of epigenesis, whereby DNA methylation and/or histone modification of specific genes is induced by environmental factors. There is now compelling experimental and growing clinical evidence that epigenetic factors play a major role in individual susceptibility to obesity and type-2 diabetes/insulin resistance [11].

Experimentally there is now a large amount of work showing that environmental manipulation in early life can lead to obesity, insulin resistance and endothelial dysfunction and that this is associated with epigenetic changes. Most work has been conducted in rodents, where maternal undernutrition (balanced or a low protein diet) or maternal glucocorticoid administration

3

lead to offspring who develop insulin resistance and/or hyperinsulinemia, leptin resistance, hyperphagia, sarcopenia, obesity (visceral), endothelial dysfunction, reduced nephron number and hypertension [12]. These rats also have alterations in their hypothalamic-pituitary-adrenal axis, altered rate of maturation (earlier puberty, as also seen in humans [13]) and altered behaviors in open field testing. This is analogous to the metabolic syndrome complex seen in humans. These changes are associated with specific epigenetic and/or gene expression changes in the liver, fat and muscle of the offspring [11]. Components of the hypothalamic-pituitary-adrenal axis are particularly affected, including changes both in the glucocorticoid receptor and in the enzyme which inactivates active glucocorticoids (11β-hydroxysteroid dehydrogenase type 2), with consequential changes for glucocorticoid-dependent metabolic enzymes such as phosphoenolpyruvate carboxykinase. Changes are also seen in transcriptional factors regulating fat metabolism such as peroxisome proliferator activated receptor-α, in factors associated with insulin action such as phosphoinositide 3-kinase and protein kinase-ζ, and in factors associated with endothelial function such as endothelial nitric oxide synthase and estrogen receptor-α. Recently, we have shown that reversal of the developmental induction of metabolic dysfunction by neonatal leptin administration in females is associated with reversal of the epigenetic changes [14].

There may be major gender effects that need consideration. Experimentally, females and males have differing sensitivities to maternal undernutrition and neonatal manipulation. As selection operates to optimize reproductive fitness, it is realistic to expect developmental plasticity to operate differently in males and females, reflecting their different reproductive strategies. Epidemiological and experimental data show that females respond to intrauterine undernutrition with accelerated maturation (puberty) provided that postnatal nutrition is adequate to support pregnancy [15]. This is logical in that females can only protect fitness by maximizing their reproductive lifespan – in the expectation of a threatening environment it would therefore be appropriate to put on postnatal fat to support pregnancy and lactation at a young age, and to enter puberty early. Males in most systems, including probably Paleolithic humans, rely on dominance in a narrower period of their lifespan to maximize their fitness. Thus they may protect body size differently. This is an area of fertile research.

A key question is over what period of development does metabolic plasticity exist? The work of Kwong et al. [16] suggests that periconceptional factors can lead to permanent effects on the offspring in rodents. At the other extreme, the term 'programming' was used by Lucas [17] to show long-term the effects of breastfeeding versus formula feeding, suggesting that metabolic plasticity extends well after birth in humans. Recent studies confirm that formula feeding is associated with a high risk of later obesity, insulin resistance and hypercholesterolemia [18].

4

Interaction between the Prenatal and Postnatal Environments

A key factor in rodent studies is that the obesity and metabolic phenotype is dependent on the post-weaning environment. Vickers et al. [19] showed that the effect of prenatal undernutrition and that of postnatal high-fat diets were comparable on the development of obesity and insulin resistance, but that there was a clear synergistic interaction between the prenatal poor environment and the postnatal rich environment such that those antenatally undernourished were more at risk of developing obesity and insulin resistance on a high-energy diet after birth. Indeed, for some measures such as alterations in the neuroendocrine control of appetite [20], it required both elements to be present for abnormality to be seen.

A Framework for Understanding Developmental Pathways to Obesity and Insulin Resistance

The epidemiological studies of Eriksson et al. [21] in Finland showed that in a population who are now in their 60s and on whom detailed growth records exist, those who developed type-2 diabetes in their life course showed an earlier adiposity rebound (the time in childhood between 2 and 6 years of age when body fat stops falling from its high levels in infancy and starts to rise again) and progressively gained weight relative to height through later childhood and adolescence. There were different patterns for those born above the mean for birth weight and below the mean – those above did not regress to the mean (unlike the bulk of the population who did not develop diabetes) but put on weight relative to height from 1 year of age, whereas those born below the mean actually were thin at birth and put on weight for height faster than controls by 3–4 years of age [22]. As this was an unbiased sample because of the nature of the data collection in Helsinki, it suggests that the pathway to diabetes in Finland (an admittedly very homogeneous population) in individuals born in the 1930s started in infancy or before, and that there may be more than one pathway. The Finnish group also showed that there were interactions with specific polymorphisms in the risk of developing insulin resistance – the association of smaller birth size with increased risk of diabetes was seen only in carriers of the high-risk Pro12Pro allele of peroxisome proliferator activated receptor-γ2 [23]. Such studies together with the experimental work point to a nexus of genomic, developmental/epigenomic and concurrent environmental factors in determining an individual's risk of obesity and type-2 diabetes.

Current opinion [6] suggests at least two major developmental pathways to obesity and insulin resistance.

5

The Mismatch Pathway

This pathway involves the fetus/embryo/neonate sensing a level of poor nutrition and making developmental choices towards a thrifty trajectory involving both central and peripheral factors such as sarcopenia, a propensity to prefer a high-fat diet, hyperphagia, reduced energy expenditure, and insulin resistance [24]. This is probably underpinned by epigenetic processes and is based on the developing organism predicting it will live in a nutritionally challenged environment. If it meets instead a nutritionally rich environment, then it is mismatched and this mismatch is reflected in metabolic disease as its physiological settings are inappropriate. Experimentally, there is support for this paradigm. In the rat, leptin administration to the infant offspring of undernourished mothers confers life-long protection against a high-fat diet and is associated with reversal of the epigenetic changes, thus providing strong evidence for both the epigenetic underpinnings of this pathway and the predictive (mismatch) model [14, 25]. (Leptin is an adipokine, and we suggest that its administration tricks the neonate into thinking it is fat when it is not and thus induces a plastic choice appropriate for a nutritionally rich environment.) Notably, for some of the genes studied, epigenetic and expression responses to neonatal leptin exposure are directionally dependent on past maternal nutritional status [14]. This suggests that epigenetic and phenotypic responses to an environmental stimulus at one stage in development can be determined both in magnitude and in direction by past environmental exposure. Our studies with this model have also highlighted important gender influences (unpublished work). Furthermore, genomic polymorphisms may have effects on epigenetic changes in other genes [26] and it is reasonable to assume that polymorphisms will directly affect CpG islands. These layers of complexity embracing genomic, developmental and environmental factors provide a basis for considerable variation in gene expression affecting metabolic homeostasis.

In humans this pathway exists in part because of the presence of maternal and/or placental disease which limits nutrient information to the fetus, in part because a surprisingly high proportion of mothers eat imprudent diets [27, 28], but primarily because of the presence of maternal constraint [29]. This is a phenomenon of particular importance in monotocous species to limit fetal growth so that the fetus can exit the pelvic canal. Thus fetal growth is not primarily regulated by the fetal genome but by maternal-placental delivery of nutrients. Maternal constraint is particularly enhanced in first-born children (who have a greater incidence of obesity [30], and the proportion of whom rises as family size falls) and in mothers of smaller stature as in many Asian populations. Because of the constitutive nature of maternal constraint, fetal environment and growth is largely limited (with the exception below), yet postnatal nutritional environments have changed rapidly. Thus the risk of mismatch grows, driven by the lower energy expenditures and greater food intakes of children and adolescents against a background of maternal constraint favoring developmental trajectories appropriate for sparse environments.

Until recently it was assumed that maternal nutrition, unless very limited, could not affect the fetus. But nutritional variation within the normal Western dietary range can affect patterns of fetal growth [27] and cord blood IGF-1 levels [31]. A nutritional survey of women of reproductive age in the UK showed that up to 50% in the lowest educational achievement groups had diets judged as imprudent [28]. In Singapore, anecdotal evidence suggests that dieting is common in pregnancy. In Japan, the *falling* birth weight is associated with reduced maternal weight gain, in part due to dieting [32].

The Fetal Hyperinsulinemia Pathway

Whereas the mismatch pathway is physiological (in that it is the outcome of an evolutionarily appropriate mechanism), the offspring of diabetic or pre-diabetic mothers have larger fat mass and a greater lifetime risk of developing type-2 diabetes. In this case the mechanism is thought to be simply high transplacental glucose transfer leading to higher fetal insulin levels. Fetal insulin is weakly anabolic, in part through driving IGF-1 secretion, but is strongly adipogenic. Thus the offspring of diabetic mothers have inappropriately more fat cells, particularly subcutaneous fat, and as fat cell number is largely determined antenatally, postnatal growth in a high-energy environment will be associated with a higher risk of obesity and diabetes. This is therefore a simpler and single-system pathway.

It may however coexist with the mismatch pathway. Work from India shows that babies >2.9 kg at birth have mothers who have a high probability of developing type-2 diabetes within 5 years [33]. This suggests that these short mothers, themselves the outcome of a programmed pregnancy but now in a more nutritionally rich environment and pregnant (which is inherently an insulin-resistant state), give birth to smaller babies (with visceral obesity) because of maternal constraint and that these smaller babies are relatively obese because of maternal hyperinsulinemia. This combined pathway may underpin the growing and very high incidence of juvenile-onset type-2 diabetes in India.

Fat mothers give birth to fatter babies [34]. These are likely to have a life course similar to that of the infant of the diabetic mother, but the mechanism by which fat mothers give birth to fat babies is unclear.

Infant Overnutrition

Experimentally and clinically there is good evidence that infant over-nutrition (such as by formula feeding) can lead to a greater risk of obesity and insulin resistance/type-2 diabetes [18]. Similarly, there is as yet no clarity as to whether this is a distinct mechanism and pathway or reflects either the mismatch pathway (rapid switching in nutritional levels) or an extension of the fetal hyperinsulinemia pathway into the neonatal period (or both).

There is great confusion as to the significance of the infant pattern of growth. Some have argued that rapid infant weight gain is bad, others that it is good. Thus there is no consensus as to how to apply individual nutritional recommendations and growth curves to children of differing birth phenotypes.

Conclusions

If the logic of this article is sound, in time a key strategy may be individualized nutritional and growth curve recommendations for infants and children based on their size, gender, epigenetic profile and genotype. This is an area meriting urgent research. This discussion has highlighted the many gaps in our knowledge, yet points to the growing recognition that, in order to understand lifestyle disease, a developmental/epigenetic perspective needs to be added to the genetic and environmental dimensions.

References

1 Gilbert SF: Mechanisms for the environmental regulation of gene expression: ecological aspects of animal development. J Biosci 2005;30:65–74.
2 Deurenberg-Yap M, Chew SK, Lin VF, et al: Relationships between indices of obesity and its co-morbidities in multi-ethnic Singapore. Int J Obes Relat Metab Disord 2001;25: 1554–1562.
3 Pi-Sunyer FX: The epidemiology of central fat distribution in relation to disease. Nutr Rev 2004;62:S120–S126.
4 Boesch C, Machann J, Vermathen P, Schick F: Role of proton MR for the study of muscle lipid metabolism. NMR Biomed 2006;19:968–988.
5 Harrington TAM, Thomas EL, Frost G, et al: Distribution of adipose tissue in the newborn. Pediatr Res 2004;55:437–441.
6 Kuzawa CW, Gluckman PD, Hanson MA: Developmental perspectives on the origin of obesity; in Fantuzzi G, Mazzone T (eds): Adipose Tissue and Adipokines in Health and Disease. Totowa, Humana Press, 2007, pp 207–219.
7 Frayling TM, Timpson NJ, Weedon MN, et al: A common variant in the *FTO* gene is associated with body mass index and predisposes to childhood and adult obesity. Science 2007;316: 889–894.
8 Godfrey K: The 'developmental origins' hypothesis: epidemiology; in Gluckman PD, Hanson MA (eds): Developmental Origins of Health and Disease. Cambridge, Cambridge University Press, 2006, pp 6–32.
9 Gluckman PD, Hanson MA: Living with the past: evolution, development, and patterns of disease. Science 2004;305:1733–1736.
10 Bateson P, Barker D, Clutton-Brock T, et al: Developmental plasticity and human health. Nature 2004;430:419–421.
11 Burdge GC, Hanson MA, Slater-Jeffries JL, Lillycrop KA: Epigenetic regulation of transcription: a mechanism for inducing variations in phenotype (fetal programming) by differences in nutrition during early life? Br J Nutr 2007;97:1036–1046.
12 McMillen IC, Robinson JS: Developmental origins of the metabolic syndrome: prediction, plasticity, and programming. Physiol Rev 2005;85:571–633.
13 Sloboda DM, Hart R, Doherty DA, et al: Age at menarche: influences of prenatal and postnatal growth. J Clin Endocrinol Metab 2007;92:46–50.
14 Gluckman PD, Lillycrop KA, Vickers MH, et al: Metabolic plasticity during mammalian development is directionally dependent on early nutritional status. Proc Natl Acad Sci USA 2007;104:12796–12800.

15 Gluckman PD, Hanson MA: Evolution, development and timing of puberty. Trends Endocrinol Metab 2006;17:7–12.
16 Kwong WY, Wild AE, Roberts P, et al: Maternal undernutrition during the preimplantation period of rat development causes blastocyst abnormalities and programming of postnatal hypertension. Development 2000;127:4195–4202.
17 Lucas A: Programming by early nutrition in man. Ciba Found Symp 1991;156:38–50.
18 Singhal A: Early nutrition and long-term cardiovascular health. Nutr Rev 2006;64:S44–S49.
19 Vickers MH, Breier BH, Cutfield WS, et al: Fetal origins of hyperphagia, obesity and hypertension and its postnatal amplification by hypercaloric nutrition. Am J Physiol 2000;279: E83–E87.
20 Ikenasio-Thorpe BA, Breier BH, Vickers MH, Fraser M: Prenatal influences on susceptibility to diet-induced obesity are mediated by altered neuroendocrine gene expression. J Endocrinol 2007;193:31–37.
21 Eriksson JG, Forsén T, Tuomilehto J, et al: Early adiposity rebound in childhood and risk of type 2 diabetes in adult life. Diabetologia 2003;46:190–194.
22 Eriksson JG, Forsén TJ, Osmond C, Barker DJP: Pathways of infant and childhood growth that lead to type 2 diabetes. Diabetes Care 2003;26:3006–3010.
23 Eriksson JG, Osmond C, Lindi V, et al: Interactions between peroxisome proliferator-activated receptor gene polymorphism and birth length influence risk for type 2 diabetes. Diabetes Care 2003;26:2476–2477.
24 Gluckman PD, Hanson MA, Beedle AS: Early life events and their consequences for later disease: a life history and evolutionary perspective. Am J Hum Biol 2007;19:1–19.
25 Vickers MH, Gluckman PD, Coveny AH, et al: Neonatal leptin treatment reverses developmental programming. Endocrinology 2005;146:4211–4216.
26 Linglart A, Gensure RC, Olney RC, et al: A novel STX16 deletion in autosomal dominant pseudohypoparathyroidism type Ib redefines the boundaries of a cis-acting imprinting control element of GNAS. Am J Hum Genet 2005;76:804–814.
27 Godfrey K, Robinson S, Barker DJ, et al: Maternal nutrition in early and late pregnancy in relation to placental and fetal growth. BMJ 1996;312:410–414.
28 Robinson SM, Crozier SR, Borland SE, et al: Impact of educational attainment on the quality of young women's diets. Eur J Clin Nutr 2004;58:1174–1180.
29 Gluckman PD, Hanson MA: Maternal constraint of fetal growth and its consequences. Semin Fetal Neonatal Med 2004;9:419–425.
30 Stettler N, Tershakovec AM, Zemel BS, et al: Early risk factors for increased adiposity: a cohort study of African American subjects followed from birth to young adulthood. Am J Clin Nutr 2000;72:378–383.
31 Javaid MK, Godfrey KM, Taylor P, et al: Umbilical venous IGF-1 concentration, neonatal bone mass, and body composition. J Bone Miner Res 2004;19:56–63.
32 Gluckman PD, Chong YS, Fukuoka H, et al: Low birthweight and subsequent obesity in Japan. Lancet 2007;369:1081–1082.
33 Yajnik CS, Joglekar CV, Pandit AN, et al: Higher offspring birth weight predicts the metabolic syndrome in mothers but not fathers 8 years after delivery. Diabetes 2003;52:2090–2096.
34 Ahlsson F, Gustafsson J, Tuvemo T, Lundgren M: Females born large for gestational age have a doubled risk of giving birth to large for gestational age infants. Acta Paediatr Scand 2007; 96:358–362.

Discussion

Dr. Isolauri: Regarding the current practice that particularly obese pregnant women should try to lose weight during pregnancy and they are advised to gain less weight, significantly less weight, than the normal weight women. What are the consequences on the child?

Dr. Gluckman: I think the first thing is when they are losing weight. The available evidence, and I refer you to a meta-analysis [1] published recently, is that the most important determinant of pregnancy outcome, if birth weight and gestational length are used as the measures of outcome, is of course the weight and body mass index of the woman at conception. There is a lot of advantage in trying to encourage women who are obese to think about their body composition before they conceive. I know it is difficult to ask but increasingly I think that it is needed. If genetic mechanisms are involved, we are still to learn the extent to which early nutritional stimuli, such as around the periconceptional period, are potentially more dramatic in their long-term effects than later nutritional stimuli, but that may or may not be the case. All the work is still pointing a lot to late effects as much as early effects, so I just don't know the answer. When I worked with the World Health Organization committee on optimizing the outcomes of pregnancy a couple of years back, we came to the conclusion that there must be a minimal weight gain during pregnancy that must be recommended, and that would appear to be at least 10 kg, potentially 12 kg. I do believe therefore the issue of dieting in pregnancy is very complex, very poorly understood, and needs to be supported by appropriate research, for instance using epigenetic biomarkers as one of the outcomes because birth weight is such a crude index. So at the moment my personal bias, which is bias without data, is women should be encouraged to lose weight before they conceive, certainly not right at the beginning of pregnancy, and that they should not be so severely undernourished that they don't gain 10–12 kg during pregnancy.

Dr. Walker: I am fascinated by the persistence of change that goes from one generation to the other which you alluded to, which has been shown in humans by Dick Guerrant in Brazil and Andrew Prentice in Africa. Do you have any thoughts about the potential mechanisms by which this occurs?

Dr. Gluckman: It is difficult because we have to separate female and male effects if we are talking about more than one generation. If we are talking about females we can go to F2 without any particularly complex mechanisms needing to be involved because the egg of F2 is actually exposed to the F0 environment because it was formed at the time the fetus of F1 was in fact in utero. In terms of males it is a bit more complicated. F2 transmission but not F3 generation has been shown through both the male and female. Then there is this business in the male with fungicide toxin going through the F3 and F4 generation by male line transmission. How is trans-generational transmission of epigenetic marks maintained? It does not need to be through methylation marks themselves being maintained, although for some genes the methylation mark is not entirely wiped out at meiosis, for many it is, but there are data showing that, even at the 2-cell stage, methylation marks are still present on H19, for example, despite the claims of others that it is completely wiped out. My own bias is more likely to involve, in particular, small RNAs. Small RNAs can transfer across generations, small RNAs may be the way in which the epigenetic markers are maintained from generation to generation. Again the data don't exist; it is a hot topic.

Dr. Koletzko: You alluded to the observation in India that people born with low birth weight and growing fast tend to have a very high rate of abdominal obesity, high body fat content with the same BMI, and a high risk of type-2 diabetes. It is very plausible that this has to do with early life events. You also showed the fascinating results from Eriksson and coworkers clearly showing that in this case the Pro12α-polymorphism of PPARγ2 has a huge predictive effect on birth weight association. When this is seen, would there not be an enormous opportunity to better understand what is really happening if we were able to apply some of these new developments, even doing genome-wide association studies comparing populations in India and the Western world to try to decipher the extent to which these associations are modified by genetic variation? One would expect that there should be very different susceptibility sub-groups.

Dr. Gluckman: I will be honest and the answer is you might be right. The first problem is there has been remarkable inconsistency in these SNP relationships. For example Eriksson himself cannot confirm that relationship in the different populations of Finns, and it has certainly not been confirmed elsewhere. On the other hand, SNPs in some populations do show relationships to obesity, insulin resistance, hyperphagia, the MC4 receptor polymorphisms, the perilipin polymorphisms, other PPARα polymorphisms, and so forth. I have done a lot of work in Singapore because Indians and Chinese live along side each other there and have a differential incidence of 3 times: the Indians have 3 times the incidence of type-2 diabetes in Singapore compared to the ethnic Chinese. It comes no where near explaining the differences in incidence despite the large amount of full genome-wide scanning that has been done in Singapore across the so-called Singaporese diabetes studies to look at this. Yes, it may be there, and yes, there might be polymorphisms defined, I have no doubt they will exist. But I see no reason why they would have evolved because the change in environment leading to these diseases has to be sustained, and it doesn't exist. It has to have been there for founder effects and these populations haven't been isolated long enough for founder effects to be clear. In my opinion, in evolutionary terms, it is actually very hard to find an explanation. On the other hand, if you buy into the concept of the development of plasticity that says it is a fundamental thing of all plants and most lower animals, that one changes one's phenotype in later life in a physiological and adaptive sense in relationship to early signals, and at least part of that is mediated by epigenetic processes, then one would expect to find epigenetic processes at the heart of it. But there is another overlay and that is where I think the polymorphisms come back into play, most polymorphisms we look at in terms of those within the expressed region of the gene. Of course many genes have a lot of polymorphisms in the promoter regions of the genes, we haven't looked at those to nearly the same extent, and the extent to which they will alter the capacity of epigenetic processes to lead to one outcome or another is not at all known. There are actually very little data in the literature which relate polymorphisms in promoter regions to alterations in epigenetic expression. To follow this through we first have to understand more about the epigenetic processes, but in doing so we are clearly going to have to understand a lot more about polymorphic variation, not just expressed sequences but non-expressed sequences of the genome which we have not been looking at to nearly the same extent, and that is where I think your question is probably correct.

Dr. Lagercrantz: I strongly believe in and support the Barker hypothesis. But if you look at the curve for birth weight and metabolic syndrome, it is U-shaped, therefore if a child has a very high birth weight it will also develop metabolic syndrome. There are strong data supporting that the famine in Holland resulted in metabolic syndrome, but what about the famine in Leningrad?

Dr. Gluckman: The answer is look at the literature. Part of the problem is everybody has focused on the extremes. If one looks at the normal range of birth weight in good studies, there is a consistent relationship between birth weight within the normative range for that population and outcomes. The problem is the U-shaped curve is real in the modern world. 150 years ago there were not many gestational diabetics and therefore there was not this large number of very large birth weight babies. If you look at older populations versus modern populations, multiple pathways come into play. Just imagine a U; a U can have a narrow shape or a broad shape. In the United States or New Zealand or, I suspect, Finland or Sweden, below about 2,800 g birth weight the risks of later obesity and type-2 diabetes rise as birth weight falls. That is also true in India. But looking at the other end of the U, the right-hand shape, in your country and mine, up to a birth weight of about 3,600–3,800 g there is no increased risk, that seems to be a reasonably optimal birth weight. Above 4,000 g, perhaps 4,200 g, the risks change but they have a different pattern; it is now a pattern due to maternal gestational diabetes and all the effects of maternal obesity through mechanisms we don't understand.

But in India at 2,900 g where the mothers are very short, the risk starts to rise again. In other words the U has a very narrow base and above a birth weight of 2,950 g the mother has a very high risk of having undiagnosed gestational diabetes and has a greater than 60% chance of developing type-2 diabetes within 4 years of the pregnancy, and that of course reflects the fact that she herself was born small, has now grown up in a nutritionally enriched environment, and is at greater risk of getting disease. The evidence is pretty overwhelming that the relationships exist if you understand them within a population context regarding the history of that population. Now the outcome issue, if you look at obesity and type-2 diabetes in sarcopenia, the evidence is pretty strong, because fundamentally they are related on a life history concept to the outcome. Gillman et al. [2] recently did calculations suggesting that 50% of the attributable risk of obesity relates to pregnancy, lactational and early infant factors. There is no doubt if one looks at the Eriksson data that by the age of 3 to 4 to 5 years these children are behaving differently and at birth these children already had visceral obesity. But when you come to cardiovascular disease, which is of course where Dr. Barker first started, it is much more complex. Proximate factors like smoking and other lifestyle factors appear to be much more important because cardiovascular disease is a lot further from metabolic programming than in fact are metabolic studies in metabolism itself. I agree with others that for cardiovascular disease what Dr. Barker originally stated is probably more difficult to tease out.

References

1 Kramer MS: The epidemiology of adverse pregnancy outcomes: an overview. J Nutr 2003;133: 1592–1596S.
2 Gillman MW, Rifas-Shiman S, Berkey CS, et al: Maternal gestational diabetes, birth weight, and adolescent obesity. Pediatrics 2003;111:e221–e226.

Bier DM, German JB, Lönnerdal B (eds): Personalized Nutrition for the Diverse Needs of Infants and Children.
Nestlé Nutr Workshop Ser Pediatr Program, vol 62, pp 13–33,
Nestec Ltd., Vevey/S. Karger AG, Basel, © 2008.

Factors Influencing the Establishment of the Intestinal Microbiota in Infancy

Ingegerd Adlerberth

Department of Clinical Bacteriology, Göteborg University, Göteborg, Sweden

Abstract

The establishment of the intestinal microbiota commences at birth and new bacteria establish in succession during the first years of life until an adult-type highly complex microbiota has been achieved. The first bacteria to establish in the neonatal gut are usually aerobic or facultatively anaerobic bacteria, like enterobacteria, enterococci and staphylococci. During their growth they consume oxygen and change the intestinal milieu making it suitable for the proliferation of anaerobic bacteria. *Bifidobacterium, Clostridium* and *Bacteroides* are among the first anaerobes establishing in the microbiota. As more oxygen-sensitive species establish and the complexity of the microbiota increases, the population sizes of aerobic and facultative bacteria decline. This phenomenon is thought to result from oxygen depletion, substrate competition and the accumulation of toxic metabolites. A wide range of factors influence the intestinal microbiota and its establishment, including delivery and feeding mode, antibiotic treatment, and contacts with parents, siblings, and hospital staff. Differences in colonization pattern can be observed between vaginally and sectio-delivered infants, and between infants in industrialized and developing countries, reflecting the importance of maternal microbiota and the environment as sources of colonizing bacteria. This article describes the intestinal colonization pattern in human infants, and reviews factors affecting this process.

Sequential Establishment of the Intestinal Microbiota

As the neonate leaves the sterile environment of the womb and encounters a world full of microbes, colonization of the skin and mucosal membranes begins immediately. With time, diversified bacterial ecosystems establish at these sites, of which the intestinal microbiota is the most complex.

The first bacteria to establish in the gut are usually aerobic or facultative anaerobic bacteria, since the neonatal gut is rich in oxygen. Such bacteria

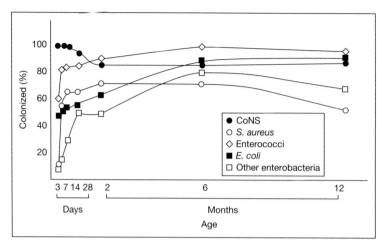

Fig. 1. Frequency of colonization by various facultative bacteria in Swedish vaginally delivered infants at different time points after birth. Adapted from Adlerberth et al. [7] and Lindberg et al. [10].

include *Escherichia coli* and other enterobacteria, enterococci and staphylococci [1–7]. As these early colonizers do not have to compete with other bacteria, they may reach population levels of 10^{9-11} colony forming units (CFU)/g feces early in life, which is roughly 1,000 times higher than their population levels in adults [6–11].

We have recently reported the longitudinal colonization pattern in more than 100 Swedish infants [7]. The colonization by facultative bacteria is shown in figure 1. Coagulase-negative staphylococci are the first bacteria to establish in the infantile gut, colonizing practically 100% of the infants from 3 days of age. Enterococci also rapidly colonize most infants. *E. coli* colonizes half of the infants within the first week of life, but the colonization frequency increases slowly, and *Staphylococcus aureus* is, actually, equally or more common than *E. coli* in Swedish infants between 1 week and 2 months of age (fig. 1). Members of the *Enterobacteriaceae* family other than *E. coli*, e.g. *Klebsiella, Enterobacter* and *Proteus*, do not colonize the infants at birth, but become increasingly common in the microbiota over the first 6 months of life (fig. 1). The colonization frequency of coagulase-negative staphylococci decline after some weeks and colonization by *S. aureus* and enterobacteria other than *E. coli* decline after the 6th month of life. This phenomenon can be regarded as a reflection of their relatively poor adaptation to the more complex intestinal ecosystem which develops over the first year of life.

The population counts of the facultative bacteria are shown in figure 2. *E. coli*, a species well adapted to the human gut, display high population numbers initially which decrease only moderately over the first year of life. In contrast,

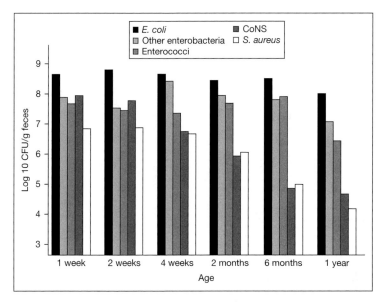

Fig. 2. Population levels of various facultative bacteria in culture-positive Swedish infants at different time points after birth. Adapted from references Adlerberth et al. [7] and Lindberg et al. [10].

the population levels of staphylococci decline substantially after the first weeks of life (fig. 2), indicating the poor fitness of staphylococci in an increasingly complex microbiota.

As facultative bacteria consume oxygen the intestinal milieu becomes more suitable for strictly anaerobic bacteria [8, 9]. *Bifidobacterium*, *Clostridium* and *Bacteroides* are examples of anaerobic bacteria which colonize young infants in population levels reaching 10^{9-11} CFU/g feces [6–9, 12]. The same groups dominate the early microbiota in recent studies using non-culture-dependent molecular methods for analyses of the intestinal microbiota [13–17].

The colonization pattern with anaerobic bacteria in Swedish infants is shown in figure 3. Bifidobacteria are the earliest anaerobes, colonizing two thirds of the 1-week-old infants. Clostridia are initially less common, but rapidly catch up with bifidobacteria. In contrast, *Bacteroides* appears much later, colonizing only one third of Swedish 2-month-old infants (fig. 3). The mean population counts of different anaerobic bacteria in colonized infants are shown in figure 4.

Among bifidobacterial species, *B. breve, B. bifidum* and *B. infantis* seem to be especially apt to colonize the infantile intestine (table 1). Clostridia are a poorly defined accumulation of Gram-positive anaerobic sporeformers,

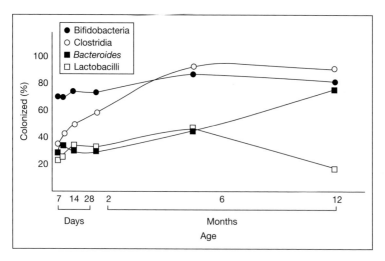

Fig. 3. Frequency of colonization by various anaerobic bacteria in Swedish vaginally delivered infants at different time points after birth. Adapted from references Adlerberth et al. [7] and Ahrne et al. [18].

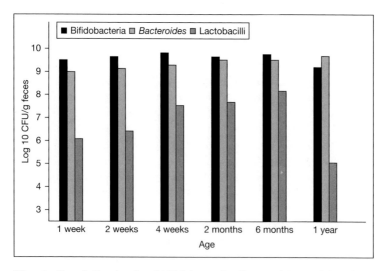

Fig. 4. Population levels of bifidobacteria, *Bacteroides* and lactobacilli in culture-positive Swedish infants at different time points after birth. Vegetative clostridial bacterial levels were not determined. Clostridial spores amounted to 10^5–10^6 CFU/g feces. Adapted from references Adlerberth et al. [7] and Ahrne et al. [18].

Table 1. Species of bifidobacteria, clostridia and *Bacteroides* colonizing infants and adults

	Infants	References	Adults	References
Bifidobacterium	B. breve B. bifidum B. infantis B. longum	4, 16	B. catenulatum B. adolescentis B. longum	4, 16
Clostridium	C. perfringens C. difficile C. paraputrificum C. tertium	5, 21	C. perfringens C. ramosum C. bifermentans C. inocuum	19
Bacteroides	B. vulgatus B. thetaiotamicron B. distasonis B. fragilis B. ovatus	21, 100	B. vulgatus B. thetaiotamicron B. distasonis B. fragilis B. ovatus	19

many of which are not genetically related to one another. *C. perfringens* and *C. difficile* belong to group I that is common in the infantile microbiota (table 1). *C. difficile* is found in less than 4% of healthy adult individuals. Among *Bacteroides* species, the *B. fragilis* group are common inhabitants of the gut microbiota throughout life (table 1).

Lactobacilli are quite infrequent colonizers of the infant gut and their population numbers are low compared to many other anaerobes [6, 9, 18] (fig. 3, 4). Approximately one third of Swedish infants acquire lactobacilli in the first month (fig. 3), but persistent colonization by lactobacilli is quite uncommon [18]. Furthermore, lactobacilli show much lower population counts than, e.g., *Bacteroides* and bifidobacteria (fig. 4). The species most commonly isolated in the first 6 months of life are *L. rhamnosus* and *L. gasseri*, which are later replaced by *L. paracasei, L. plantarum, L. acidophilus* and *L. delbruckeii* [18].

Eubacterium, Veillonella, Fusobacterium, Peptostreptococcus and *Ruminococcus* are examples of anaerobes that are frequent in the intestinal microbiota of adults [19], but less commonly isolated from infants. This could be related either to a lack of exposure to such bacteria in early life, or to poor fitness of such bacteria in the intestinal milieu during the first period of life. *Eubacterium* species are isolated from less than half of infants in the first year of life [3, 9, 20]. Peptostreptococci appear when solid foods are introduced [9, 21], and most infants harbor these bacteria at 12 months of age [3, 9]. *Ruminococcus* and *Fusobacterium* species are rarely isolated from infants in the first year of life [3, 21, 22]. In contrast, *Veillonella* may be isolated from up to 50% of 1-month-old infants [4, 5, 21, 23] and when present they often reach high population counts [9, 24].

Many of the above-mentioned bacteria are extremely sensitive to oxygen and are therefore difficult to culture, and this might have underestimated their prevalence in the infantile microbiota. Recent studies using non-culture-dependent DNA-based methods have indicated that *Eubacterium* and *Ruminococcus* are present quite early in the microbiota [25–27]. In addition, many of the bacterial DNA sequences identified especially in fecal samples obtained after some months of age show little homology with known bacteria, indicating the presence of bacteria not detectable by culture [25].

Anaerobic bacteria establish successively until a highly diverse 'adult' type of microbiota has developed at a few years of age [24, 28]. The increasingly complex anaerobic microbiota provides selective pressure on the facultative bacteria and suppresses their growth. The mean ratio of strict to facultative anaerobes is approximately 1:10 at one week, 4:1 at one month and 60:1 at one year of age using culture-based identification [6]. In the adult microbiota the strict anaerobes are hundred- or thousand-fold more numerous than the facultative bacteria.

The ability of the microbiota to suppress the growth of the facultative bacteria, such as *E. coli*, enterococci and staphylococci, or certain anaerobes, e.g. *C. difficile,* is termed 'colonization resistance'. It also implies resistance to the implantation of new bacterial strains into the ecosystem. The exact mechanisms leading to colonization resistance are not defined, but are likely to include competition for nutrients and binding sites, and production of toxic metabolites [29, 30].

Source of Bacteria Colonizing Infants

Staphylococci, which are the first colonizers of the infant gut, are ubiquitously present on the skin and mucosal membranes of most individuals. Strains colonizing the neonatal intestine may be acquired from any individual in close contact with the baby, e.g. parents or hospital staff. The parental skin flora is the most important source of *S. aureus* strains colonizing the neonatal gut [31]. Bacteria may be transferred during general care, but breastfeeding may be another important source as the nipples are frequently colonized by staphylococci, and staphylococci are isolated from breast milk in large numbers [32].

Most infants acquire enterococci within the first week of life. Enterococci, especially *E. faecalis* and *E. faecium,* are typical fecal bacteria, but they are also sturdy bacteria that resist most hygienic measures, which makes them spread easily in, e.g., the hospital milieu [33]. Infants may acquire enterococci from their mother's fecal microbiota during delivery (vertical transfer) or from environmental sources (horizontal transfer), although this has not been specifically studied. As both infants delivered vaginally and infants delivered by cesarean section acquire enterococci very early [7], it is evident that contact with fecal material is not necessary for acquisition of these bacteria.

E. coli was previously the first colonizer of the infant gut [34, 35]. *E. coli* is present in the gut of almost all adult individuals, and approximately one third of babies acquire *E. coli* from the mother's fecal microbiota during delivery [35–39]. The remainder of infants previously became colonized by the spread of *E. coli* strains between infants in the maternity wards by the hospital staff [35, 37]. 'Rooming in', short hospital stays and strict hygiene have reduced such exposure, and today it takes 6 months before 80% of the infants have acquired *E. coli* [6, 7], indicating a very limited spread of *E. coli* not only in the hospital, but also in families and homes in modern Western societies.

Enterobacteria other than *E. coli*, e.g. *Klebsiella* and *Enterobacter*, that are common colonizers of the infantile gut [1, 2, 7, 40] rarely derive from the mother [36, 41], because they are uncommon in the adult fecal microbiota [19]. Instead they may spread in maternity and neonatal wards between infants carried by the staff [36, 41]. As these bacteria are present in soil and other natural environments they may also be acquired from foods [39]. We recently showed that early introduction of solid foods was associated with colonization by *Klebsiella* species [6].

The origin of the anaerobic bacteria colonizing neonates has been little studied. Transfer of bifidobacteria from mother to infant may occur during a vaginal delivery [42] but horizontal transfer is probably also common. Infants' intestinal carriage of different bifidobacterial species or subgroups varies between different maternity wards, indicating transfer between infants [4, 40, 43]. Bifidobacteria are not restricted to the intestine but are also part of the oral microbiota of healthy adults [44], which could be another source of strains colonizing neonates.

Bacteroides are usually restricted to the gut and are not part of the oral microbiota. They are strict anaerobes which do not survive long in the presence of oxygen, which hampers their spread. Few Swedish infants acquire *Bacteroides* in the first week of life and they most likely acquire these bacteria from their mother during delivery [7]. The colonization frequency increases only slowly with age [7], reflecting a low level of exposure to these typical fecal bacteria in modern Western societies.

Clostridial spores resist disinfectants and are ubiquitous in the hospital milieu and other environments [45], and these bacteria are therefore quite easily acquired by the neonate [12, 46–49]. The gut microbiota of the mother is probably less important as a source of colonizing strains. Thus, strains of *C. difficile* colonizing neonates are rarely of maternal origin [49].

Lactobacilli of the species *L. crispatus*, *L. gasseri*, *L. iners* and *L. jensenii* dominate the vaginal microbiota of healthy women [50], and maternal vaginal lactobacilli may transiently colonize the intestine of the baby [51]. In accordance, we found that *L. gasseri* was the commonest *Lactobacillus* species in the first month of life in Swedish infants [18]. Another source of lactobacilli may be breast milk, as lactobacilli may be found in human milk [52]. Furthermore, as lactobacilli are part of the oral microbiota, these bacteria may be transferred via saliva from parent to infant. *L. rhamnosus* is a common oral colonizer and the dominant *Lactobacillus* species in the infantile gut in the first 6 months of life [18]. *Lactobacillus* species that appear later in the microbiota, like *L. paracasei, L. plantarum, L. acidophilus* and *L. delbruckeii*, may be picked up from foods [18].

The origin of the wide range of other anaerobic bacteria successively establishing in the infantile gut has not been determined. Possibly, many of these bacteria are acquired from the maternal gut microbiota during normal vaginal delivery, although their proliferation is restricted during the first period after birth. Alternatively, they are acquired from other yet not identified sources at later time points.

Influence of Delivery Mode on Intestinal Colonization Pattern

An infant born by cesarean section is not exposed to maternal intestinal and vaginal microbiota during delivery and, thus, the first bacteria establishing in the gut are derived exclusively from other sources. The acquisition of several of the common early colonizers is delayed, especially colonization by *Bacteroides*, but also bifidobacteria and *E. coli* [6, 7, 15, 47, 53–55]. As seen in figure 5, infants delivered by cesarean section do not catch up within the first year of life with respect to colonization by *Bacteroides* and *E. coli*, an illustration of the low exposure to these fecal bacteria in the society [7]. Furthermore, infants delivered by cesarean section have a lower ratio of anaerobic to facultative bacteria at 1 year of age, which might be regarded as a sign of a poorly developed anaerobic microbiota, unable to suppress the growth of facultative bacteria [6].

Infants born by cesarean section commonly show increased colonization with enterobacteria other than *E. coli*, e.g. *Klebsiella* and *Enterobacter* species [6, 7, 56, 57], suggesting that these bacteria may take the place of *E. coli*, whose colonization is reduced due to lack of contact with fecal bacteria. Furthermore, the lack of competition from anaerobic bacteria probably enables their establishment and persistence, a sign of reduced colonization resistance in infants delivered by cesarean section [58].

Clostridia, including *C. perfringens* and *C. difficile* are also more common in the gut microbiota of infants born by cesarean section than in vaginally delivered infants [6, 7, 15, 47]. Clostridial spores are ubiquitous in the environment and might easily expand in the poorly developed anaerobic microbiota of neonates delivered by cesarean section.

Neonatal Intensive Care and Treatment with Antibiotics

Infants cared for at neonatal intensive care units (NICUs) have few bacterial species in their gut microbiota [59–62]. Coagulase-negative staphylococci,

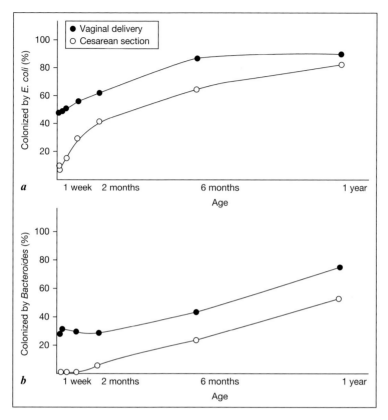

Fig. 5. Frequency of colonization by (**a**) *E. coli* and (**b**) *Bacteroides* at different time points after birth in Swedish infants delivered vaginally or by cesarean section. Adapted from reference Adlerberth et al. [7].

enterobacteria and enterococci are the bacteria most frequently isolated from these infants and anaerobes are almost completely absent [59–61]. Parenteral nutrition and use of broad-spectrum antibiotics selecting for coagulase-negative staphylococci, enterococci and non-*E. coli* enterobacteria, which frequently have resistance mechanisms, may be responsible for this quite 'unnatural' colonization pattern.

Breastfeeding and Intestinal Colonization Pattern

It is often stated that breastfeeding has a profound influence on the gut microbiota, but many studies from the 1980s and onwards report only minor differences in the colonization pattern of breast- and formula-fed infants (table 2). Bifidobacteria are mostly found equally often and in similar counts

Table 2. Results of studies performed from 1980 and onwards comparing the intestinal microbiota of breastfed and formula-fed infants

Bacterial group	Number of studies		
	↑ in breastfed	no clear difference	↓ in breastfed
Bifidobacteria	7/27	20/27	–
Bacteroides	2/19	9/19	8/19
Clostridia	–	4/17	13/17
Lactobacilli	2/16	10/16	4/16
Enterobacteria	1/21	9/21	11/21
Enterococci	–	5/16	11/16
Staphylococci	5/12	7/12	–

Data from references [12, 15, 67–71, 81–85].

in breast- and formula-fed infants using conventional culture- [2, 9, 21, 23, 40, 63–66] or non-culture-dependent methods [15, 67–71]. Previous reports of marked differences in the colonization frequency of bifidobacteria between breast- and formula-fed infants may be explained by the use of older types of infant formulas with higher protein and phosphate content.

Bacteroides are isolated less frequently from breastfed than from formula-fed infants in many studies [2, 15, 21, 72, 73], but others find no differences regarding colonization by *Bacteroides* [14, 23, 40, 65, 66, 74]. Clostridia, including *C. difficile*, are usually more prevalent in formula-fed infants [2, 9, 15, 21, 23, 69, 72, 73, 75].

Among facultative bacteria, some studies report higher counts of staphylococci in breastfed than bottle-fed infants, especially during the first weeks of life [2, 40, 65, 66, 76]. As mentioned earlier, these bacteria might be acquired from the mother during breastfeeding. In contrast, breastfed infants may have lower counts of enterococci [2, 9, 21, 72, 73, 77] and enterobacteria [9, 15, 21, 69, 73] than formula-fed infants.

It is commonly stated that breastfeeding promotes the expansion of lactobacilli in the neonatal gut. This might relate to the fact that bifidobacteria were included earlier in the genus *Lactobacillus*, as *L. bifidus*, and not until 1986 were they transferred to the genus *Bifidobacterium* in Bergey's Manual of Systematic Bacteriology [78]. Clearly, most studies find no differences regarding *Lactobacillus* colonization between breast- and formula-fed infants, or even more lactobacilli in formula-fed infants [15, 21, 23, 72]. However, we recently reported that *L. rhamnosus* was more common in 6-month-old Swedish infants if they still received breast milk than if they had been weaned by that age [18], indicating that certain species of lactobacilli may be favored by breastfeeding.

Infant formulas have been adapted in several ways in order to induce a colonization pattern similar to breastfed infants. For example, addition of lactoferrin or nucleotides to infant formulas has been tested, but does not seem to change the microbiota of bottle-fed infants towards the 'breastfed' pattern [63, 74, 79, 80]. Supplementation with galactooligosaccharides and fructooligosaccharides may increase bifidobacterial counts [68, 81–85], although it is doubtful if this would represent a 'breastfed' pattern as high bifidobacterial counts are common in both formula-fed and breastfed infants. Most studies find no effect of supplementation with galacto- and fructooligosaccharides on colonization by *Bacteroides*, clostridia, enterococci, *E. coli* or other *Enterobacteriaceae* [81, 82, 84, 86, 87], although one study reported reduced colonization by facultative bacteria [85] and another reduced counts of clostridia [88] in infants receiving supplemented formula. Intake of a formula supplemented with fructo- but not galactooligosaccharides led to decreased counts of *E. coli* and enterococci but increased counts of *Bacteroides* in one study [89], and to increased counts of clostridia and *Bacteroides* in another [90]. In summary, the effects of oligosaccharides on intestinal bacteria other than bifidobacteria are inconclusive and probably minor.

Effects of Lifestyle on the Intestinal Microbiota

The effect of family, home environment and lifestyle on the establishment of the intestinal microbiota has been little studied. When examining the colonization pattern of 300 Swedish, Italian and British infants over the first year of life, we noted an effect of lifestyle on some colonization parameters [6]. Infants with older siblings were less often colonized by non-*E. coli* enterobacteria and clostridia than single children and had a higher ratio of anaerobic over facultative bacteria at 12 months of age, suggesting a more mature colonization pattern. The colonization pattern of single children, thus, showed some resemblance to that of infants born by cesarean section, although the observed effects were weaker. Thus, both delivery by cesarean section and being firstborn may result in an anaerobic microbiota of low complexity, unable to suppress the growth of facultatives [6]. In accordance, another study found that infants with older siblings tended to have higher counts of bifidobacteria in the gut at 1 month of age compared to firstborn infants [15]. Whether this results from a spread of bacteria between siblings, or results from differences in transfer of bacteria during first and subsequent deliveries is not known. Usually, second and third deliveries are more rapid, and it is possible that contamination of the baby with fecal bacteria occurs more often compared with first deliveries.

Having pets in the home does not seem to influence the colonization pattern of neonates [6, 15]. However, in a recent study including more than 200 Swedish and Italian neonates, having pets was associated with decreased colonization by *S. aureus* early in life [Lindberg et al., in preparation].

Penders et al. [15] also examined the effect of farm residence on the intestinal microbiota, i.e. colonization by bifidobacteria, *Bacteroides*, *E. coli*, lactobacilli and *C. difficile* by 1 month of age. No statistically significant associations were found, but there was a tendency towards lower counts of *C. difficile* in infants in farming families [15], which could indicate a generally more complex microbiota in these infants. Clearly, further studies are needed to address the effects of various lifestyle factors on intestinal colonization pattern in infancy.

Colonization Pattern of Infants in Non-Western Societies

Whereas Western infants are born in hospitals with high hygienic standards and grow up in households with excellent sanitary conditions, infants in developing countries are often delivered and raised under poor and crowded conditions. It is not surprising that these conditions influence the early colonization pattern. Although few direct comparative studies have been performed, it is clear that infants in developing countries are colonized earlier by *E. coli* and other enterobacteria, enterococci and lactobacilli and have a more varied microbiota early in life than infants in Western societies [1, 3, 39, 91, 92]. Furthermore, in developing countries, also infants delivered by cesarean section acquire gut bacteria, including the anaerobes bifidobacteria and *Bacteroides*, very early [1, 92], a testimony to the circulation of fecal bacteria in the hospital.

The heavy exposure to a wide variety of bacteria in developing countries leads to a rapid turnover of strains in the microbiota. Pakistani infants harbor 8–9 different *E. coli* strains in their microbiota over the first 6 months of life [39], compared with two strains in Swedish infants followed over the first year of life [11].

'Opportunistic' colonizers are less common in the gut microbiota of infants in developing countries than in Western societies, as a sign of a much earlier acquisition of a complex microbiota. Skin bacteria like coagulase-negative staphylococci are common in the gut flora of European infants but uncommon in Ethiopian infants [6, 91]. *S. aureus* is less common in the gut microbiota of infants in developing as compared to Western countries, as evident when comparing isolation rates in different studies [3, 10]. Although Pakistani infants frequently become colonized by enterobacteria other than *E. coli* in the first week of life, they disappear from the microbiota already after some weeks, probably in response to overwhelming competition [1, 39]. In contrast, Swedish infants display increasing colonization by enterobacteria other than *E. coli* over the first 6 months of life [7].

Differences in colonization pattern have also been observed between infants in Western societies and infants in the former socialist countries of Eastern Europe, the latter being colonized earlier with lactobacilli and eubacteria [20, 93]. At 1 year of age Estonian children less frequently harbor *C. difficile* than Swedish infants [20]. Interestingly, colonization by *S. aureus* is more common in Swedish than in Italian infants in the first year of life [Lindberg et al., in preparation], possibly indicating an earlier maturation of the intestinal microbiota in Italian infants.

Possible Consequences to Health of the 'Non-Western' and 'Western' Colonization Patterns

In developing countries, the early and diverse gut microbiota containing, e.g., various enterobacterial strains may be an important source of bacteria causing septicemia in the neonatal period, as bacteria may reach the blood stream by direct translocation over the intestinal epithelial barrier when reaching high population counts in the gut [94]. The incidence of neonatal septicemia is much higher in developing as compared to industrialized societies (20/1,000 vs. 4/1,000) [12], and a majority of these infections is caused by intestinal bacteria such as *E. coli, Klebsiella* and other enterobacteria, enterococci and *Pseudomonas* [12, 95, 96].

The consequences for health of the 'Western' colonization pattern are not known. It is interesting to note that staphylococci are today the most common cause of neonatal septicemia in Sweden and many other Western societies [97], and the intestinal microbiota may well be a source of infecting strains [59].

Intestinal commensal bacteria are a major stimulus for the gut immune system [98], and a late acquisition of typical fecal bacteria or a delay in the establishment of a complex and diverse intestinal microbiota may have profound effects on the developing immune system. In accordance, Pakistani infants show a strong salivary IgA response against a pool of *E. coli* O antigens at 2 months of age, while similar levels are not reached by Swedish infants until 1–2 years of age [99].

Whether the rising incidence of immunoregulatory disorders such as allergies, Crohn's disease and type-1 diabetes in Western countries depends on a paucity of immune stimulation, e.g. by gut bacteria, remains to be investigated.

References

1   Adlerberth I, Carlsson B, de Man P, et al: Intestinal colonization with Enterobacteriaceae in Pakistani and Swedish hospital delivered infants. Acta Paediatr Scand 1991;80:602–610.
2   Balmer SE, Wharton BA: Diet and faecal flora in the newborn: breastmilk and infant formula. Arch Dis Cild 1989;64:1672–1677.
3   Mata LJ, Urrutia JJ: Intestinal colonization of breastfed children in a rural area of low socio-economic level. Ann NY Acad Sci 1971;176:93–109.
4   Mitsuoka T, Kaneuchi C: Ecology of the bifidobacteria. Am J Clin Nutr 1977;30:1799–1810.
5   Rotimi VO, Duerden BI: The development of the bacterial flora in normal neonates. J Med Microbiol 1981;14:51–62.
6   Adlerberth I, Strachan DP, Matricardi PM, et al: Gut microbiota and development of atopic eczema in 3 European birth cohorts. J Allergy Clin Immunol 2007;120:343–350.

7 Adlerberth I, Lindberg E, Aberg N, et al: Reduced enterobacterial and increased staphylococcal colonization of the infantile bowel: an effect of hygienic lifestyle? Pediatr Res 2006;59:96–101.

8 Hoogkamp-Korstanje JAA, Lindner JGGM, Marcelis JH, et al: Composition and ecology of the human intestinal flora. Antonie Van Leeuwenhoek 1979;45:35–40.

9 Stark PL, Lee A: The microbial ecology of the large bowel of breast-fed and formula-fed infants during the first year of life. J Med Microbiol 1982;15:189–203.

10 Lindberg E, Nowrouzian F, Adlerberth I, Wold AE: Long-time persistence of superantigen-producing strains of *Staphylococcus aureus* in the intestinal microflora of healthy infants. Pediatr Res 2000;48:741–747.

11 Nowrouzian F, Hesselmar B, Saalman R, et al: *Escherichia coli* in infants' intestinal microflora: colonization rate, strain turnover, and virulence gene carriage. Pediatr Res 2003; 54:8–14.

12 Adlerberth I, Hanson LÅ, Wold AE: The ontogeny of the intestinal flora; in Sanderson IR, Walker WA (eds): Development of the Gastrointestinal Tract. Hamilton, Decker, 1999, pp 279–292.

13 Favier CF, de Vos WM, Akkermans AD: Development of bacterial and bifidobacterial communities in feces of newborn babies. Anaerobe 2003;9:219–229.

14 Hopkins MJ, Macfarlane GT, Furrie E, et al: Characterisation of intestinal bacteria in infant stools using real-time PCR and northern hybridisation analyses. FEMS Microbiol Ecol 2005;54:77–85.

15 Penders J, Thijs C, Vink C, et al: Factors influencing the composition of the intestinal microbiota in early infancy. Pediatrics 2006;118:511–521.

16 Matsuki T, Watanabe K, Tanaka R, et al: Distribution of bifidobacterial species in human intestinal microflora examined with 16S rRNA-gene-targeted species-specific primers. Appl Environ Microbiol 1999;65:4506–4512.

17 Harmsen HJ, Wildeboer-Veloo AC, Raangs GC, et al: Analysis of intestinal flora development in breast-fed and formula-fed infants by using molecular identification and detection methods. J Pediatr Gastroenterol Nutr 2000;30:61–67.

18 Ahrne S, Lönnermark E, Wold AE, et al: Lactobacilli in the intestinal microbiota of Swedish infants. Microbes Infect 2005;7:1256–1262.

19 Finegold SM, Sutter VL, Mathisen GE: Normal indigenous intestinal flora; in Hentges DJ (ed): Human Intestinal Microflora in Health and Disease. London, Academic Press, 1983, pp 3–31.

20 Sepp E, Julge K, Vasar M, et al: Intestinal microflora of Estonian and Swedish infants. Acta Paediatr 1997;86:956–961.

21 Benno Y, Sawada K, Mitsuoka T: The intestinal microflora of infants: composition of the fecal flora in breastfed and bottlefed infants. Microbiol Immunol 1984;28:975–986.

22 George M, Nord KE, Ronquist G, et al: Faecal microflora and urease activity during the first six months of infancy. Ups J Med Sci 1996;101:233–250.

23 Kleessen B, Bunke H, Tovar K, et al: Influence of two infant formulas and human milk on the development of the faecal flora in newborn infants. Acta Paediatr Scand 1995;84:1347–1356.

24 Ellis-Pegler RB, Crabtree C, Lambert HP: The faecal flora of children in the United Kingdom. J Hyg Camb 1975;75:135–142.

25 Favier CF, Vaughan EE, de Vos VM, Akkermans AD: Molecular monitoring of succession of bacterial communities in human neonates. Appl Environ Microbiol 2002;68:219–226.

26 Harmsen HJ, Wildeboer-Veloo AC, Grijpstra J, et al: Development of 16S rRNA-based probes for the Coriobacterium group and the Atopobium cluster and their application for enumeration of Coriobacteriaceae in human feces from volunteers of different age groups. Appl Environ Microbiol 2000;66:4523–4527.

27 Wang M, Ahrné S, Antonsson M, Molin G: T-RFLP combined with principal component analysis and 16S rRNA gene sequencing: an effective strategy for comparison of fecal microbiota in infants of different ages. J Microbiol Methods 2004;59:53–69.

28 Midtvedt A-C: The establishment and development of some metabolic activities associated with the intestinal microflora in healthy children; thesis, Karolinska Institute, Stockholm University, 1994.

29 Freter R: Factors affecting the microecology of the gut; in Fuller R (ed): Probiotics – The Scientific Basis. London, Chapman & Hall, 1992, pp 111–144.

30 Hentges DJ: Role of intestinal flora in host defence against infection; in Hentges DJ (ed): Human Intestinal Microflora in Health and Disease. New York, Academic Press, 1983, pp 311–331.

31 Lindberg E, Adlerberth I, Hesselmar B, et al: High rate of transfer of *Staphylococcus aureus* from parental skin to infant gut flora. J Clin Microbiol 2004;42:530–534.

32 Boo NY, Nordiah AJ, Alfizah H, et al: Contamination of breast milk obtained by manual expression and breast pumps in mothers of very low birthweight infants. J Hosp Infect 2001;49: 274–281.

33 Kearns AM, Freeman R, Lightfoot NF: Nosocomial enterococci: resistance to heat and sodium hypochlorite. J Hosp Infect 1995;30:193–199.

34 Bettelheim KA, Breadon A, Faiers MC, et al: The origin of O-serotypes of *Escherichia coli* in babies after normal delivery. J Hyg Camb 1974;72:67–70.

35 Bettelheim KA, Lenox-King SMJ: The acquisition of *Escherichia coli* by newborn babies. Infection 1976;4:174–179.

36 Fryklund B, Tullus K, Berglund B, Burman LG: Importance of the environment and the faecal flora of infants, nursing staff and parents as sources of Gram-negative bacteria colonizing newborns in three neonatal wards. Infection 1992;20:253–257.

37 Gothefors L, Carlsson B, Ahlstedt S, et al: Influence of maternal gut flora and colostral and cord serum antibodies on presence of *Escherichia coli* in faeces of the newborn infant. Acta Paediatr Scand 1976;65:225–232.

38 Murono K, Fujita K, Yoshikawa M, et al: Acquisition of nonmaternal Enterobacteriaceae by infants delivered in hospitals. J Paediatr 1993;122:120–125.

39 Adlerberth I, Jalil F, Carlsson B, et al: High turn over rate of *Escherichia coli* strains in the intestinal flora of infants in Pakistan. Epidemiol Infect 1998;121:587–598.

40 Lundequist B, Nord CE, Winberg J: The composition of faecal microflora in breastfed and bottlefed infants from birth to 8 weeks. Acta Paediatr Scand 1985;74:54–58.

41 Shinebaum R, Cooke EM, Brayson JC: Acquisition of *Klebsiella aerogenes* by neonates. J Med Microbiol 1979;12:201–205.

42 Tannock GW, Fuller R, Smith SL, Hall MA: Plasmid profiling of members of the family Enterobacteriaceae, lactobacilli, and bifidobacteria to study the transmission of bacteria from mother to infant. J Clin Microbiol 1990;28:1225–1228.

43 Bezirtzoglou E, Romond C: Occurrence of Bifidobacterium in the feces of newborns delivered by cesarean section. Biol Neonate 1990;58:247–251.

44 Sutter VL: Anaerobes as normal oral flora. Rev Infect Dis 1984;6(suppl 1):S62–S66.

45 Wilson KH: The microecology of *Clostridium difficile*. Clin Infect Dis 1993;16(suppl 4): s214–s218.

46 el-Mohandes AE, Keijser JF, Refat M, Jackson BJ: Prevalence and toxigenicity of *Clostridium difficile* isolates in fecal microflora of preterm infants in the intensive care nursery. Biol Neonate 1993;63:225–229.

47 Neut C, Bezirtzoglou E, Romond C, et al: Bacterial colonization of the large intestine in newborns delivered by caesarean section. Zbl Bakt Hyg A 1987;266:330–337.

48 Kato H, Kato N, Watanabe K, et al: Application of typing by pulsed-field gel electrophoresis to the study of *Clostridium difficile* in a neonatal intensive care unit. J Clin Microbiol 1994;32:2067–2070.

49 Martirosian G, Kuipers S, Verbrugh H, et al: PCR ribotyping and arbitrarily primed PCR for typing strains of *Clostridium difficile* from a Polish maternity hospital. J Clin Microbiol 1995; 33:2016–2021.

50 Vasquez A, Jacobsson T, Ahrné S, et al: Vaginal lactobacillus flora of healthy Swedish women. J Clin Microbiol 2002;40:2746–2749.

51 Matsumiya Y, Kato N, Watanabe K, Kato H: Molecular epidemiological study of vertical transmission of vaginal Lactobacillus species from mothers to newborn infants in Japanese, by arbitrarily primed polymerase chain reaction. J Infect Chemother 2002;8:43–49.

52 Martin R, Langa S, Reviriego C, et al: Human milk is a source of lactic acid bacteria for the infant gut. J Pediatr 2003;143:754–758.

53 Bennet R, Nord CE: Development of the faecal anaerobic microflora after caesarean section and treatment with antibiotics in newborn infants. Infection 1987;15:332–336.

54 Grönlund MM, Lethonen OP, Eerola E, Kero P: Fecal microflora in healthy infants born by different methods of delivery: permanent changes in intestinal microflora after cesarean delivery. J Pediatr Gastroenterol Nutr 1999;28:19–25.

55 Hall MA, Coole CB, Smith SL, et al: Factors influencing the presence of faecal lactobacilli on early infancy. Arch Dis Child 1990;65:185–188.

56 Bennet R, Eriksson M, Nord CE, Zetterström R: Fecal bacterial microflora of newborn infants during intensive care management and treatment with five antibiotic regimens. Pediatr Infect Dis 1986;5:533–539.

57 Long SS, Swenson RM: Development of anaerobic fecal flora in healthy newborn infants. J Pediatr 1977;91:298–301.

58 Bennet R: Relationship between anaerobic bacteria and enterobacteria in feces of newborn infants. Pediatr Infect Dis J 1987;6:426.

59 el-Mohandes AE, Keiser JF, Johnson LA, et al: Aerobes isolated in fecal microflora of infants in the intensive care nursery: relationship to human milk use and systemic sepsis. Am J Infect Control 1993;21:231–234.

60 Gewolb IH, Schwalbe RS, Taciak VL, et al: Stool microflora in extremely low birthweight infants. Arch Dis Child Fetal Neonatal Ed 1999;80:F167–F173.

61 Hallstrom M, Eerola E, Vuento R, et al: Effects of mode of delivery and necrotising enterocolitis on the intestinal microflora in preterm infants. Eur J Clin Microbiol Infect Dis 2004;23:463–470.

62 Magne F, Suau A, Pochart P, Desleux JF: Fecal microbial community in preterm infants. J Pediatr Gastroenterol Nutr 2005;41:386–392.

63 Balmer SE, Hanvey LS, Wharton BA: Diet and faecal flora in the newborn: nucleotides. Arch Dis Child 1994;70:F137–F140.

64 Langhendries JP, Detry J, Van-Hees J, et al: Effect of a fermented infant formula containing viable bifidobacteria on the fecal flora composition and pH of healthy fullterm infants. J Pediatr Gastroenterol Nutr 1995;21:177–181.

65 Simhon A, Douglas JR, Drasar BS, Soothill JF: Effect of feeding on infants faecal flora. Arch Dis Child 1982;57:54–58.

66 Cooke G, Behan J, Clarke N, et al: Comparing the gut flora of Irish breastfed and formula-fed neonates aged between birth and 6 weeks old. Microb Ecol Health Dis 2005;17:163–168.

67 Bakker-Zierikzee AM, Alles MS, Knol J, et al: Effects of infant formula containing a mixture of galacto- and fructo-oligosaccharides or viable Bifidobacterium animalis on the intestinal microflora during the first 4 months of life. Br J Nutr 2005;94:783–790.

68 Haarman M, Knol J: Quantitative real-time PCR assays to identify and quantify fecal Bifidobacterium species in infants receiving a prebiotic infant formula. Appl Environ Microbiol 2005;71:2318–2324.

69 Penders J, Vink C, Driessen C, et al: Quantification of Bifidobacterium spp., Escherichia coli and Clostridium difficile in faecal samples of breast-fed and formula-fed infants by real-time PCR. FEMS Microbiol Lett 2005;243:141–147.

70 Sakata S, Tonooka T, Ishizeki S, et al: Culture-independent analysis of fecal microbiota in infants, with special reference to Bifidobacterium species. FEMS Microbiol Lett 2005;243: 417–423.

71 Satokari RM, Vaughan EE, Favier CF, et al: Diversity of Bifidobacterium and Lactobacillus spp. in breast-fed and formula-fed infants as assessed by 16S rDNA sequence differences. Microb Ecol Health Dis 2002;14:97–105.

72 Mevissen-Verhage EAE, Marcelis JH, Harmsen-Van Amerongen WCM, et al: Effect of iron on neonatal gut flora during the first three months of life. Eur J Clin Microbiol 1985;4:273–278.

73 Yoshioka H, Iseki K, Fujita J: Development and differences of intestinal flora in the neonatal period in breastfed and bottlefed infants. Pediatrics 1983;72:317–321.

74 Roberts AK, Chierici R, Sawatzki G, et al: Supplementation of an adapted formula with bovine lactoferrin: 1. Effect on the infant faecal flora. Acta Paediatr Scand 1992;81:119–124.

75 Tullus K, Aronsson B, Marcus S, et al: Intestinal colonization with Clostridium difficile in infants up to 18 months of age. Eur J Clin Microbiol Infect Dis 1989;8:390–393.

76 el-Mohandes AE, Keiser JF, Johnson LA, et al: Aerobes isolated in fecal microflora of infants in the intensive care nursery: relationship to human milk use and systemic sepsis. Am J Infect Control 1993;21:231–234.

77 Balmer SE, Scott PH, Wharton BA: Diet and faecal flora in the newborn: casein and whey proteins. Arch Dis Child 1989;64:1678–1684.

78 Scardovi V: Genus Bifidobacterium Orla-Jensen 1924; in Sneath PHA, Mair NS, Sharpe ME, Holt JG (eds): Bergey's Manual of Systematic Bacteriology. Baltimore, Williams & Wilkins, 1986, pp 1418–1434.

79 Balmer SE, Scott PH, Wharton BA: Diet and fecal flora in the newborn: lactoferrin. Arch Dis Child 1989;64:1685–1690.

80 Gil A, Corall E, Martínez A, Molina JA: Effects of the addition of nucleotides to an adapted milk formula on the microbial pattern of faeces in at term newborn infants. J Clin Nutr Gastroenterol 1986;1:127–132.
81 Boehm G, Lidestri M, Casetta P, et al: Supplementation of a bovine milk formula with an oligosaccharide mixture increases counts of faecal bifidobacteria in preterm infants. Arch Dis Child Fetal Neonatal Ed 2002;86:F178–F181.
82 Moro G, Minoli I, Mosca M, et al: Dosage-related bifidogenic effects of galacto- and fructooligosaccharides in formula-fed term infants. J Pediatr Gastroenterol Nutr 2002;34:291–295.
83 Schmelzle H, Wirth S, Skopnik H, et al: Randomized double-blind study of the nutritional efficacy and bifidogenicity of a new infant formula containing partially hydrolyzed protein, a high beta-palmitic acid level, and nondigestible oligosaccharides. J Pediatr Gastroenterol Nutr 2003;36:343–351.
84 Rinne MM, Gueimonde M, Kalliomaki M, et al: Similar bifidogenic effects of prebiotic-supplemented partially hydrolyzed infant formula and breastfeeding on infant gut microbiota. FEMS Immunol Med Microbiol 2005;43:59–65.
85 Knol J, Boehm G, Lidestri M, et al: Increase of faecal bifidobacteria due to dietary oligosaccharides induces a reduction of clinically relevant pathogen germs in the faeces of formula-fed preterm infants. Acta Paediatr Suppl 2005;94:31–33.
86 Brunser O, Figueroa G, Gotteland M, et al: Effects of probiotic or prebiotic supplemented milk formulas on fecal microbiota composition of infants. Asia Pac J Clin Nutr 2006;15:368–376.
87 Brunser O, Gotteland M, Cruchet S, et al: Effect of a milk formula with prebiotics on the intestinal microbiota of infants after an antibiotic treatment. Pediatr Res 2006;59:451–456.
88 Costalos C, Kapiki A, Apostolou M, Papathoma E: The effect of a prebiotic supplemented formula on growth and stool microbiology of term infants. Early Hum Dev 2007;84:45–49.
89 Kapiki A, Costalos C, Oikonomidou C, et al: The effect of a fructooligosaccharide supplemented formula on gut flora of preterm infants. Early Hum Dev 2007;83:335–339.
90 Euler AR, Mitchell DK, Kline R, Pickering LK: Prebiotic effect of fructooligosaccharide supplemented term infant formula at two concentrations compared with unsupplemented formula and human milk. J Pediatr Gastroenterol Nutr 2005;40:157–164.
91 Bennet R, Eriksson M, Tafari N, Nord CE: Intestinal bacteria of newborn ethiopian infants in relation to antibiotic treatment and colonization with potentially pathogenic Gram-negative bacteria. Scand J Infect Dis 1991;23:63–69.
92 Rotimi VO, Olowe SA, Ahmed I: The development of bacterial flora in premature neonates. J Hyg Camb 1985;94:309–318.
93 Sepp E, Naaber P, Voor T, et al: Development of the intestinal microflora during the first month of life in Estonian and Swedish infants. Microb Ecol Health Dis 2000;12:22–26.
94 Van Camp JM, Tomaselli V, Coran AG: Bacterial translocation in the neonate. Curr Opin Pediatr 1994;6:327–333.
95 Bhutta ZA, Naqvi SH, Muzaffar T, Farooqui BJ: Neonatal sepsis in Pakistan. Presentation and pathogens. Acta Paediatr Scand 1991;80:596–601.
96 Salamati P, Rahbarimanesh AA, Yunesian M, Naseri M: Neonatal nosocomial infections in Bahrami Children Hospital. Indian J Pediatr 2006;73:197–200.
97 Kallman J, Kihlstrom E, Sjoberg L, Schollin J: Increase of staphylococci in neonatal septicaemia: a fourteen-year study. Acta Paediatr 1997;86:533–538.
98 Cebra JJ: Influences of microbiota on intestinal immune system development. Am J Clin Nutr 1999;69:1046S–1051S.
99 Mellander L, Carlsson B, Jalil F, et al: Secretory IgA antibody response against Escherichia coli antigens in infants in relation to exposure. J Pediatr 1985;107:430–433.
100 Rotimi VO, Duerden BI: Bacteroides species in the normal neonatal faecal flora. J Hyg Camb 1981;87:299–304.

Discussion

Dr. Isolauri: You mentioned two points of confusion: one was that not constantly breastfeeding seems to promote bifidobacteria in the infant. I think that is not very confusing if one accepts that breast milk is not a standard product, also in terms of prebiotics as well as bifidobacteria; breast milk is a reflection of the mother. You also mentioned another point that the addition of oligosaccharides increases bifidobacteria and sometimes it doesn't. At the same time you said that not all infants are colonized with bifidobacteria early on. I don't see a confusion here either because bifidogenic agents probably do not promote bifidobacteria if the baby is not colonized early with bifidobacteria. Somebody needs to be stimulated; so the early days appear to be very important. Do you agree?

Dr. Adlerberth: I agree with you. Clearly, prebiotics need to have some bacteria present from the start to be able to support their growth. The data concerning promotion of bifidobacterial growth by those oligosaccharides are quite convincing, but the results are less convincing regarding lactobacilli [1–7]. As you said, this could well have to do with a low colonization frequency with lactobacilli from the beginning.

Dr. Björkstén: I would like to have your comments on microbial diversity. Most studies, including most of our studies and those of our chairperson, have looked at single species rather than using a holistic approach. You used a different approach comparing variations in *Escherichia coli* strains in Pakistani and Swedish children, showing that the Pakistani children had a constant change in strains while in Sweden the same strains remained for long periods of time in the individual child. We have seen the same thing looking for lactobacilli in Estonia as compared to Sweden, all species are present in both countries but the Estonians often change strains while the diversity is less in Swedish children. I think it is a major difference from an immunological point of view if one is continuously exposed to hundreds of strains or keeps the same strains over long periods of time. Have you looked at diversity in your recent studies?

Dr. Adlerberth: Yes, for example we have done strain typing of all *E. coli* stains from Swedish infants in the Allergyflora Study, and it is clear that infants in Sweden encounter very few *E. coli* stains and commonly keep a single strain over prolonged periods. Thus, there is little immune stimulation provided by *E. coli,* for instance, since the immune system is activated by each new strain that colonizes, but this activation ceases as soon as a secretory IgA response against the strain has developed, as S-IgA prevents translocation of the strain and further interactions with the immune system [8]. But if one is constantly exposed to new strains they will have constant stimulation of the immune system.

Dr. Björkstén: Benn et al. [9] in Copenhagen showed that the presence of staphylococci in the vaginal flora in mid-pregnancy is associated with a more than twofold increased risk of asthma medication at age 5 years, so it seems to be a very early event indeed.

Dr. Walker: As I look at the literature there are some questions that come up that I find difficult to explain in the context of bacterial flora and clinical disease. For example, there are number of studies suggesting that in inflammatory bowel disease there is a difference in the composition of flora compared to non-inflammatory bowel disease patients and the same thing has been reported for allergic patients. What I don't quite understand is if one is dealing with a billion organisms in the gut, if some strains are reduced by a couple of logs, how does that potentially influence the pathophysiology the diseases or is it just a marker of the disease?

Dr. Adlerberth: There are great variations between gut bacteria, for instance regarding their ability to evoke an inflammatory response. To start with, gram-positive and gram-negative bacteria differ with regard to the cytokine patterns and proinflammatory mediators they induce, so one could expect differences between a flora dominated by gram-positive and one dominated by gram-negative bacteria [10]. Furthermore, at the species level, there may be great variations between different strains in their inflammatogenic and immunogenic properties. For example, it has been very nicely shown for *E. coli* that certain strains are very potent in evoking inflammatory responses depending on their expression of toxins and other virulence factors [11]. However, we know very little about the properties of most bacteria residing in the gut. I believe that the composition of the microflora could be very important for the emergence of a range of diseases, but we know very little about it yet.

Dr. Walker: Is there a corollary to that observation, e.g., can we extrapolate from culturing stools to what is going on at the surface of the colon and small intestine with regard to disease? Is there an association?

Dr. Adlerberth: There is clearly an association, but in the mucosa there are proportionally more aerobic bacteria than in the gut lumen and in the fecal sample. So very much the same species are present but in different proportions, and there are also bacteria in the gut which are not in association with the mucosa and which feed mostly from dietary substances, although most bacteria are likely to feed from the mucous layer.

Dr. Salminen: I found your presentation quite intriguing especially when you compared the older and the newer studies which I sometimes think are not really comparable. To the best of my knowledge the only published studies for bifidobacteria are from Benno et al. [12] who have followed the Japanese bifidobacterial numbers and species composition in infants since 1970. They also used a similar culturing method which was upgraded along the line to the neomolecular methods. I think their results in Japanese infants actually point out that there is no change in the concentration over the decades, but there is a significant change in the species composition, and therefore the metabolic activity of bifidobacteria in breastfed infants indicates that it is either environmental or dietary due to the mother's diet. So it is quite difficult to actually interpret whether there is a change. But to actually put them into the perspective of the method used, I think the traces are perhaps not as significant within the gut.

Dr. Adlerberth: Of course, methodological differences between studies make it difficult to compare the results, but still we can get indications pointing towards changes in the microbiota over the last decades. Regarding bifidobacteria, colonization today is as frequent as in earlier studies, but it would be very interesting to look at the species variation in the bifidobacterial flora of Western infants to see if it is as diverse today as it has been, and if the same species predominate.

Dr. Salminen: That poses an additional question because not very many differences were seen; the country differences haven't been shown yet. As Dr. Björkstén also pointed out, if we look at our studies no differences are seen with the use of the traditional culture method, and I think the culture method is just not sensitive enough. When molecular methods are used, and when you go to species composition and start measuring the metabolic activity of the different species, then significant differences are actually seen: differences between different birth methods and, most significantly, early differences in microbiota between the children who later develop the atopic disease. I understand that you are continuing on the molecular methods with your recent cohort, is that right?

Dr. Adlerberth: Yes we are. I agree with you, we need to go over these molecular methods but still today I think that both culturing and molecular methods are needed, since most molecular methods detect only the dominant bacterial populations. For instance, with T-RLFP you can only detect bacteria which are present in populations above 10^6 or 10^7/g, whereas culture on selective media may detect much smaller bacterial populations. With time, however, I think that the molecular methods will take over completely.

Dr. Salminen: I completely agree with you, they complement each other, but when we take modern molecular methods coupled with metabolic activity and bioavailability measurement, that is perhaps the best outcome so far.

Dr. Saavedra: This was a great summary with regard to what we are seeing from the point of view of colonization in the distal bowel and colon. One thing we always neglect to consider is that there are different populations in the gut depending on where we look in the gut: close to the mucosa or closer to the lumen, or the proximal gut versus the distal gut. When we examine stool we are of course looking at the very distal end of things. If we compare what the differences today might be with the differences yesterday, it is likely that bigger differences are happening in the small bowel. Today most of the intervention studies suggest that anything from 10^6, 10^8, or higher colonies be given orally as an intervention to correct what might be the difference between today's flora in the proximal gut rather than the distal gut. If an endoscopy is done today in an average child to obtain a duodenal aspirate and 10^6 colony-forming units of bacteria are found, it would be called abnormal bacterial overgrowth, and that is really what we are giving orally in all these intervention studies. So aren't we looking at the wrong thing from the point of view of really trying to understand what the immunologic potential is that dietary microbes might have?

Dr. Adlerberth: I agree with you in that what happens in the small intestine is of prior importance for stimulation of the immune system. This is where most of the antigen uptake is going on. However, also in the colon there are lymphoid patches and also translocation and induction of immune responses, although the events in the small intestine are probably most important. It is not so easy, however, to study the microbiota of the small intestine.

Dr. Hernell: I think it is true that when you start to introduce complementary food the microbiota becomes more diversified as the diet becomes more diversified. When we now postpone the introduction of complementary foods to 6 months, how would that affect the flora and the stimulation of the immune system? Actually, that hasn't been discussed much.

Dr. Adlerberth: Many classical studies have clearly shown that at weaning there is a major change in the microbiota, for example the studies by Mata and Urratia [13] and Stark and Lee [14] from Guatemala and Australia. However, in a recent study in which molecular methods were applied to study infantile microbiota, there were actually very little changes detected in the flora in connection to weaning [15]. So perhaps today weaning does not have a great impact on the microbiota.

Dr. Corthésy: Among all the factors that can influence early gut colonization you didn't mention bacterial translocation. There is evidence that bacteria can translocate from the gut of mothers via the milk to the children. What are your views on the impact that this can have on early colonization?

Dr. Björkstén: It has been known for more than 30 years that gut bacteria are present in human milk, but there is still no evidence that they are translocated. We don't know how they got there, though. One of the currently marketed probiotic strains (*Lactobacillus reuteri*) was actually isolated from the breast milk of a Peruvian woman.

Dr. Isolauri: Currently we agree that breast milk is not sterile like infant formulas.

References

1   Boehm G, Lidestri M, Casetta P, et al: Supplementation of a bovine milk formula with an oligosaccharide mixture increases counts of faecal bifidobacteria in preterm infants. Arch Dis Child Fetal Neonatal Ed 2002;86:F178–F181.
2   Moro G, Minoli I, Mosca M, et al: Dosage-related bifidogenic effects of galacto- and fructooligosaccharides in formula-fed term infants. J Pediatr Gastroenterol Nutr 2002;34: 291–295.

3 Schmelzle H, Wirth S, Skopnik H, et al: Randomized double-blind study of the nutritional efficacy and bifidogenicity of a new infant formula containing partially hydrolyzed protein, a high beta-palmitic acid level, and nondigestible oligosaccharides. J Pediatr Gastroenterol Nutr 2003;36:343–351.

4 Rinne MM, Gueimonde M, Kalliomaki M, et al: Similar bifidogenic effects of prebiotic-supplemented partially hydrolyzed infant formula and breastfeeding on infant gut microbiota. FEMS Immunol Med Microbiol 2005;43:59–65.

5 Knol J, Boehm G, Lidestri M, et al: Increase of faecal bifidobacteria due to dietary oligosaccharides induces a reduction of clinically relevant pathogen germs in the faeces of formula-fed preterm infants. Acta Paediatr Suppl 2005;94:31–33.

6 Brunser O, Figueroa G, Gotteland M, et al: Effects of probiotic or prebiotic supplemented milk formulas on fecal microbiota composition of infants. Asia Pac J Clin Nutr 2006;15:368–376.

7 Costalos C, Kapiki A, Apostolou M, Papathoma E: The effect of a prebiotic supplemented formula on growth and stool microbiology of term infants. Early Hum Dev 2007;84:45–49.

8 Shroff KE, Meslin K, Cebra JJ: Commensal enteric bacteria engender a self-limiting humoral mucosal immune response while permanently colonizing the gut. Infect Immun 1995;63: 3904–3913.

9 Benn CS, Thorsen P, Jensen JS, et al: Maternal vaginal microflora during pregnancy and the risk of asthma hospitalization and use of antiasthma medication in early childhood. J Allergy Clin Immunol 2002;110:72–77.

10 Hessle CC, Andersson B, Wold AE: Gram-positive and Gram-negative bacteria elicit different patterns of pro-inflammatory cytokines in human monocytes. Cytokine 2005;30:311–318.

11 Oelschlaeger TA, Dobrindt U, Hacker J: Virulence factors of uropathogens. Curr Opin Urol 2002;12:33–38.

12 Benno Y, Sawada K, Mitsuoka T: The intestinal microflora of infants: composition of fecal flora in breast-fed and bottle-fed infants. Microbiol Immunol 1984;28:975–986.

13 Mata LJ, Urrutia JJ: Intestinal colonization of breastfed children in a rural area of low socioeconomic level. Ann NY Acad Sci 1971;176:93–109.

14 Stark PL, Lee A: The microbial ecology of the large bowel of breast-fed and formula-fed infants during the first year of life. J Med Microbiol 1982;15:189–203.

15 Magne F, Hachelaf W, Suau A, et al: A longitudinal study of infant faecal microbiota during weaning. FEMS Microbiol Ecol 2006;58:563–571.

Bier DM, German JB, Lönnerdal B (eds): Personalized Nutrition for the Diverse Needs of Infants and Children.
Nestlé Nutr Workshop Ser Pediatr Program, vol 62, pp 35–49,
Nestec Ltd., Vevey/S. Karger AG, Basel, © 2008.

Genetically Determined Variation in Polyunsaturated Fatty Acid Metabolism May Result in Different Dietary Requirements

Berthold Koletzko[a], Hans Demmelmair[a],
Linda Schaeffer[a,b], Thomas Illig[b], Joachim Heinrich[b]

[a]Division of Metabolic Diseases and Nutritional Medicine, Dr. von Hauner Children's Hospital, University of Munich, Munich, [b]Helmholtz Institute of Epidemiology, Neuherberg, Germany

Abstract

Tissue availability of polyunsaturated fatty acids (PUFAs) is of major relevance for health, and it depends on both dietary intake and metabolic turnover. We found close associations between variants in the human genes of Δ5- and Δ6-desaturase, *FADS1* and *FADS2*, and serum phospholipid contents of PUFAs and long-chain PUFAs (LC-PUFAs). Polymorphisms and reconstructed haplotypes of *FADS1* and the upstream region of *FADS2* showed strong associations with levels of the n-6 LC-PUFA arachidonic acid (20:4n-6). Carriers of the less common polymorphisms and their respective haplotypes also had a lower prevalence of allergic rhinitis and atopic eczema. Our data demonstrate for the first time that the fatty acid composition of serum phospholipids is genetically controlled by the *FADS1 FADS2* gene cluster. The investigated single nucleotide polymorphisms in this cluster explain 28% of the variance of serum phospholipid arachidonic acid and up to 12% of its precursor acids. Based on this genetic variation, individuals may require different amounts of dietary PUFAs or LC-PUFAs to achieve comparable biological effects. We strongly recommend including analyses of *FADS1* and *FADS2* polymorphism in future cohort and intervention studies addressing the biological effects of PUFAs and LC-PUFAs, which should enhance the sensitivity and precision of such studies.

The metabolic availability of polyunsaturated fatty acid acids (PUFAs) has a major impact on human health. PUFA status has been related, among other outcomes, to early visual, cognitive and motor development [1, 2], mental

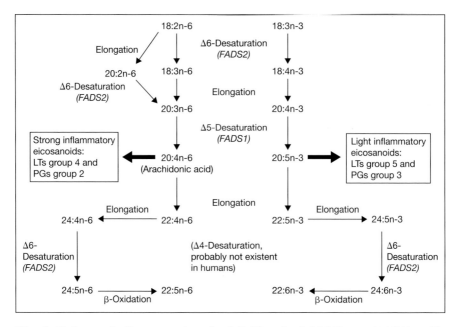

Fig. 1. Pathways for the conversion of n-6 (left) and n-3 (right) essential fatty acids into LC-PUFAs by enzymatic desaturation and chain elongation. Modified from Schaeffer et al. [15].

health and psychiatric disorders [3], cardiovascular disease mortality [4], immunological and inflammatory responses as well as related diseases such as allergies [5, 6]. These and other biological effects of PUFAs appear to be mediated to a large part by the availability of the long-chain PUFAs (LC-PUFAs) with $\geq$20 carbon atoms and $\geq$3 double bonds, such as the n-6 LC-PUFA arachidonic acid (20:4n-6), and the n-3 LC-PUFAs eicosapentaenoic acid (20:5n-3) and docosahexaenoic acid (22:6n-3; fig. 1). Preformed LC-PUFAs are also supplied with some foods (e.g. arachidonic acid with meats and eggs; eicosapentaenoic acid and docosahexaenoic acid with marine foods). Dietary LC-PUFA supply has a marked effect on blood and tissue contents which has been documented in numerous studies [7]. LC-PUFAs can also be derived in human metabolism from the precursor essential fatty acids, linoleic acid (18:2n-6) and α-linolenic acid (18:3n-3), by consecutive desaturation and chain elongation (fig. 1).

The activity of PUFA desaturation and chain elongation appears to be very limited in humans [8], but there are numerous indications for considerable inter-individual variation in the capacity for endogenous formation of LC-PUFAs. For example, in a study published almost 2 decades ago, we found a

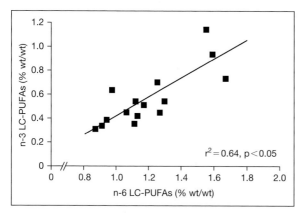

Fig. 2. Correlation of n-3 and n-6 LC-PUFA contents in mature human milk, suggesting inter-individual differences in the ability to form LC-PUFAs. Modified from Koletzko et al. [9].

rather close correlation of n-6 and n-3 LC-PUFA contents in mature human milk [9] (fig. 2), even though the main dietary sources of the two LC-PUFA families are very different. Thus, it appears that some women have a higher ability to synthesize and secrete milk LC-PUFAs of both the n-6 and the n-3 series than others.

A similar conclusion was drawn by Innis et al. [10] who observed a positive correlation of docosahexaenoic acid and n-6 docosapentaenoic acid in red blood cell phosphoglycerides of preschool children, in contrast to the reciprocal relationship found in animals where high n-6 docosapentaenoic acid levels are a marker of low docosahexaenoic acid availability. The authors concluded that the positive relationship of n-6 and n-3 LC-PUFA levels observed in these children may reflect different activity levels of desaturases between individuals affecting the conversion of both the n-6 and the n-3 fatty acids.

Recently we repeatedly studied the dietary intake and fatty acid composition of plasma phospholipids in a group of healthy children at the ages of 24, 36 and 60 months. As one might expect, dietary fatty acid intake patterns changed markedly over time from the age of 2 to 5 years, and there was no correlation or 'tracking' of dietary intakes of saturated, monounsaturated and polyunsaturated fatty acid over time. In contrast, there was a significant correlation ('tracking') over the 3 time points of plasma phospholipid levels of n-6 LC-PUFA ($r = 0.67$) and the arachidonic acid/linoleic acid ratio ($r = 0.64$), and to a lesser degree also of n-3 LC-PUFA ($r = 0.32$) and of the docosahexaenoic acid/α-linolenic acid ratio ($r = 0.32$) [11]. This tracking of plasma LC-PUFA levels in the absence of tracking of dietary intake patterns leads us to conclude that there is inter-individual variation in the ability to endogenously synthesize LC-PUFAs among these children, which persists over time and could most likely be due to genetically determined differences in metabolic turnover. Considerable inter-individual differences in endogenous PUFA conversion have also been demonstrated in stable isotope studies [12, 13], but these data do not reveal to which extent such differences in PUFA conversion may be due to moderating nutritional, metabolic and endocrine factors [8], or due to genetic variation.

The enzymes Δ5- and Δ6-desaturase are considered rate-limiting for the enzyme-mediated conversion steps of this pathway [8]. Both desaturases are expressed in the majority of human tissues, with the highest levels in liver but considerable activity also found in the brain, heart, and lung. The hypothesis that they play a key role in inflammatory diseases is strengthened by functional studies in mice, in which selective Δ5- and Δ6-desaturase inhibitors induced marked anti-inflammatory effects [14].

In human tissue, the regulatory mechanisms of Δ5- and Δ6-desaturases have scarcely been examined. The human desaturase cDNAs were first cloned in 1999 and identified in 2000 as fatty acid desaturase-1 (*FADS1*, encoding Δ5-desaturase) and fatty acid desaturase-2 (*FADS2*, encoding Δ6-desaturase) in the human genome [15]. The two genes are located in a cluster on chromosome 11 (11q12–13.1) with a head-to-head orientation. The sequence of the *FADS1 FADS2* gene cluster can be identified as a region of conserved synteny to the mouse genes *Fads1* and *Fads2* coding for the homologous enzymes on mouse chromosome 18, with the same head-to-head orientation and the same homologous adjacent genes (http://www.ensembl.org/Homo_sapiens/syntenyview). Linkage was previously reported between or nearby the human chromosomal region 11q12–13.1 and complex diseases like type-1 diabetes, osteoarthritis, and bipolar disorders, as well as asthma, atopy and allergy-related quantitative traits such as total and specific IgE levels [15].

Evaluation of the Effects of *FADS1* and *FADS2* Polymorphisms on LC-PUFA Status in Humans

In an attempt to explore the genetic determinants of PUFA metabolism, we performed an analysis of 18 single nucleotide polymorphisms (SNPs) of the *FADS1 FADS2* gene cluster in 727 adult volunteers participating in the European Community Respiratory Health Survey I (ECRHS I) [15]. In 1991–1992 a population-based sample of randomly selected, mainly Caucasian subjects aged between 20 and 64 years, was recruited in the city of Erfurt, Germany. Of the cohort of 1,282 participants who answered the main questionnaire, samples from 727 participants were available for genetic testing of DNA, and deep frozen (−80°C) serum samples were used for analysis of phospholipid fatty acid contents. The study protocol was approved by the Ethics Committee of the Bavarian Board of Physicians at Munich. The analyzed SNPs were chosen from data reported in public databases on the basis of positional and functional aspects to enhance the chance of detecting associations [15]. Genotyping of SNPs in the *FADS1 FADS2* cluster was performed using matrix-assisted laser desorption/ionization time-of-flight mass spectrometry (MALDI-TOF MS) to detect allele-specific primer extension products (Mass Array, Sequenom, San Diego, Calif., USA).

The results of genotyping confirmed that 18 SNPs reported in public databases in the *FADS1 FADS2* cluster were polymorphic, with a mean genotyping success rate of 97.4%. The distributions of genotypes for all analyzed SNPs were consistent with Hardy-Weinberg equilibrium. Redundant markers (rs174545, rs174546, and rs174568) were left out of the analyses. Association analysis of SNPs with fatty acids showed highly significant results for the majority of the SNPs in the *FADS1 FADS2* cluster and the n-6 and n-3 fatty acids (p values $<1.0*10^{-13}$) except for n-6 docosapentaenoic acid (22:5n-6) and docosahexaenoic acid (22:6n-3). Subjects carrying the minor alleles of the SNPs rs174544, rs174553, rs174556, rs174561, rs174568, rs968567, rs99780, rs174570, rs2072114, rs174583, and rs174589 exhibited enhanced levels of the precursor fatty acids linoleic acid (18:2n-6), eicosadienoic acid (20:2n-6), dihomo-γ-linolenic acid (20:3n-6), and α-linolenic acid (18:3n-3), and decreased levels of the product fatty acids γ-linolenic acid (18:3n-6), arachidonic acid (20:4n-6; fig. 3), adrenic acid (22:4n-6), eicosapentaenoic acid (20:5n-3), and n-3 docosapentaenoic acid (22:5n-3) [15].

Haplotypes were statistically reconstructed for two different windows (table 1). To avoid large reconstruction errors resulting from missing data, the reconstruction was based only on persons from whom all genotypes were available. The strongest associations were found in the first part of the gene cluster. The second window was restricted to the first five strongly correlated SNPs with $r^2 > 0.7$, for which complete genotype data of 637 subjects was available. For the 5-locus haplotypes, only two haplotypes had a frequency >5%, with the most common haplotype carrying the major alleles at all loci (frequency 68%), and with the next frequent haplotype carrying only minor alleles (frequency 26%). Haplotype association analysis indicated highly significant associations also after correction for multiple testing (p values multiplied by 17 for the 17 tested outcomes) between the haplotypes and the fatty acid levels (examples for linoleic and arachidonic acid are shown in table 2). Virtually all haplotypes carrying minor alleles were associated (p $<1.0*10^{-13}$) with increased levels of linoleic acid (18:2n-6), eicosadienoic acid (20:2n-6), dihomo-γ-linolenic acid (20:3n-6), and α-linolenic acid (18:3n-3), and with decreased levels of γ-linolenic acid (18:3n-6), arachidonic acid (20:4n-6), adrenic acid (22:4n-6), eicosapentaenoic acid (20:5n-3), and n-3 docosapentaenoic acid (22:5n-3), which was in line with the findings of the SNP analysis. For n-6 docosapentaenoic acid (22:5n-6, after correction for multiple testing) and docosahexaenoic acid (22:6n-3, uncorrected and corrected), haplotype analysis – as the previous SNP association analysis – showed no significant result, presumably because the effect of desaturation activity on

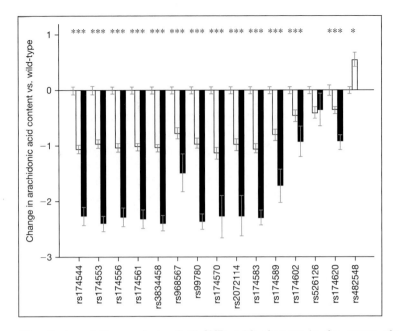

Fig. 3. Association analysis of 15 SNPs with changes in the serum phospholipid contents of the major n-6 LC-PUFA arachidonic acid (20:4n-6) versus mean values for subjects carrying the respective major SNP on both alleles [major A major A]. □ = Changes in fatty acid composition for heterozygous carriers of the minor SNP (level [major A, minor a] minus level [major A, major A]); ■ = homozygotes of the minor allele (level [minor a, minor a] minus level [major A, major A]). Heterozygotes for the minor allele of the SNP rs174544 have a lower level of arachidonic acid (9.2%) in comparison to homozygotes for the major allele (10.2%), whereas those homozygous for that minor allele exhibit only 8% arachidonic acid (means ± SE). *p < 0.05; ***p < 0.01. Adapted from Schaeffer et al. [15].

their plasma concentration is moderated by the indirect synthesis via peroxisomal β-oxidation.

Genotypes or haplotypes were not associated with total or specific IgE levels, but carriers of the minor alleles of several SNPs had significantly reduced odds ratios (ORs) for allergic rhinitis and atopic eczema: allergic rhinitis, rs174544 (OR = 0.59, 95% CI 0.36, 0.99), and rs2072114 (OR = 0.45, 95% CI 0.23, 0.88), and atopic eczema, rs174556 (OR = 0.49, 95% CI 0.25, 0.94). The 5-locus haplotype consisting only of minor alleles showed protective ORs with allergic rhinitis (OR = 0.46, 95% CI 0.26, 0.83) as well as with atopic eczema (OR = 0.46, 95% CI 0.22, 0.94). The 11-locus haplotypes also showed a tendency towards protective ORs. Thus, in this population-based sample we found that minor alleles of SNPs in the *FADS1* gene and the promoter region of the *FADS2* gene, the

Table 1. Haplotype characteristics for 11-locus and 5-locus haplotypes

Haplotype		Alleles[a]	Frequency, %
11-locus haplotype (rs174544–rs174589)			
MaA[b]	CACTTGCCACG	11111111111	68.8
Haplo.1	AGTCdelATCATC	22222221122	10.6
Haplo.2	AGTCdelGTTGTG	22222122221	7.8
Haplo.3	CGCTdelGTTATC	12112122122	2.9
Haplo.4	AGTCdelGTCGTG	22222121221	2.6
Haplo.5	AGTCdelATCGTG	22222221221	1.2
Haplo.6	AGTCdelATCATG	22222221121	1.0
Haplo.rare (frequency <1%)			5.0
5-locus haplotype (rs17544–rs3834458)			
MaA	CACTT	11111	68.6
MiA[c]	AGTCdel	22222	25.7
Haplo.1	CGCTdel	12112	3.5
Haplo.rare (frequency <1%)			2.3

Adapted from Schaeffer et al. [15].
[a]1 = Major allele; 2 = minor allele.
[b]MaA = Major allele, haplotype carrying only common alleles.
[c]MiA = Minor allele, haplotype carrying only rare allele.

two genes encoding the two relevant desaturases on the metabolic pathway leading to arachidonic acid (20:4n-6) production, as well as their corresponding haplotypes were highly associated with an increase in levels of linoleic acid (18:2n-6), eicosadienoic acid (20:2n-6), dihomo-γ-linolenic acid (20:3n-6), and α-linolenic acid (18:3n-3), and with a decrease in the levels of γ-linolenic acid (18:3n-6), arachidonic acid (20:4n-6), adrenic acid (22:4n-6), eicosapentaenoic acid (20:5n-3), and n-3 docosapentaenoic acid (22:5n-3), and less pronounced in n-6 docosapentaenoic acid (22:5n-6) in human serum phospholipids. The most significant associations and the highest proportion of genetically explained variability (28%) were found for arachidonic acid (20:4n-6; table 3).

Implications of the Observed Genetic Effects on PUFA and LC-PUFA Status in Humans

Our findings highlight the contribution of the desaturation pathways on n-6 and n-3 PUFA and LC-PUFA levels in serum phospholipids, and the major importance of its genetic control. Not only arachidonic acid (20:4n-6), but also

Table 2. Examples of associations of *FADS1 FADS2* haplotypes with the major dietary essential fatty acid, linoleic acid (18:2n-6), and the major n-6 LC-PUFA, arachidonic acid (20:4n-6)

Haplotype		C18:2n-6	C20:4n-6
Haplo.1	p	$8.5*10^{-6}$	$3.7*10^{-15}$
	Coefficient	1.18	−1.03
Haplo.2	p	0.0066	$<1.0*10^{-14}$
	Coefficient	0.95	−1.48
Haplo.3	p	0.0060	$3.2*10^{-7}$
	Coefficient	1.518	−1.266
Haplo.4	p	0.086	$9.4*10^{-5}$
	Coefficient	1.311	−1.124
Haplo.5	p	1.0	0.045
	Coefficient	−0.29	−1.066
Haplo.6	p	0.16	0.22
	Coefficient	1.907	−0.955
Haplo.rare	p	0.079	0.068
	Coefficient	1.067	−0.564
MiA-Haplotype	p	$1.2*10^{-13}$	$<1.0*10^{-14}$
	Coefficient	1.18	−1.17
Haplo.1	p	0.024	$1.3*10^{-7}$
	Coefficient	1.177	−1.122
Haplo.rare	p	0.32	0.70
	Coefficient	1.067	−0.482

p values and β-coefficients (change of fatty acid or change of log of fatty acid per copy of the haplotype) are given. p values that exceed 1.0 after correction for multiple testing have been marked down to 1.0. Adapted from Schaeffer et al. [15].

Table 3. Percentage of variations in the fatty acid levels explained by the SNPs for the models containing the SNPs of the 5-locus and 11-locus haplotypes

Fatty acid	R^2 5 SNPs %	R^2 11 SNPs %
Linoleic acid (C18:2n-6)	8.6	9.2
γ-Linolenic acid (ln C18:3n-6)	7.9	7.9
Eicosadienoic acid (C20:2n-6)	10.1	12.3
Dihomo-γ-linolenic acid (C20:3n-6)	7.4	10.8
Arachidonic acid (C20:4n-6)	27.7	28.5
Adrenic acid (C22:4n-6)	6.3	5.9
n-6 Docosapentaenoic acid (ln C22:5n-6)	1.2	1.5
α-Linolenic acid (C18:3n-3)	3.9	5.4
Eicosapentaenoic acid (ln C20:5n-3)	5.2	6.9
n-3 Docosapentaenoic acid (C22:5n-3)	5.5	5.1
Docosahexaenoic acid (C22:6n-3)	1.4	2.9

its precursors, linoleic acid (18:2n-6), γ-linolenic acid (18:3n-6) and dihomo-γ-linolenic acid (20:3n-6), showed strong associations with the genetic variants. In free-living individuals with self-selected diets, the reconstructed haplotypes explain a major proportion of the variation in plasma phospholipid content, particularly of arachidonic acid where about 28% of variation of blood levels is due to genetic variation (table 3), whereas the value is in the order of 10% for the precursor fatty acids of arachidonic acid. Smaller percentage values are found for n-3 fatty acids, which may reflect a higher importance and a larger degree of variation in dietary intakes of both the precursor α-linolenic acid primarily from vegetable oils and the products eicosapentaenoic acid and docosahexaenoic acid primarily from marine foods.

Conclusion

(1) Blood lipid levels of both PUFAs with 18 carbon atoms that are conventionally referred to as the essential fatty acids, and of their biologically active LC-PUFA derivatives, are influenced not only by diet, but to a large degree also by genetic variants commonly found in a European population.

(2) Levels of docosahexaenoic acid are not significantly affected by the SNPs studied, but dietary supply is the primary determinant of docosahexaenoic acid values.

(3) The studied SNPs for fatty acid desaturation enzymes are associated with allergic rhinitis and atopic dermatitis which supports the conclusion that the availability of PUFAs affects allergic endpoints.

(4) At the same level of dietary intake of precursor PUFAs or LC-PUFAs, the respective biological and health effects may markedly differ due to genetic differences in their metabolism.

(5) Based on genetic variation, subgroups of the population may have different requirements of dietary PUFA or LC-PUFA intakes, respectively, to achieve comparable biological effects.

(6) These relationships should be explored in more detail in different populations.

(7) We strongly recommend including analyses of *FADS1* and *FADS2* polymorphism in future cohort and intervention studies addressing the biological effects of PUFAs and LC-PUFAs, which should also lead to enhanced sensitivity and precision of such studies.

Acknowledgements

This work was partly funded by German Research Foundation (Deutsche Forschungsgemeinschaft, Bonn, Germany), research grants HEI 3294/1–1 and KO 912/8–1, BMBF (NGFN), the SFB-386 (DFG), and by a travel grant from the

Boehringer Ingelheim Fonds. B.K. is the recipient of a Freedom to Discover Award of the Bristol Myers Squib Foundation, New York, N.Y., USA.

References

1 Beblo S, Reinhardt H, Demmelmair H, et al: Effect of fish oil supplementation on fatty acid status, coordination and fine motor skills in children with phenylketonuria. J Pediatr 2007; 150:479–484.
2 Koletzko B, Cetin I, Brenna JT; the Perinatal Lipid Intake Working Group: Dietary fat intakes for pregnant and lactating women. Br J Nutr 2007;98:873–877.
3 Muskiet FA, Kemperman RF: Folate and long-chain polyunsaturated fatty acids in psychiatric disease. J Nutr Biochem 2006;17:717–727.
4 Leaf A: Prevention of sudden cardiac death by n-3 polyunsaturated fatty acids. Fundam Clin Pharmacol 2006;20:525–538.
5 Kompauer I, Demmelmair H, Koletzko B, et al: Association of fatty acids in serum phospholipids with hay fever, specific and total immunoglobulin E. Br J Nutr 2005;93:529–535.
6 Trak-Fellermeier MA, Brasche S, Winkler G, et al: Food and fatty acid intake and atopic disease in adults. Eur Respir J 2004;23:575–582.
7 Krauss-Etschmann S, Shadid R, Campoy C, et al: Effects of fish-oil and folate supplementation of pregnant women on maternal and fetal plasma concentrations of docosahexaenoic acid and eicosapentaenoic acid: a European randomized multicenter trial. Am J Clin Nutr 2007;85:1392–1400.
8 Krohn K, Demmelmair H, Koletzko B: Macronutrient requirements for growth: fat and fatty acids; in Duggan C, Watkins JB, Walker WA (eds): Nutrition in Pediatrics. Basic Science and Clinical Applications, ed 4. Hamilton, Decker, 2008, chapt 7.
9 Koletzko B, Mrotzek M, Bremer HJ: Fatty acid composition of mature human milk in Germany. Am J Clin Nutr 1988;47:954–959.
10 Innis SM, Vaghri Z, King DJ: n-6 Docosapentaenoic acid is not a predictor of low docosahexaenoic acid status in Canadian preschool children. Am J Clin Nutr 2004;80:768–773.
11 Guerra A, Demmelmair H, Toschke AM, Koletzko B: Three-year tracking of fatty acid composition of plasma phospholipids in healthy children. Ann Nutr Metab 2007;51:433–438.
12 Del Prado M, Villalpando S, Elizando A, et al: Contribution of dietary and newly formed arachidonic acid to human milk lipids in women eating a low fat diet. Am J Clin Nutr 2001;74: 242–247.
13 Demmelmair H, von Schenck U, Behrendt E, et al: Estimation of arachidonic acid synthesis in full term neonates using natural variation of 13C content. J Pediatr Gastroenterol Nutr 1995;21:31–36.
14 Obukowicz MG, Welsch DJ, Salsgiver WJ, et al: Novel, selective delta6 or delta5 fatty acid desaturase inhibitors as antiinflammatory agents in mice. J Pharmacol Exp Ther 1998;287: 157–166.
15 Schaeffer L, Gohlke H, Müller M, et al: Common genetic variants of the FADS1 FADS2 gene cluster and their reconstructed haplotypes are associated with the fatty acid composition in phospholipids. Hum Mol Genet 2006;15:1745–1756.

Discussion

Dr. Isolauri: Thank you very much for these new aspects and challenges to the food industry. Concerning the data on the effect of n-6 fatty acids and margarine in allergy: are all margarines the same in n-6 composition and how well does spread on bread reflect the whole fatty acid intake?

Dr. Koletzko: Margarine is only one of many factors affecting n-6 intake. Margarines differ quite a bit in their composition. There are more and more margarines based on rape seed oil which has less linoleic acid and more oleic acid. There is quite a variation but these were epidemiological studies which just looked at associations between dietary patterns and outcomes, and there are a number of studies with large sample sizes that found an association which might or might not be due to linoleic acid intake. We actually looked at this in an adult population, in a school-age population, and in birth cohorts. In the adult population we found that both the dietary intake of arachidonic acid and the plasma levels of arachidonic acid are to some extent associated with allergic end points, allergic sensitization and allergic disease. The data are not very clear cut and there are somewhat different results in males and females which might be explained by different dietary patterns and different reporting patterns between males and females, but there is some association. If there is such a strong effect of genetic variation, dietary data alone will not give the full picture.

Dr. Prescott: Thank you very much for your very important work which clearly illustrates that we need to look at this in our studies. In our work in Perth we have recently shown that fatty acid supplementation in pregnancy can modify T-cell signaling pathways, particularly protein kinase C isozymes which we also showed had a protective effect on allergic disease. Clearly we need to talk about looking at potential polymorphisms and how that might modulate these effects. We also have another larger cohort of 400 children in which we are looking at the effect of fish oil supplementation on early immune function and allergy prevention. My question is how do you think that high dose fish oil in pregnancy may have epigenetic effects on the baby?

Dr. Koletzko: Those are obviously issues that one might want to study and you clearly have populations to look at that. If I recall correctly your first study was in 100 mothers who had a very high dose of long-chain n-3, which is a huge dose relative to the potential impact on endogenous metabolism. We have done a similar study with 300 women using a lower dose of 500 mg DHA and the results are very similar to yours in terms of modification of immune phenotypes in the newborn infants. I am very excited about the potential of using omega-3 fatty acids as a preventive intervention in pregnancy. Perhaps we should join our cohorts together to search for polymorphisms. We have material left that could be used for epigenetic analysis and I think this would be an exciting opportunity.

Dr. Waterland: You spoke of these different haplotypes consisting of clusters of SNPs, but where were the SNPs located? Were they within the coding regions or within the regulatory regions of the genes? The contra-oriented juxtaposition position of FADS1 and FADS2 suggests the potential for a shared regulatory region. I wonder if you have explored the potential epigenetic regulation of those two genes?

Dr. Koletzko: We certainly did not look at epigenetic aspects in this study. We just had DNA available from these subjects and we looked at the polymorphisms. The SNPs were primarily exon SNPs with functional relevance although exon SNPs without known functional relevance were not fully excluded.

Dr. Hofstratt: Is there a kind of market for having a genetic test go with a margarine or other food stuffs?

Dr. Koletzko: That is the whole question behind personalized nutrition, where we come to a situation in which people choose their food products and make dietary choices according to differences in biological predisposition and genetic variation. At least in Europe I am not sure that in the near future people will go into a supermarket and take a quick blood test and then look for the products that are labeled green, blue and red. I am not sure this is within reach for the general consumer market, but it is certainly in reach for clinical nutrition. For example fish oil interventions are now used in intensive care with the concept that an inflammatory response can be reduced and outcome improved. In a clinical setting I can see that happening with the rapidly advancing methodology. With pharmacological agents we test for genetic polymorphisms before we give a drug we could do the same with the fatty acid polymorphisms to dose the fish oil intervention. Will this be happening with respect to the general consumer market? What would consumer research at Nestlé say? Is this something that we can expect in the next 15 or 20 years?

Dr. Rinaldo: I work in a biochemical genetics laboratory and in recent years we have faced a dramatic increase in requests to measure polyunsaturated fatty acids (PUFAs) for all sorts of studies beyond my primary area of interest which is inherited disorders of fatty acid oxidation. We are testing patients who are under lipid-restricted diets. A major issue that came up in these studies was that historically plasma PUFA results have been expressed as a percent of the total amount. Once I showed our collaborators and colleagues results expressed using absolute amounts, and some of the variabilities in plasma you mentioned earlier disappeared. In your presentation, your results were expressed as a percent of a total, so I would like to know if the reported differences between genders and other variabilities could be a confounding factor in the evaluation of this polymorphism?

Dr. Koletzko: A number of people have looked at that comparing absolute concentrations, milligrams per liter for example, to percentage of fatty acids in e.g. phospholipids or total lipids. It is a complex question but my understanding of the literature and also my experience with our own measurements is that the percentage data show much less variation than the absolute data. If there is a change in the total concentration of lipid fractions, if the lipoproteins go up and down, the relative proportion of fatty acids does not necessarily change. Moreover, there are a number of studies which have associated end points with plasma levels, and it was clearly shown that the correlation to phospholipid percentage data was much closer than to the absolute data, and also much closer than to the red blood cell levels, which are often considered the best determinant of fatty acid status but I have considerable doubts. With respect to the inborn errors I agree with you that there are a number of unresolved questions. We also looked at samples from β-oxidation disorder patients and we have often found extremely low DHA values and patterns with classical essential fatty acid deficiency with an increased Mead acid, which is clearly a problem that needs to be looked at in further detail. We have indications from a population of children with phenylketonuria (PKU) that the supply matters. Both our group [1] and the group in Milan [2] have shown that DHA supplementation to children with PKU improves electrophysiology, latency time, and speed of information processing. In the *Journal of Pediatrics* we also published that supplementation with DHA in PKU children improves fine motor coordination and some other simpler behavioral responses [3]. Yes, there is really room to look at this in further detail in children on restricted diets.

Dr. Rinaldo: That is exactly the point; in some patients with long-chain fatty acid oxidation disorders the percent estimate indicated a DHA deficiency when the values were looked at as absolute amounts, where actually comfortably within what we had defined as the age-matched reference range, which was really the type of discrepancy I was referring to. What would be your advise; should we overrule a normal absolute amount because as a percent it appears to be low?

Dr. Koletzko: I am not claiming that I have the final answer and we probably need to look at this in further detail, particularly under extreme conditions such as a severely restricted diet which might be very different from other situations. However, the data that are available indicate that percentage values are more predictive of functional response, and in a way it is plausible because if you think of circulating plasma lipids they would be exchanged presumably as a lipid with tissue and not selectively as one fatty acid. This is somewhat speculative and I really suggest we need to look at this further. In the animal world, however, there are also data relating tissue composition much closer to percentage values in plasma.

Dr. Haschke: I would like to comment on what consumer researchers at Nestlé should do in the future. This is not a subject for consumer research. The matter is much too complex and complicated. If you look at the pharma industry where poly-morphisms are clearly associated with different drug metabolisms, the message is not even understood by most medical doctors. There are a few who are focused and apply the methods. As we have learned from the pharma industry, the future for the nutri-tion industry will be to develop research organizations like the pharma diagnostic sec-tions, which are the most rapidly developing sections in the pharma industry. If you look at Roche or Bayer, for example, their diagnostic sections are just booming. The message must be focused, and the outcome must be affordable because if nobody can pay for the findings, it will be very difficult to transfer them to a consumer message. The prices for chips have come down, one thousand-fold within half a year now. If there is a future for this kind of research, then the nutrition companies are well advised to establish diagnostic sections and also focus on the product outcome just as the pharma industry is doing.

Dr. Koletzko: As you alluded to, the price barrier will no longer be a barrier for diagnostic testing in the foreseeable future, and it will depend on consumers who understand that there is a clear advantage to applying this. If, for example, the results from this first study on the predictive effects on allergic end points are confirmed, then I am sure many families will want to know this and will probably adapt the dietary pattern for their children if there is evidence that this is of benefit for them. In a way we are not far away from that. It is very clear that for a child with inborn errors the dietary pattern can be adapted by focusing on the phenotype or genotype. Many peo-ple will also do this if they have a high cholesterol value; they will take dietary advice based on their high cholesterol value and will buy a margarine with phytostanols based on that finding. So I don't see that this is very far away. If people find the information that this is of benefit for them, then I am sure it will happen.

Dr. Gluckman: In our rodent studies we find that FADS1 and FADS2 are two of the most sensitive genes, a life-long expression from fetal undernutrition. So there are probably genes that are already subject to quite a lot of direct or indirect epigenetic regulation. They tend to move together.

Dr. Koletzko: That is exciting information that I would like to hear more about. The question then also rises can we study that in humans and can we find similar pat-terns?

Dr. Gluckman: The dilemma is what tissue, because this is a matter of the meta-bolic reactive tissues. I would doubt that you see it just by studying blood. I think that is the dilemma of epigenetics; that it is so often tissue-specific effects as opposed to global effects.

Dr. Koletzko: We assume that most of the desaturation in humans occurs in the liver, and liver biopsies are actually done in humans. If you don't need much material perhaps there are opportunities.

Dr. Laitinen: You started your talk by showing the scheme on n-3 and n-6 fatty acids and their immunological effects, and you also presented the thought that n-3 fatty acids are the good ones: they have a lot of beneficial effects in immunological terms, and this has indeed led to supplementation studies with interesting results as well. But there are also some studies showing that there might be some risks, for example one study looking at n-3 fatty acids in breast milk showed an increased risk of atopy. So what are your thoughts on this increased trend of supplementing with n-3 fatty acids and could these new results of yours on genetic variation contribute to this?

Dr. Koletzko: Obviously we have very little information so far on the effects of the supplementation in the perinatal period in pregnancy and in the lactation period on allergic end points. The studies that Dr. Prescott and our group have done do not give sufficient evidence yet to really draw firm conclusions, and we need to look at this further. However, the early nutrition programming project together with the perinatal lipid nutrition project and seven international scientific societies have just brought out a position paper recommending that pregnant and breastfeeding women should aim at achieving a dietary DHA intake averaging at least 200 mg/day based on reduction of early preterm birth, and also based on the reported benefits on outcomes in child development [4]. This is already a very strong data set which this group of 50 international scientists looked at in an evidence-based way, supporting that some supply of long-chain n-3 during pregnancy is beneficial, not necessarily for allergy though, and there we need more good studies.

Dr. Isolauri: At the enterocyte level the effect of n-6 fatty acids appears to be suppression of T-cell proliferation and an increase in IL-10 production, and that of n-3 is also associated with dendritic cells producing IgA. Therefore we do not have enough data to support one over the other.

Dr. Koletzko: Everybody in science knows that the world is usually not as simple that there is just good and evil. In the real world, particularly in biology, things are usually more complex and to say arachidonic acid is bad and eicosapentanoic acid is good is probably an over-simplification. It doesn't reflect what is really happening in biology.

Dr. German: Actually now this population has been identified, wouldn't it be a very valuable resource to discover what else is affected by arachidonic acid and therefore likely be beneficially sensitive to things like n-3? You talked about allergic rhinitis; what else do they get?

Dr. Koletzko: This is a cohort that was recruited in 1991 and 1992, and it was recruited with this specific perspective to look at respiratory health and respiratory allergy. So the phenotyping in that area is very good and that is why we took that population because it was convenient: the blood was there, DNA was there, the phenotyping was there, but we don't have a very good description of other outcomes in this population. However, there are other cohorts, we are now working on a cohort of children trying to look at the same question and with different phenotype descriptions. Again I would like to reiterate if any of you is embarking on either cohort or intervention studies grab the opportunity and look at those polymorphisms. If you can't do them yourself we will be happy to collaborate and do it because it is a very simple, high throughput measurement. It would be worthwhile to look at in many different populations and see what the effects might be.

Dr. Gluckman: Are there any gender-specific effects in these studies? I mention this because quite gender-specific effects of other polymorphisms, such as PPARα polymorphisms, and the relationship between PUFA intake and, e.g., plasma cholesterol or other lipoprotein-related levels in blood have been seen.

Dr. Koletzko: We can't really draw conclusive evidence from the our population. But in the epidemiological studies by Trak-Fellermeier et al. [5] for example, there are differences in the relationship between dietary fatty acid intake and allergic response between men and women. It is very difficult from an epidemiological study to decide why that is. Obviously women have a different food intake pattern, less energy and less fat intake, and they also tend to be more conscious about the food selection in general. They may be better in reporting dietary patterns than many men. So it is very difficult to understand to which extent this is a biological difference, and to which extent it is a behavioral or other difference.

Dr. German: Does this polymorphism predict sensitivity to n-3 supplementation for anti-inflammatory effects?

Dr. Koletzko: It needs to be studied and perhaps with Dr. Prescott's data one could actually make a first step towards that.

Dr. Nassar: Based on the anticipated benefits and despite the hazards, do you recommend supplementation of n-3 to patients with protein energy malnutrition?

Dr. Koletzko: Obviously n-3 fatty acids are essential substrates which one wants to include in a dietary supply. We tend to think that, at least in children, DHA is an essential substrate based on the observation that in children with PKU and a restricted intake of DHA, functional disturbances can be overcome with DHA supplementation. Probably children generally should have some supply of DHA. However, in a situation of nutritional rehabilitation after malnutrition, I would suggest that this should be closely studied. There are potential benefits similar to the situation in the critically ill. But once it has been studied, I think one would feel much more comfortable because one could not totally exclude that there might also be adverse effects. Obviously in a state of protein energy malnutrition there is often a reduction in anti-oxidative protection and it is conceivable that there might be more oxidative stress if omega 3 fatty acids are supplied, particularly in a combination with ascorbic acid, iron or other prooxidants. The other question regards a situation with a high risk of infection; if a high dose of an immunosuppressant substrate is given, there is a potential that infectious risk increases. I am not sure this would happen, I am not saying one should not do it, I am just saying in my view it would be worthwhile to study in a controlled fashion: supplement one group and another group not, and see what the effects are on such end points.

References

1   Koletzko B, Sauerwald T, Demmelmair H, et al: Dietary long-chain polyunsaturated fatty acid supplementation in infants with phenylketonuria: a randomized controlled trial. J Inherit Metab Dis 2007;30:326–332.
2   Agostoni C, Harvie A, McCulloch DL, et al: A randomized trial of long-chain polyunsaturated fatty acid supplementation in infants with phenylketonuria. Dev Med Child Neurol 2006;48: 207–212.
3   Beblo S, Reinhardt H, Demmelmair H, et al: Effect of fish oil supplementation on fatty acid status, coordination, and fine motor skills in children with phenylketonuria. J Pediatr 2007;150:479–484.
4   Koletzko B, Cetin I, Brenna JT, et al: Dietary fat intakes for pregnant and lactating women. Br J Nutr 2007;98:873–877.
5   Trak-Fellermeier MA, Brasche S, Winkler G, et al: Food and fatty acid intake and atopic disease in adults. Eur Respir J 2004;23:575–582.

Bier DM, German JB, Lönnerdal B (eds): Personalized Nutrition for the Diverse Needs of Infants and Children.
Nestlé Nutr Workshop Ser Pediatr Program, vol 62, pp 51–54,
Nestec Ltd., Vevey/S. Karger AG, Basel, © 2008.

Discussion on '(Molecular) Imaging: Developments Enabling Evidence-Based Medicine'

H. Hofstraat

Healthcare Strategic Partnerships, Philips Research Laboratories/CTMM, Eindhoven,
The Netherlands

Discussion

Dr. Nassar: Is a magnetic resonance spectroscopy (MRS) very sensitive in detecting mild derangements in the metabolism of the cell or does the cell have to be rapidly growing, such as a malignant or tumor cell, to be detected?

Dr. Hofstraat: The problem with magnetic resonance imaging (MRI) is that it is not very sensitive. Typically with MRI a little bit less than millimolar quantities are measured; 7-Tesla is more sensitive. Of course this limits application to those constituents of a body with rather abundant cells. If you are looking for the first signs of a disease for instance, it is impossible to do so with MRI. There you need to apply nuclear imaging if you want to measure a surface marker which is present in very low quantities. It is impossible to do that with MRI, with the techniques I just discussed.

Dr. Nassar: We performed MRS on protein energy malnutrition patients and the actual curves of the metabolites were not sensitive so we calculated the ratios between the metabolites for more information, but the primary curves did not help us much.

Dr. Hofstraat: Perhaps what you were doing should be looked at in more detail. At present we are doing MRS on the brain and we have been able to measure a number of active substances in the brain at millimolar concentrations. This is relevant, but sensitivity is also a problem, as is quantification.

Dr. Bier: You brought up the issue of cost which we would like to pursue because at least the development of MRI was facilitated to some degree in that it was able to answer clinical questions that could not be answered in any other way, and one could actually charge quite a lot for the service. But we are talking about nutrition where a great fraction of the questions are never going to generate any revenue. How does one approach this and what is happening with the cost of instruments? Many people in this room would love to have the 7-Tesla instrument, but can't afford.

Dr. Hofstraat: Indeed cost is an issue particularly for nutritional applications and this is a fundamental question. We are presently finishing some discussions with the Dutch government about healthcare, not about nutrition. The questions are about medical technology and imaging instruments costing EUR 2.5 million. The questions are what does it bring, what does it replace, how does healthcare become less costly?

Of course the answer is that in the short-term it does add to the cost, but one needs to have a long-term view and not look only at medical technology assessment in the sense of one method being replaced by another and what does that mean, but looking at the intergrowth of the cost of healthcare. It is not about cost but about investment and return on investment, and at the moment we are very slow in making the transition. People are presently investing more in taking their car to a garage every year so that nothing goes wrong somewhere along the road, than in their own healthcare.

Dr. Bier: One of the issues with regard to MRIs originally being applied clinically actually resulted in a neologism in English called the 'incidentaloma', that is what is found incidentally that turned out to raise the cost of medical care for a lot of very healthy people. So it is hard factoring in where money can actually be saved and gets to be a difficult issue in prevention.

Dr. Hofstraat: Absolutely, this is a fundamental question. It is not just a matter of introducing an instrument but also introducing a solution rather than an instrument. This is an essential question which can basically only be addressed by collaboration between a company, like Phillips or Siemens, and clinicians.

Dr. Brandtzaeg: I like your imaging ideas for the future very much, but I wonder if your ultimate goal is to get rid of the pathologists. Since all these techniques are non-invasive, they are an attractive idea. However, also pathology as such is now using imaging more and more. How do you see the future of combining the noninvasive and invasive molecular imaging in the evaluation of biomarkers?

Dr. Hofstraat: That is very much the future. Let's take the example of nodule detection. You can find extremely small nodules with CT imaging. But many of these nodules that are found need not actually be treated because there is no problem with them. So pathology is needed to get additional information perhaps from biomarkers, from in vitro diagnostics, to work jointly with imaging to provide the right answer. However, this is sometimes difficult because tumors can be heterogeneous for instance. It is important to get the biopsy from the right position which may not be so easy, and here again imaging can help pathology by locating the tumor for biopsy. When the tumor biopsy has been obtained, it is brought to the pathologist who diagnoses the disease, and here also imaging and pathology go hand in hand.

Dr. Gluckman: Our particular concern of course is neonates and children. The issue for us is that, certainly in the neonatal period, one can do a quantification of body fat by MRI and DEXA because the child can lie still. But between about 3 or 4 weeks of age and about 5 years of age without sedation, we have a problem because of the time of movement. Do you see any techniques on the horizon that are going to be so rapid that it may be possible to get better measures of the metabolic state in a child without sedation? I think the combination of the sedation issue and the radiology issue, particularly if one is using a radiation-based technique, is really limiting our ability to ask the questions we really need to ask.

Dr. Hofstraat: That is certainly an issue. I showed the typical speed at which we can now take an MRI. For an adult of 2 m height, it takes 40 s, but for a child it means a period of 10 s in which no movement should be made. We can correct for some movements, but it is very difficult to correct for erratic movements and that is really a problem. At the moment we are experimenting with an approach in which a scanner is introduced in what we call an ambient experience environment. Children, starting at 3 or 4 years of age, are guided by a dolphin and that helps to keep the children lying extremely still, even during a relatively long procedure. At the moment there is a tremendous improvement in the number of children who need to be sedated. It only helps, of course, as soon as the children are able to interact with their environment. It works, but it is not the solution for the whole problem.

Dr. Gluckman: Can you comment about the measurement of intrahepatic fat given the particular interest in hepatic fat as a measure in relation to the metabolic syndrome and the new non-invasive technology for the measurement of hepatic fat?

Dr. Hofstraat: In principle it is also possible to measure hepatic fat. I am not a nutritionist so I am not able to comment on the importance of hepatic or other fats. There is also some literature on blood-borne markers, proteins in particular, that also may give some information. I am also interested in in vitro diagnosis and recently a group in Tubingen [1] f published an article on that. So imaging is not necessarily the answer to all problems; in vitro diagnosis can also be of help.

Dr. Simell: In addition to the exposure time in small children, another big problem is the organ size. For instance the pancreatic islets have turned out to be tremendously difficult to visualize by any means. The other one is the gut which, from our point of view, is a very important organ. Do you have any ideas about how to do that?

Dr. Hofstraat: It is a matter of optimizing the instrumentation for the right application. For instance with CT or MRI, a rather high special resolution can be obtained, but generally that is at the expense of increasing the exposure time. For example, the rapidly moving bed scan gives sufficient data for adults, but I doubt whether the resolution would be enough for a small infant. We need to investigate that. We have developed a special MRI tool to measure small animals, rodents, where we can go down to a resolution of below 100 μm^2, I think it is 70–80 μm^2. It is a matter of optimizing for the right application, and the question of course remains whether somebody is willing to invest the money to do it. CT has the disadvantage that X-ray is needed, and to get a volumetric measurement you have to scan around. Even though we now have a 20-slice CT instrument it still takes some time and I am not sure whether one would want do that repeatedly in small infants. With MRIs it is not as much a problem.

Dr. Walker: Along the same line of thinking there is a lot of interest in metabolomics and proteomics as a screening tool for biomarkers. Can you combine a less expensive technique such as that with your own more expensive techniques to define an early biomarker? Let's say, for example, for a cardiovascular lesion because that is what we are looking for. We need to diagnose diseases much earlier so we can begin to prevent them.

Dr. Hofstraat: That is our ambition in this high risk initiative. It is based on 6,000 patient samples that are screened particularly for metabolites and proteins by BG Medicine. At the same time we do CT and MRI measurements on a subset of the same patients. The idea is that at some point you come to a screening approach in which the in vitro and in vivo diagnoses are combined, in vitro for early warning and in vivo for confirmation and to aid treatment. So that is exactly what is happening.

Dr. German: Since you are developing contrast agents as nanoparticles, could you actually use bacteria that would simultaneously be contrast agents and imaging metabolic markers? Further, since basically they go right through, they could be used in more of a surveillance mode and potentially even look at cross-talk with other bacteria in the intestinal mucus?

Dr. Hofstraat: Yes, very feasible. At the moment we are also developing tools to follow stem cells in the body and there will be no problem at all to follow bacteria as well. The question of course is under what circumstances you would be able to use these bacteria for diagnostic purposes. So there might be some requirements in order to do that.

Dr. German: We know little about that initial colonization of infants and how, for example, milk causes stimulation of appropriate bacteria. So if you could actually image using molecular contrast you could determine that particular bacteria are interacting?

Dr. Hofstraat: In principle that is very feasible. Indeed we followed stem cells which were labeled with nanoparticles or with very small ion oxide particles that can easily be followed with MRI. Then you can even see a concentration of cells, even counting the individual cells, because in that case relatively large particles can be imaged.

Dr. Polberger: Do you think there is a future for imaging techniques of the brain as an evaluation of protein and/or nutrition?

Dr. Hofstraat: At the moment we are doing functional MRI of the brain. It enables us to see processes in the brain; you can actually see somebody think in principle. We have done some tests at the John Hopkins in Baltimore where children are doing things, such as looking at cartoons or they have a display with which they interact, and different spaces in the brain can be seen to become active. It is not on the average MR machine; some changes must be made to do that. It has been used for instance to identify children with attention deficit/hyperactive disorder. So in principle there are a lot of things that can be done with MRI to see the impact of chemistry or directly measure chemistry. The question though is what is the effect; is it a measurable signal or does it involve a material concentration that is sufficient for direct measurement in the case of MRI, or is it appropriate to use a radioactive analogon, so you can give a drug but at the same time have the radioactive analogon at a concentration of a few nanomolars present to enable detection? That is the question.

References

1 Kantartzis K, Fritsche A, Machicao F, et al: Upstream transcription factor 1 gene polymorphisms are associated with high antilipolytic insulin sensitivity and show gene-gene interactions. J Mol Med 2007;85:55–61.

Bier DM, German JB, Lönnerdal B (eds): Personalized Nutrition for the Diverse Needs of Infants and Children.
Nestlé Nutr Workshop Ser Pediatr Program, vol 62, pp 55–80,
Nestec Ltd., Vevey/S. Karger AG, Basel, © 2008.

Metabolic Profiling

Gerard T. Berry

Children's Hospital, Boston, MA, USA

Abstract

The concept of chemical individuality was introduced by Garrod in 1908. Inheritance of Mendelian traits including disease states has finally reached a new level of understanding based on the modern principles of gene expression coupled with new insight into the metabolism of RNA species and protein. Over 300 different perturbations in metabolite profiles with their identifying alteration(s) in protein and/or gene structure and/or function have been identified in the past 100 years. With the realization in 1953 that the sentinel disease, phenylketonuria, can be effectively treated by nutritional manipulation tailored to the needs of each individual, we have essentially entered a new phase in metabolic medicine, namely that of nutritional therapeutics. The infant destined for a lifetime of cognitive and motoric handicaps may be rescued by the implementation of a nutritional prescription in early development. Patients with inherited defects that impact on intermediary metabolism need to receive nutritional therapy on an individualized basis. Metabolic profiling, i.e., the array of small molecules or analytes, as well as large macromolecules, measured with precision in body fluids or tissues, can be used to devise a nutritional therapeutic plan, as well as serve as endpoints to evaluate the biochemical efficacy of intervention.

Metabolic profiling has revealed biochemical individuality and hereditable states that require unique nutritional prescriptions for therapy [1, 2]. In the past 100 years, the number of aberrant biochemical profiles in man has grown exponentially largely due to the multiplicity of analytical biochemical methods and sophisticated instrumentation such as ion exchange liquid chromatography, gas chromatography, diverse mass spectrometry techniques, Edman degradation method of peptide sequencing, the Sanger dideoxy-termination method of DNA sequencing, recombinant technology and gene cloning, amplification of dsDNA via thermostabile DNA polymerase and thermal cycling, and nuclear magnetic resonance spectroscopy. However, the flourishing of analytical chemical and molecular biological methodologies would never have risen and met its raison d'être in the field of biochemical genetics were it not for the great insight into the relationships between clinical disease and human biochemistry or intermediary metabolism by the metabolic pioneers in the previous century.

Biochemical Individuality: Beyond Garrod

The Next Phase: Nutritional Therapeutics

In 1908 Archibald Garrod ushered in a new mode of thinking in the medical world [3]. He introduced the topic of biochemical individuality, in retrospect, the biochemical side of genetic diseases and variations in human intermediary metabolism. The list of important biochemical observations, including the respective inborn errors of metabolism, are shown in table 1. Of course, Garrod's four original landmark observations begin this list of ever-growing biochemical genetic diseases. [3, 4]. The four original autosomal recessive disorders included alkaptonuria, cystinuria, albinism and pentosuria. The last of the disorders as of 2007 is phosphoserine aminotransferase deficiency [5]. Yet, the one disease that so greatly illustrates not only chemical individuality, but also personalized nutrition is phenylketonuria or PKU. This entity was discovered in 1934 by Følling [6]. Approximately 20 years later an effective treatment was born, and it was only then that a new phase of individualized biochemical therapy became a reality. In 1953, Bickel et al. [7] showed that it was possible to selectively reduce phenylalanine in the diet of patients with PKU, an idea originally envisioned by Penrose [8].

The Paradigm of PKU Dietary Management

The use of a medical food, a nutritional mixture of all of the non-offending amino acids, yet devoid of the potentially poisonous amino acid, phenylalanine, brought this new phase in medicine to fruition. This was to be the astounding new and effective phase of nutritional therapeutics. The beauty is in its simplicity and adherence to the principles of intermediary metabolism and modern nutrition. For example, patients with severe PKU due to a complete absence of phenylalanine hydroxylase (PAH) enzyme activity may be safely given a medical food, a sound nutritional mixture of amino acids except for phenylalanine. However, it must be emphasized that careful and frequent metabolic profiling must be performed to assure safety. Concomitant administration of whole protein containing just the right amount of phenylalanine to satisfy age-dependent requirements for endogenous protein synthesis will enable normal growth and development while maintaining the plasma phenylalanine level within or close to the normal range. Thus, a patient with a potentially devastating disease that could result in severe mental retardation and lifelong institutionalization may

Table 1. Metabolic disturbances in man

Year	Author	Disease	Laboratory findings	Protein defect [E.C.]	Gene (OMIM)	Inheritance/ chromosome/ frequency
1902	Garrod[4]	Alkaptonuria	Increased concentration of homogentisic acid in urine	Homogentisate 1,2 – dioxygenase [E.C. 1.13.11.5]	HGD (203500)	AR/3q 21–q23/ 1/250,000– 1/1,000,000
1908 1951 1994	Garrod [18] Dent & Rose Calonge et al.	Cystinuria	Increased cystine and dibasic amino acids in urine	Type A (Type I), heavy subunit, rBAT	SLC3A1 (220200)	AR/2p16.3
				Type B (non-Type I), light subunit, $b^{0,TAT}$	SLC7A9 (220200)	Incompletely recessive /19q13.1
				Type AB	SLC3A1 and SLC7A9	Incompletely recessive Overall frequency of 1/7,000
1908 1961 1996	Garrod Witkop et al. Schnur et al.	Oculocutaneous Albinism (Type 1A and 1B)	–	Tyrosinase [E.C. 1.14.18.1]	TYR (SHEP5) (606933)	AR/11q14–q21/ 1/18,000
1908	Garrod	Essential Pentosuria	Increased L-xylulose in urine	L-xylulose reductase (xylitol dehydrogenase) [E.C. 1.1.1.10]	DCXR (260800)	AR/17
1908 1917 1935	Von Reuss [19] Göppert [20] Mason & Turner[21]	Galactosemia	Increased galactose in urine/ plasma and galactose-1-phosphate in red blood cells	galactose-1-phosphate uridyltransferase [E.C. 2.7.7.12]	GALT (606999)	AR/9p13/ 1/40,000– 1/60,000
1912 1948	Wilson [31] Cumings [32]	Wilson disease	Increased free copper and decreased	Polypeptide that acts as a membrane	ATP7B (606882)	AR/13q 14.3–q21.1

Table 1. (continued)

Year	Author	Disease	Laboratory findings	Protein defect [E.C.]	Gene (OMIM)	Inheritance/chromosome/frequency
1993 1994	Tanzi et al. Thomas et al.		ceruloplasmin in plasma	copper-transport protein		1/30,000
1924	Lignac	Cystinosis	Increased lysosomal cystine	Cystinosin	CTNS (606272)	AR/17p13/ 1/100,000– 1/200,000
1929 1952 1977 1978 1983 1995	von Gierke Cori and Cori Bialek et al. Narisawa et al. Nordlie et al. Lei et al.	Glycogen Storage Disease, Type 1 (a,b,c)	Ketotic hypoglycemia and increased plasma lactate, urate and triglycerides	Glucose-6-phosphatase [E.C. 3.1.3.9]	G6PC (232200)	AR/17q21
1932 1957	Medes Sakai [41]	Tyrosinemia type I	Increased tyrosine in plasma and urine. Increased succinylacetone in plasma and urine	Fumaryl acetoacetate hydrolase	FAH	AR/15q23–q25/ 1/100,000
1934	Følling	Phenylke-tonuria	Increased phenylalanine in plasma and phenylalanine metabolites in urine	Phenylalanine hydroxylase [E.C. 1.14.3.1]	PAH (261600)	AR/12q24.1/ 1/12,000
1954	Menkes et al.	Maple Syrup Urine Disease	Increased leucine, isoleucine and valine in plasma	Branched-chain 2-keto acid dehydrogenase (BCKD) complex	BCKDHA (608348) BCKDHB (248611) DBT	AR/19q13.1–q13.2 AR/7q31–q32 AR/1p31

58

Year	Reference	Disease	Biochemical feature	Protein / Enzyme	Gene (248610) DLD (238331)	AR/6q14 Overall frequency 1/250,000
1956	Baron [35]	Hartnup's disease	Increased neutral amino acids in urine	B(0) AT1 protein	SLC6A19	AR/5p15
1958	Smith and Strang [36]	Oasthouse Disease	Increased methionine and alpha-hydroxybutyric acid in urine			
1958	Allan et al.	Arginino-succinate Lyase Deficiency	Elevated argininosuccinate and citrulline in plasma and urine	Argininosuccinic acid lyase	ASL	AR/7q11.2 1/70,000
1961	Childs et al.	Propionic Acidemia	Increased propionic acid and 2-methylcitrate in plasma and urine	Propionyl-CoA carboxylase	PCCA PCCB	AR/13q32 AR/13q21-q22
1961 1962	Ghadimi & Partington [44] Auerbach [45]	Histidinemia	Increased histidine in plasma	Histidine ammonia-lyase	HAL	AR/12q22-q23
1962	Russell et al.	Ornithine Trans-carbamylase Deficiency	Elevated NH_4^+ and orotate in plasma and urine, respectively	Ornithine transcarbamylase	OTC	X-linked/X
1962	Carson & Neill [38] Gerritsen et al. [46]	Homo-cystinuria	Increased total and free homocysteine in plasma and urine	cystathionine beta-synthase	CBS	AR/21q22.3
1963	McMurray et al.	Citrullinemia	Elevated citrulline in plasma and urine	Argininosuccinate synthetase	ASS	AR/9q34.1
1963	Frimpter [39]	Cystathioninuria	Increased cystathionine in urine	cystathionine gamma-lyase	CTH	AR/1p31.1

Table 1. (continued)

Year	Author	Disease	Laboratory findings	Protein defect [E.C.]	Gene (OMIM)	Inheritance/chromosome/frequency
1964 1993	Smith[27] Irons et al.	Smith-Lemli-Opitz	Increased 7-dehydrocholesterol and decreased cholesterol in plasma	3β-hydroxy-cholesterol Δ^7-reductase	DHCR7	AR/11q12–q13
1995 1964	Shefer [28] Drummond [37]	Blue-Diaper Syndrome	Increased indoles in urine in Blue-Diaper Syndrome			
1965	Gerristsen	Nonketotic Hyperglycinemia (NKH)	Increased glycine in plasma and/or CSF	P protein T protein H protein	GLDC GCST GCSH	AR/16q24, 9p22, AR/3p21.2–p21.1
1966	Tanaka et al. [22]	Isovaleric Acidemia	Increased isovaleric acid in plasma and isovalerylglycine in urine	Isovaleryl-CoA dehydrogenase	IVCD (243500)	AR/15q14–q15
1967	Oberholzer et al. [23]	Methylmalonic Acidemia	Increased methylmalonic acid and 2-methylcitrate in plasma and urine	L-methylmalonyl-CoA mutase	MUT	AR/6p21
1967	Mudd et al.	Sulfite Oxidase Deficiency	Increased S-sulfo-L-cysteine and absent sulfate in urine	Sulfite oxidase [E.C. 1.8.3.1]	SUOX (606887)	AR/12
1969	Terheggen et al.	Argininemia	Elevated arginine in plasma	Liver arginase	ARG1	AR/6q23
1969 1999	Shih et al. Camacho et al.	Hyperornithinemia-Hyperammonemia-Homocitrullinuria (HHH)	Increased ammonium and ornithine in plasma and increased homocitrulline in urine	Mitochondrial ornithine transporter	SLC25A15 (603861)	AR/13q14
1971	Daum et al.	Beta-Ketothiolase Deficiency	Increased 2-methyl-3-hydroxybutyrate, 2-	Mitochondrial acetoacetyl-CoA	ACAT1 (607809)	AR/11q22.3–q23.1

Year	Reference	Disorder	Metabolite findings	Enzyme	Gene (OMIM)	Inheritance/Locus
			methylacetoacetate and tiglylglyine in urine	thiolase (T2) [E.C. 2.3.1.9]		
1972	Higgins et al.	Trimethylaminuria	Increased trimethylamine in urine	Flavin-containing monooxygenase-3	FMO 3 (136132)	AR/1q23-q25
1972	Fellman et al.	Tyrosinemia, Type II	Increased tyrosine in plasma and PHPPA, PHPLA,PHAA and p-tyramine in urine	Tyrosine aminotransferase, cytosolic	TAT	AR/16q22.1-q22.3
1973 1977	Simell et al. Valle et al.	Hyper-ornithinemia with gyrate atrophy of choroid and retina	Increased ornithine in plasma	Ornithine aminotransferase [E.C. 2.6.1.13]	OAT (258870)	AR/10q26
1982	Beemer et al.	3-Methylcrotonyl-CoA carboxylase deficiency	Increased 3-methylcrotonylglycine in urine	3-methylcrotonyl-CoA carboxylase	MCCA MCCB (210200)	AR/3q25-q27 AR/5q12-q13.1 (1:40,000 in Germany and Australia)
1974	Goodman et al.	Glutaric Aciduria, Type 1	Increased glutarate and 3-hydroxyglutarate in plasma and urine	Glutaryl-CoA dehydrogenase [E.C.1.3.99.7]	GCDH	AR/19p13.2
1976 1982 1983 1983 1983 1990	Gregersen et al. Kolvraa et al. Stanley et al. Rhead et al. Divry et al. Matsubara et al.	Medium-chain-acyl-CoA Dehydrogenase Deficiency	Hypoketotic hypoglycemia, octanoic acidemia, urinary n-hexanoylglycine, suberylglycine and C6-C10 dicarboxylic aciduria	Acyl-CoA dehydrogenase, medium chain [E.C. 1.3.99.3]	ACADM (MCAD) (607008)	AR/1p31/ 1/15,000
1978	Duran et al.	Molybdenum Cofactor Deficiency	Decreased plasma urate and increased urine S-sulfo-L-cysteine	Early steps: MOCS1A MOCS1B Molybdopterin synthase Molybdopterin synthase sulfurylase	MOCS1A MOCS1B Molybdopterin synthase MoeB (252150)	AR/ AR/ AR/6p21.3 AR/

Table 1. (continued)

Year	Author	Disease	Laboratory findings	Protein defect [E.C.]	Gene (OMIM)	Inheritance/ chromosome/ frequency
1980 2004	Duran et al. Topcu et al.	L-2-hydroxy-glutaric Aciduria	Increased L-2-hydroxyglutaric acid in Urine	L-2-hydroxyglutarate hydroxyglutarate dehydrogenase	Duranin, L2HGDH (609584) (C14ORF160)	AR/14q22.1
1981 1983 1998	Jakobs et al. [34] Gibson et al. Chambliss et al.	Succinate Semi-Aldehyde Dehydrogenase (SSADH) Deficiency (4-hydroxybutyric aciduria)	Increased γ-hydroxybutyric acid in urine	SSADH enzyme [E.C. 1.2.1.24]	ALDH5A1 (271980)	AR/6p22
1983 1983	Giardini [42] Endo [43]	Tyrosinemia Type III	Increased tyrosine in Plasma	4-hydroxyphenyl-pyruvate dioxygenase	HPD	AR/12q24-qter
1983 1990 1994	Glasgow et al. Rocchiccioli et al. Ijest et al.	Long-Chain 3-hydroxyacyl-CoA Dehydrogenase Deficiency	Hypoglycemia, increased plasma 3-hydroxypalmitate and 3-hydroxypalmitoyl-carnitine	Hydroxyacyl-CoA dehydrogenase/ 3-ketoacyl-CoA thiolase/ enoyl-CoA Hydratase, alpha subunit [E.C. 1.1.211]	HADHA (LCHAD) (600890)	AR/2p23
1984	Bennett et al. [30]	Acetyl-CoA Acetyltransferase 2 Deficiency	Increased 3-hydroxybutyrate and acetoacetate in urine	Cystolic acetoacetyl-CoA thiolase (T1) [E.C. 2.3.1.9]	ACAT2 (100678)	AR/6q25.3-q26
1984	Brown [47]	Malonyl-CoA decarboxylase deficiency	Increased malonic acid in Urine	Malonyl-CoA decarboxylase	MLYCD (MCD)	AR/16q24
1984	Turnbull et al.	Short-Chain	Increased plasma	Acyl-CoA	ACADS	AR/12q22-qter

Year	Authors	Disease	Metabolite findings	Enzyme	Gene (OMIM)	Inheritance/Locus
1987 1990	Amendt et al. Naito et al.	Acyl-CoA Dehydrogenase Deficiency	butyrlcarnitine and urine ethylmalonate	dehydrogenase, short-chain	(SCAD) (606885)	
1985 1993 1993 1995 1995	Hale et al. Aoyama et al. Bertrand et al. Strauss et al. Aoyama et al.	Very Long-Chain Acyl-CoA Dehydrogenase Deficiency	Hypoketotic hypoglycemia, increased plasma palmitoylcarnitine and dicarboxylic aciduria	Acyl-CoA dehydrogenase, very long-chain [E.C. 1:3.99.13]	ACADVL (VLCAD) (609575)	AR/17p13
		Maple Syrup Urine Disease, Type III	Increased leucine, isoleucine and valine in plasma Increased lactate and pyruvate in plasma Increased 2-ketoglutarate in urine	Dihydrolipoamide dehydrogenase (E3 component of BCKADH, pyruvate dehydrogenase complex and 2-oxo-glutarate dehydro-genase complex)	DLD, (LAD, PHE3)	AR/7q31–q32
1991 2004	Burlina et al. Tranti et al.	Ethylmalonic Encephalopathy	Increased ethylmalonate, methylsuccinate, 2-isobutyrrylglycine, 2-methylbutyrylglycine and lactate in urine.	Loss of ETHE1 function	ETHE1 (608451)	AR/19q13.32
1992 1995 1996 1991	Wanders et al. Brackett et al. Ushikobo et al. Dionisi Vici et al.	Trifunctional Protein Deficiency	Hypoglycemia, increased plasma 3-hydroxypalmitate and 3-hydroxypalmi-toylcarnitine	hydroxyacyl-CoA dehydrogenase/ 3-ketoacyl-CoA thiolase/ enoyl-CoA hydratase, beta subunit [E.C. 2.3.1.16]	HADHB (TFP) (143450)	AR/2p23
1992 1992	Wanders [25] Jackson [26]	LCHAD deficiency	Increased long chain-3-hydroxydicarboxylic acids in urine and increased long chain-3-hydroxyacylcarnitines in plasma	3-hydroxyacyl-CoA dehydrogenase	HADHA	AR/2p23

63

Table 1. (continued)

Year	Author	Disease	Laboratory findings	Protein defect [E.C.]	Gene (OMIM)	Inheritance/ chromosome/ frequency
1994	Stöckler [24]	Creatine Deficiency	Decreased creatine in brain and increased guanidinoacetate in plasma	Guanidinoacetate methyltransferase [E.C. 2.1.1.2]	GAMT (601240)	AR/19p13.3
2000 2001	Bianchi et al. Item et al.	Creatine Deficiency	Decreased creatine in brain	L-arginine: glycine amidino-transferase [E.C. 2.1.4.1]	GATM (AGAT) (606360)	AR/15q15.3
2001	Salomons et al.	Creatine transporter deficiency	Decreased creatine in brain	Creatine transporter	CT1 (SLC6A8) (300036)	X-linked/Xq28
2005	Mills et al.	Pyridoxal phosphate-responsive seizures	Increased threonine and glycine in CSF Increased biogenic amine metabolites in CSF (e.g. 3-0-methyldopa)	pyridox(am)ine 5'-phosphate oxidase	PNPO	AR/17q21.32
2007	Hart	Phosphoserine Aminotransferase Deficiency	Decreased serine and glycine in CSF and plasma	phosphoserine aminotransferase	PSAT1	AR/9q21.21

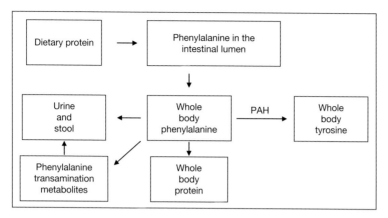

Fig. 1. Whole body nutritional model of phenylalanine metabolism. The patient with PKU and zero residual hepatic PAH enzyme activity will be in the perfect homeostatic state when the intake of phenylalanine in dietary protein is close to the amount of phenylalanine used for daily protein synthesis.

enjoy a relatively normal life because of an individualized nutritional therapeutic regimen [9]. The plasma phenylalanine level obtained at routine intervals will determine how much phenylalanine in the form of whole protein may be given each day. There is an endpoint, the plasma phenylalanine concentration, that allows the physician and nutritionist to individualize the nutritional prescription. A whole body nutritional model of phenylalanine metabolism is shown in figure 1. The purpose of this figure is to graphically depict how, in the perfect homeostatic state recreated via nutritional therapy and tailored to a particular individual with zero residual hepatic PAH activity, plasma phenylalanine levels will be in the normal range when the milligram amount of phenylalanine ingested each day in the form of biologic protein equals the amount of phenylalanine utilized for net protein synthesis (plus a small amount lost in urine and stool as phenylalanine per se or as a transamination metabolite). Please note that almost all of the PAH-mediated conversion of phenylalanine to tyrosine occurs exclusively in the liver but the toxicity of blood phenylalanine primarily occurs in the CNS. A deficiency in the product of the PAH reaction, tyrosine, will result in a secondary homeostatic imbalance, but this is largely eliminated by fortification of the medical food with tyrosine.

It is now well known that not all Mendelian autosomal recessive diseases, not even those with an identical abnormal genotype, present with the same phenotype and severity of disease expression. For example, a few uncommon patients with PKU and poor dietary therapy or compliance have had marked hyperphenylalaninemia (with levels of >20–30 mg%) but exhibit no signs of disease. This suggests that other alleles or modifier genes and/or other environmental factors are altering phenotypic expression.

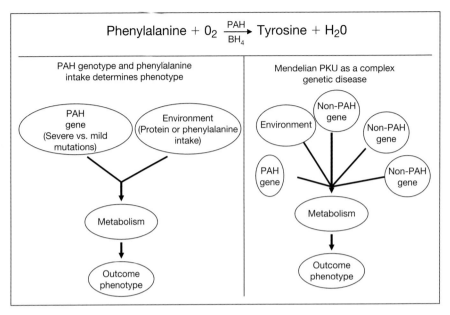

Fig. 2. PKU as a complex genetic disease versus one in which phenotypic variation is largely due to PAH genotypic heterogeneity (and thus reflected in the amount of residual PAH enzyme activity) and the main environmental factor, i.e. phenylalanine intake.

The more common mode of phenotypic variations involves basic differences in gene mutations. This is also true for PKU. A complete absence of hepatic PAH activity is likely to result in classic PKU and be due to severe PAH gene mutations whereas mild hyperphenylalaninemia would be associated with residual PAH activity and a less severe genotype. These concepts are very important when designing the nutritional therapeutic plan. A patient with hyperphenylalaninemia will be able to tolerate more biologic protein and phenylalanine per day than a patient with classic PKU. And yet there are exceptions to this 'rule'. This is why individual nutritional prescriptions are so important. The physician and nutritionist should begin by administering to the affected infant an amount of phenylalanine per day that will allow normal growth while taking into account the likely predicted residual PAH enzyme activity based on plasma phenylalanine levels in the absence of diet therapy. Then, adjustments in protein intake will need to be made based on the metabolic profiling, i.e., the levels of the amino acid, phenylalanine, in plasma in relation to the concentration of the other amino acids. This is an iterative process that may change over time and requires careful attention to achieve optimal diet therapy. The differences between PKU as a complex genetic disease vs. phenotypic variation due to genotypic heterogeneity is shown in figure 2.

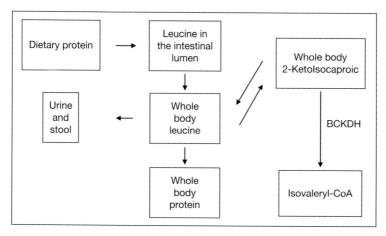

Fig. 3. Whole body nutritional model of leucine (branched-chain amino acid) metabolism. The nutritional PKU paradigm is also applicable for the patient with MSUD and zero residual BCKDH enzyme activity, even in the acute setting.

Maple Syrup Urine Disease, Another Unique Example of an Inborn Error Whose Nutritional Management Fits the PKU Paradigm

Maple syrup urine disease (MSUD) is secondary to a deficiency of the mitochondrial enzyme, the 2-keto-branched-chain dehydrogenase (BCKDH) complex [13]. It is associated with elevations in the branched-chain amino acids (BCAAs), leucine, isoleucine and valine, as well as their keto analogs and derivatives. The chronic management of patients with MSUD employs the PKU paradigm of nutrient restriction. Patients with a complete absence of BCKDH activity are given only the amount of leucine, isoleucine and valine needed for endogenous protein synthesis. Under these circumstances, the patients may have normal levels of BCAAs in plasma and demonstrate normal growth and development [14]. This is true for patients with even the most severe type of enzyme deficiency and potentially lethal disease in the newborn period such as the Mennonites of Lancaster County, Pa., USA, with homozygosity for the Y393N E1α subunit gene mutation [15].

Patients with MSUD may also be rescued from a life-threatening acute metabolic decompensation using a purely nutritional approach. In fact, the same approach used for chronic management may be employed in the care of the acutely ill patient in coma on ventilatory support. It may be used as enteral therapy such as with a nasogastric tube in the infant or as a continuous intravenous infusion [15–17]. But the principle is still the same. The simple recipe is to administer a mixture of amino acids, but without BCAAs, and a sufficient amount of total calories. As shown in figure 3, this is the PKU

67

paradigm of nutritional therapy but only in the acute setting. The guide initially is the metabolic profile. Because leucine is elevated to a much greater degree than isoleucine and valine, it is quite important to follow the metabolic profile during the entire course of acute therapy, as one or both may undergo depletion while leucine is still elevated. If isoleucine and/or valine are not administered at that point in therapy, the plasma leucine level will cease to decline. This is one of the strongest pieces of evidence that supports the hypothesis that the mode of action of this anabolic therapy is via net endogenous protein synthesis. As a mode of therapy for acutely ill patients, this treatment is still somewhat novel in the wide world of inborn errors. Most encephalopathic and critically ill patients with an 'intoxication' type of metabolic disease would be treated with a form of dialysis exclusively, not nutritional anabolic therapy. This is a testament to the power of individualized nutritional therapeutics in the intensive care setting.

As shown in table 1, metabolic profiling was crucial in the initial identification of a large number of inborn errors of metabolism. But not all of these diseases are amenable to nutritional therapy. Aside from PKU and MSUD, other examples of disorders that can be readily treated with a nutritional approach include: (1) hereditary galactosemia, lactose-restricted diet; (2) vitamin B_{12}-responsive methylmalonic acidemia, hydroxy-cobalamin; (3) biotinidase and holocarboxylase synthetase deficiencies, biotin; (4) sodium/L-carnitine transporter deficiency, L-carnitine; (5) urea cycle enzyme defects such as argininosuccinate synthetase and argininosuccinate lyase deficiencies, arginine; (6) guanidinoacetate methyltransferase deficiency, creatine; (7) homocystinuria, methionine restriction and betaine therapy; (8) GLUT1 deficiency, ketogenic diet; (9) hereditary fructose intolerance, fructose, sucrose and sorbitol restriction; (10) 3-phosphoglycerate dehydrogenase deficiency, serine and glycine therapy; (11) lysinuric protein intolerance, citrulline therapy; (12) vitamin B_6-responsive seizure disorder, pyridoxine treatment; (13) galactokinase deficiency, lactose restriction; (14) P-hydroxy-benzoatepolyprenyl transferase (COQ_2) deficiency, coenzyme Q_{10} therapy; (15) arginine:glycine amidinotransferase deficiency, creatine treatment; (16) congenital folate malabsorbption, folate megatherapy and/or folinic acid and/or 5-methyl-tetrahydrofolate (5-methyl-THF) therapy; (17) 5,10-methylenetetrahydrofolate reductase deficiency, betaine, folate megatherapy and/or 5-methyl-THF, methionine, pyridoxine, cobalamin and L-carnitine treatment; (18) hereditary orotic aciduria, uridine therapy; (19) X-linked sideroblastic anemia, pyridoxine and folate treatment; (20) Wilson disease, penicillanine or trientine and zinc treatment; (21) acrodermatitis enteropathica, zinc supplementation; (22) primary hypomagnesemia, magnesium sulfate treatment; (23) Refsum disease, phytanate-restricted diet; (24) phosphomannose-isomerase deficiency (CDGIb), mannose therapy; (25) cystinosis, cysteamine therapy, and (26) phosphoserine aminotransferase deficiency, serine and glycine therapy. The complete list of diseases

Table 2. Metabolic disturbances amenable to nutritional and/or pharmacological therapy

Disease (OMIM)	Nutritional therapy	Drug therapy
Alkaptonuria (203500)	protein restriction	2-(2-nitro-4-trifluoro-methylbenzoyl)-1,3-cyclohexanedione (NTBC) or Nitisinone
Cystinuria	high fluid intake + alkali	(penicillamine)
Galactosemia	lactose restriction	
Phenylketonuria	protein restriction phenylalanine-free medical food	tetrahydrobiopterin
Propionic acidemia	protein restriction medical food (carnitine)	(metronidazole)
Isovaleric acidemia	protein restriction glycine, carnitine	
Methylmalonic acidemia	protein restriction medical food cobalamin (carnitine)	(metronidazole)
Homocystinuria	protein restriction medical food and cystine vitamin B6	betaine
Methylmalonic acidemia and Homocystinuria (primary cobalamin defect)	protein restriction cobalamin vitamin B6 folate	betaine
Biotinidase	biotin	
Urea Cycle Enzyme Defects: Ornithine Transcarbamylase deficiency	protein restriction citrulline (medical food)	sodium phenylbutyrate
Arginase deficiency	protein restriction medical food	phenylbutyrate
Argininosuccinic Acid Synthetase deficiency (Citrullinemia type 1)	protein restriction arginine	phenylbutyrate
N-Acetylglutamate Synthetase deficiency	protein restriction	carbamoylglutamate
Argininosuccinate Lyase deficiency (Argininosuccinic Aciduria)	protein restriction arginine	phenylbutyrate
Carbamyl Phosphate Synthetase deficiency	protein restriction citrulline	phenylbutyrate

Table 2. (continued)

Disease (OMIM)	Nutritional therapy	Drug therapy
Citrullinemia, Type 2	protein restriction (alkali)	
Hyperornithinemia-Hyperammonemia-Homocitrullinemia disease	protein restriction (ornithine)	
Lysinuric protein intolerance	protein restriction citrulline	
Ornithine aminotransferase deficiency	arginine restriction	
Holocarboxylase Synthetase deficiency	biotin	
3-methylcrotonyl-CoA carboxylase deficiency	(protein restriction) (carnitine)	
Glutaric aciduria, type 2	protein restriction long-chain fat restriction riboflavin	
Hartnup disease	nicotinamide therapy	
Primary carnitine deficiency	carnitine	
Guanidinoacetate methyltransferase deficiency	protein restriction creatine (ornithine)	
GLUT1 deficiency	ketogenic diet	
Hereditary fructose intolerance	fructose, sucrose and sorbitol restriction	
3-phosphoglycerate dehydrogenase deficiency	serine glycine	
Short-chain acyl-CoA dehydrogenase deficiency	acute glucose provision long-chain fat restriction (riboflavin)	
Medium-chain acyl-CoA dehydrogenase deficiency	acute glucose provision (carnitine)	
Very long-chain acyl-CoA dehydrogenase deficiency	acute glucose provision long-chain fat restriction MCT oil	
Long-chain 3-hydroxy acyl-CoA dehydrogenase deficiency	long-chain fat restriction docosahexaenoic acid MCT oil	

Table 2. (continued)

Disease (OMIM)	Nutritional therapy	Drug therapy
Trifunctional protein deficiency	long-chain fat restriction docosahexaenoic acid MCT oil	
Vitamin B6-responsive seizure disorder	pyridoxine	
Galactokinase deficiency	lactose restriction	
Para-hydroxy-benzoatepolyprenyl transferase deficiency	coenzyme Q_{10}	
Arginine:glycine amidinotransferase deficiency	creatine	
Congenital folate malabsorbption	folate folinic acid 5-methyl tetrahydrofolate	
5,10-methylene-tetrahydrofolate reductase deficiency	folate folinic acid 5-methyl THF methionine pyridoxine cobalamin carnitine	betaine
Succinic semialdehyde dehydrogenase deficiency		vigabatrin
Guanosine triphosphate cyclohydrolase-I deficiency		tetrahydrobiopterin
X-linked sideroblastic anemia	pyridoxine folate	
Erythropoietic protoporphyria	β-carotene	
Porphyria cutanea tarda	acute glucose provision	
Acute intermittent porphyria	acute glucose provision	hematin
Wilson disease	zinc	penicillanine trietine
Menkes disease	copper chloride or copper histidine	
Acrodermatitis enteropathica	zinc	
Primary hypomagnesimia	magnesium sulfate	
Refsum disease	phytanate restricted diet	
Phosphomannose-isomerase deficiency	mannose	

Table 2. (continued)

Disease (OMIM)	Nutritional therapy	Drug therapy
Cystinosis	cysteamine	
3-hydroxy-3-methylglutaryl-CoA lyase deficiency	acute glucose provision (protein restriction)	
Hyperprolinemia Type II		
Hyperprolinemia Type I		
Galactose epimerase deficiency	lactose restriction galactose provision	
Familial hypercholesterolemia	long-chain fat restriction	HMG – CoA reductase inhibitor (statin)
Dihydropyrimidine dehydrogenase deficiency	5-Fluorouracil restriction	
Glycogen storage disease Type Ia	acute glucose provision alkali starch frequent feeding	
Glycogen storage disease Type Ib	acute glucose provision alkali starch frequent feeding	GCSF
Glycogen storage disease Type III	acute glucose provision alkali starch	
Glycogen storage disease Type VII	acute glucose provision alkali starch	
Fanconi-Bickel syndrome	acute glucose provision frequent feeding lactose restriction alkali starch	
Mitochondrial acetoacetyl-CoA thiolase deficiency	acute glucose provision (protein restriction)	
Isobutryl-CoA dehydrogenase deficiency	acute glucose provision protein restriction (carnitine)	
Nonketotoic hyperglycinemia		sodium benzoate dextromethorphan
Phosphoserine aminotransferase deficiency	serine glycine	

whose treatment is nutritional in nature, at least in part, is shown in table 2.

In summary, there is ample evidence that nutritional therapeutics play an important role in medicine. The number of instances in which a heritable disorder may be corrected or, at least ameliorated, in terms of disease expression, continues to grow. The paradigm is still the PKU mode of nutritional therapy. As employed in the neonatal period, it has the capacity to control the disease, enable normal growth and development and save the patient from serious complications. This type of intervention best exemplifies the principle of nutritional therapeutics: metabolic profiling delineates the biochemical perturbations (in plasma) and guides in the establishment of the therapeutic plan, a medical food devoid of the offending biochemical compound is administered along with a necessary, albeit small, amount of the offending nutrient (in the form of whole protein) to allow adequate endogenous biosynthesis (of body proteins) and the adequacy of the treatment is followed by serial metabolic profiling. It is expected that newer modes of individually tailored nutritional therapies will emerge as our diagnostic techniques and instrumentation capabilities, coupled with upgraded newborn screening surveillance, continue to advance.

References and Literature

1 Scriver CR, Beaudet AL, Valle D, Sly WS: The Metabolic and Molecular Bases of Inherited Disease, ed 8. New York, McGraw-Hill, 2001. (Also see the online Metabolic and Molecular Bases of Inherited Disease).
2 Fernandes J, Saudubray J-M, van den Berghe G, Walter JH (eds): Inborn Metabolic Diseases, ed 4. Berlin, Springer, 2006.
3 Harris H: Garrod's Inborn Errors on Metabolism. Oxford, Oxford University Press, 1965.
4 Garrod AE: The incidence of alkaptonuria, a study in chemical individuality. Lancet 1902;ii: 1616–1620.
5 Hart CE, Race V, Achouri Y, et al: Phosphoserine aminotransferase deficiency: a novel disorder of the serine biosynthesis pathway. Am J Hum Genet 2007;80:931–937.
6 Folling A: Über Ausscheidung von Phenylbrenztraubensäure in den Harn als Stoffwechselanomalie in Verbindung mit Imbezillität. Z Physiol Chem 1934;227:169–176.
7 Bickel H, Gerrard J, Hickmans EM: Influence of phenylalanine intake of phenylketonuria. Lancet 1953;265:812–813.
8 Penrose LS: Phenylketonuria a problem in eugenics. Ann Hum Genet 1998;62:193–202.
9 National Institutes of Health Consensus Development Panel: National Institutes of Health Consensus Development Conference Statement: phenylketonuria: screening and management. Pediatrics 2001;108:972–982.
10 Scriver CR: The PAH gene, phenylketonuria, and a paradigm shift. Hum Mutat 2007;28: 831–845.
11 Kayaalp E, Treacy E, Waters PJ, et al: Human phenylalanine hydroxylase mutations and hyperphenylalaninemia phenotypes: a metanalysis of genotype-phenotype correlations. Am J Hum Genet 1997;61:1309–1317.
12 Levy HL, Shih VE, Karolkewicz V, et al: Persistent mild hyperphenylalaninemia in the untreated state. A prospective study. N Engl J Med 1971;285:424–429.
13 Menkes JH, Hurst PL, Craig JM: A new syndrome: progressive familial infantile cerebral dysfunction associated with an unusual urinary substance. Pediatrics 1954;14:462–467.
14 Synderman SE, Norton PM, Roitman E, et al: Maple syrup urine disease with particular reference to dietotherapy. Pediatrics 1964;34:454–472.

15 Morton DH, Morton CS, Strauss KA, et al: Pediatric medicine and the genetic disorders of the Amish and Mennonite people of Pennsylvania. Am J Med Genet C Semin Med Genet 2003;15: 121:5–17.

16 Berry GT, Heidenreich R, Kaplan P, et al: Branched-chain amino acid-free parenteral nutrition in the treatment of acute metabolic decompensation in patients with maple syrup urine disease. N Engl J Med 1991;324:175–179.

17 Parini R, Sereni LP, Bagozzi DC, et al: Nasogastric drip feeding as the only treatment of neonatal maple syrup urine disease. Pediatrics 1993;92:280–283.

18 Harris H, Garrod AE: Croonian lectures on inborn errors of metabolism. Lecture 1. Lancet 1908;ii:1–7.

19 von Reuss A: Zuckerausscheidung in Säuglingsalter. Wien Med Wochenschr 1908;58:799–800.

20 Goppert F: Galaktosurie nach Milchzuckergabe bei angeborenem, familiärem chronischem Leberleiden. Klin Wochenschr 1917;54:473–477.

21 Mason HH, Turner ME: Chronic galactosemia. Am J Dis Child 1935;50:359–374.

22 Tanaka K, Budd MA, Efron ML, Isselbacher KJ: Isovaleric acidemia: a new genetic defect of leucine metabolism. Proc Natl Acad Sci USA 1966;56:236–242.

23 Oberholzer VG, Levin B, Burgess EA, Young WF: Methylmalonic aciduira. An inborn error of metabolism leading to chronic metabolic acidosis. Arch Dis Child 1967;42:492–504.

24 Stöckler S, Holzbach U, Hanefeld F, et al: Creatine deficiency in the brain: a new, treatable inborn error of metabolism. Pediatr Res 1994;36:409–413.

25 Wanders RJ, Ijist L, Poggi F: Human trifunctional protein deficiency: a new disorder of mitochondrial fatty acid beta-oxidation. Biochem Biophys Res Commun 1992;188:1139–1145.

26 Jackson S, Singh Kler R, Bartlett K, et al: Combined enzyme defect of mitochondrial fatty acid oxidation. J Clin Invest 1992;90:1219–1225.

27 Smith SW, Lemli L, Opitz JM: A newly recognized syndrome of congenital nomalies. J Pediatr 1964;64:210–221.

28 Shefer S, Salen G, Batta AK, et al: Markedly inhibited 7-dehydrocholesterol-delta(7)-reductase activity in liver microsomes from Smith-Lemli-Opitz homozygotes. J Clin Invest 1995;96: 1779–1785.

29 Online Mendelian Inheritance in Man. Baltimore, Johns Hopkins University, 2008.

30 Bennett MJ, Hosking GP, Smith MF, et al: Biochemical investigations on a patient with a defect in cytosolic acetoacetyl-CoA thiolase, associated with mental retardation. J Inherit Metab Dis 1984;7:125–128.

31 Wilson AK: Progressive lenticular degeneration: a familial nervous disease associated with cirrhosis of the liver. Brain 1912;34:295–507.

32 Cumings JN: The copper and iron content of brain and liver in the normal and in hepatolenticular degeneration. Brain 1948;71:410–415.

33 Childs B, Nyhan WL, Borden M, et al: Idiopathic hyperglycinemia and hyperglycinuria: a new disorder of amino acid metabolism I. Pediatrics 1961;27:522–538.

34 Jakobs C, Bojasch M, Monch E, et al: Urinary excretion of gamma-hydroxybutyric acid in a patient with neurological abnormalities: the probability of a new inborn error of metabolism. Clin Chim Acta 1981;111:169–178.

35 Baron DN, Dent CE, Harris H, et al: Hereditary pellagra-like skin rash with temporary cerebellar ataxia, constant renal amino-aciduria and other bizarre biochemical features. Lancet 1956;ii:421–433.

36 Smith AJ, Strang LB: An inborn error of metabolism with the urinary excretion of alpha-hydroxy-butyric acid and phenylpyruvic acid. Arch Dis Child 1958;33:109–113.

37 Drummond KN, Michael AF, Ulstrom RA, Good RA: The blue diaper syndrome: familial hypercalcemia with nephrocalcinosis and indicanuria. A new familial disease, with definition of the metabolic abnormality. Am J Med 1964;37:928–948.

38 Carson NAJ, Neill DW: Metabolic abnormalities detected in a survey of mentally backward individuals in Northern Ireland. Arch Dis Child 1962;37:505–513.

39 Frimpter GW, Haymovitz A, Horwith M: Cystathioninuria. N Engl J Med 1963;268:333–339.

40 Medes G: A new error of tyrosine metabolism: tyrosinosis. The intermediary metabolism of tyrosine and phenylalanine. Biochem J 1932;26:917–940.

41 Sakai K, Kitagawa T: An atypical case of tyrosinosis. Part 1. Jikei Med J 1957;2:1–10.

42 Giardini O, Cantani A, Kennaway NG, D'Eufemia P: Chronic tyrosinemia associated with 4-hydroxyphenylpyruvate dioxygenase deficiency with acute intermittent ataxia and without visceral and bone involvement. Pediatr Res 1983;17:25–29.

43 Endo F, Kitano A, Uehara I, et al: Four-hydroxyphenylpyruvic acid oxidase deficiency with normal fumarylacetoacetase: a new variant form of hereditary hypertyrosinemia. Pediatr Res 1983;17:92–96.
44 Ghadimi H, Partington MW, Hunter A: A familial disturbance of histidine metabolism. N Engl J Med 1961;265:221–224.
45 Auerbach VH, DiGeorge AM, Baldridge RC, et al: Histidinemia: a deficiency in histidase resulting in the urinary excretion of histidine and of imidazolepyruvic acid. J Pediat 1962;60:487–497.
46 Gerritsen T, Kaveggia EG, Waisman HA: A new type of idiopathic hyperglycinemia with hypo-oxaluria. Pediatrics 1965;36:882–891.
47 Brown GK, Scholem RD, Bankier A, Danks DM: Malonyl coenzyme A decarboxylase deficiency. J Inherit Metab Dis 1984;7:21–26.

Discussion

Dr. Simell: As many of you probably know Finland has a very peculiar genetic background. We have a number of diseases which are practically absent, for instance phenylketonuria (PKU) is extremely rare in Finland, and not a single case of galactosemia as far as I know. At the same time there are about 30 known diseases which are much more common here than anywhere else and many of these diseases are really spectacular. For example, lysinuric protein intolerance, which is caused by a transporter defect at the cellular membranes, especially on the basolateral side of the polar cells as in the gut and the kidney tubule as well. The disease has very difficult symptoms. It is interesting because the basic problem is in the transport of lysine, arginine and ornithine through the membranes causing a deficiency of all 3 amino acids in the body. This causes hyperammonemia episodes so it behaves like any hyperammonemic disease as such. Some of the patients develop alveolar proteinosis, they may develop end-stage renal disease, some of them have very severe osteoporosis, so the clinical picture is highly variable in these cases. We really don't understand why these different types of symptoms develop in some patients and others are totally without any at least. Have you any good suggestions for that?

Dr. Berry: That is one of the enigmas in metabolic diseases and most of us in the United States have never seen a patient with lysinuric protein intolerance. I wonder whether the defective basolateral transporter, which is also expressed in other cells, might be leading to kwashiorkor-like states but just involving the dibasic amino acids within certain tissues, even those involving the immune system, and that really the patients have an unusual deficiency of arginine, lysine and ornithine that perturbs protein synthesis within certain tissues. I think this disease exemplifies better than anything else the cell autonomous problem in the inborn errors, which is a very difficult problem for us. The fact is that different tissues show the abnormality and the defect resides with them, and sometimes the therapy we use, which might help at the intestinal level, really doesn't work for those particular target tissues. But it is an interesting example of where a protein deficiency state can reside just within a few cells that are target tissues within the body. I am not sure that citrulline therapy will be beneficial because the citrulline transporter may not be expressed on those target cells.

Dr. German: In those metabolic disorders in which acylcarnitines are one of the means to excrete metabolites, does that mean these individuals have heightened requirements for carnitine to facilitate that? If so, if you get a broader metabolic profile analysis, can you fine tune the nutritional therapeutics better to actually get closer to a phenotype appropriate for the genetic background?

Dr. Berry: That is a very controversial area for us. Carnitine therapy definitely plays a role in the inborn errors of metabolism. The one disease where carnitine administration can be lifesaving and is absolutely beneficial is the sodium carnitine co-transporter defect. That has been worked out at the molecular level, and with this disease one may be able to rescue a severely ill newborn with cardiomyopathy, ventricular dysrhythmia, severe liver disease, fasting hypoglycemia and skeletal muscle problems. There are other diseases though where a secondary carnitine deficiency develops, and these include the fatty acid oxidation defects and many of the branched chain amino acid disorders that involve the organic acid pathway. The secondary carnitine deficiency occurs for at least two reasons in these disorders, and in some of them reason No. 1 overshadows reason No. 2 and vice versa. For example in propionic acidemia due to propionyl-CoA carboxylase deficiency, when propionyl-CoA accumulates within the mitochondrial matrix that excess leads to increased production of propionyl carnitine which is then excreted. It exits the cell and it is excreted in the urine. So one way of thinking is that it is helping to rid the body of the excess of potentially poisonous propionate metabolites, but it is also causing a reduction in the free carnitine levels. This is such a great question because it gets to this issue as how low can a metabolate drop before problems develop. I look at this as one of the major issues in metabolism and in nutrition because there are some patients who have reductions of 50% of normal in plasma and they have no obvious abnormalities that relate to carnitine deficiency. But in our field most of the individuals around the world would treat patients with carnitine for this, and I usually support it with propionic acidemia and a few other disorders because I think that carnitine is relatively harmless (may produce loose stools or diarhea) and it may benefit the patients because of the detoxification phenomena. The second reason why carnitine levels can drop in these disorders is because the accumulation of the acylcarnitine itself in renal tubular cells can lead to defective handling of free carnitine; it is filtered, but its reapsorption is inhibited by an unknown factor, presumably by acylcarnitine as in the defects in long-chain fatty acid oxidation. But the thing that we fear most with the use of carnitine is in the long-chain fatty acid oxidation disorders because the long-chain carnitine ester theoretically might lead to a ventricular dysrhythmia. We still don't know the basis for why ventricular fibrillation sometimes occurs in patients with the very long-chain acyl-CoA dehydrogenase deficiency and the long-chain 3-hydroxy acyl-CoA dehydrogenase deficiency. It is probably more related to defects in energy metabolism or accumulation of the CoA ester itself, but one cannot rule out the possibility that long-chain acylcarnitines are playing a role in the pathogenesis of potentially lethal ventricular rhythm disturbances. I think Dr. Rinaldo who has spent a considerable amount of time studying this metabolism probably feels the same way that I do. Dr. Rinaldo, do you want to make a comment about this?

Dr. Rinaldo: There was a beautiful editorial in *Lancet* about 25 years ago actually postulating that carnitine deficiency in fatty acid oxidation disorders is a defense mechanism because when there is less carnitine, there will be fewer substrates where the enzyme deficiency is. That idea was incredibly controversial, but I think it still has some merit.

Dr. Walker: There is something about the field of metabolic disease that is a little bit different than other disease states. Usually what happens is that something at the cellular level is identified using cell lines or in an animal model by either knocking out or adding enzymes, and then determining at what happens. In the case of a metabolic disease, the patient is the subject in most instances and although that is wonderful and metabolic nutrition therapy is important, the mechanism of disease isn't really determined. Have attempts been made to knock out these enzymes in animals to look at what happens, or look at organ culture to try to find what the subcellular bases for these observations are?

Dr. Berry: Yes, there has been a great interest in this, and a number of investigators have been working to answer these questions. This is another controversial point as there are suggestions in the literature that if one uses proton NMR spectroscopy to assess phenylalanine content in brain that in some patients the levels aren't elevated even though their plasma levels are high. The large neutral amino acid transporter plays a key role in the movement of those monoamino, monocarboxylic amino acids across the blood-brain barrier. The leading hypothesis in the neurotoxicity of PKU is that high phenylalanine levels will competitively inhibit the movement of those other species into brain, not only at the blood-brain barrier, but also at the neuronal transporter level as well, so PKU really could possibly be another one of these cell curious problems where there is a "nutritional deficiency" but selectively within the neuron, oligodendroglial cell or another glial element in brain. That may be a biochemical basis for toxicity, leading to white matter abnormalities. It is possible that the modifier gene in the patient with PKU, who has no serious phenotype, actually is because there is a perturbation in their neutral amino acid transporter. There is interest in the PKU knockout model of having a large neutral amino acid perturbation transgene coupled together in a cross model to try to answer some of these questions. That is a great illustration of transport and metabolism and how the phenotype is produced. Yet, while we talk about modifier genes and epigenetic phenomenon, the ability to actually demonstrate a cause-and-effect relationship in a clear way is not always there.

Dr. Walker: Because we both examined patients who don't express a phenotype, this sometimes confuses the issue.

Dr. Berry: One thing I have to say is that I am a little disappointed that the medical community has not embraced the inborn errors of metabolism. What we have learned from these unfortunate experiments of nature about normal metabolism in nutrition has been just tremendous, and some of those examples have been lost in the general medical community.

Dr. Saavedra: You have very nicely have summarized the whole series of metabolic abnormalities leading to disease. This may be a peripheral topic and I want to know what your perspective would be on the use of ketogenic diets, which is the opposite, which is inducing a metabolic disorder in this case with the purposes of managing intractable seizures. In the experience at John Hopkins, there is clearly a subset of patients who magically seem to respond positively. Do you have you any thoughts on this?

Dr. Berry: That is another fascinating topic and there are definitely a few patients with inborn errors that tremendously respond to a ketogenic diet. An example is the transport defect, the Glut1 transporter abnormality. Glut1 is a blood-brain barrier membrane transporter that allows glucose to move from the blood into the brain In these patients there are a low glucose level within the spinal fluid, but blood glucose levels, are normal. Because humans have the ability of using β-hydroxybutyrate and acetylacetate as fuel in brain cells, one can resort to a ketogenic diet to keep those patients largely healthy, but it is not a cure. The ketogenic diet is a real mystery. Over the years I had thought it was a potentially very dangerous therapy. We have been asked whether mitochondrial patients with lesions in the mitochondrial electron transport chain and intractable seizures should receive a ketogenic diet. I thought it would be a catastrophic procedure for them, but in a few instances where it has actually been used, it has been beneficial. I don't think we really understand well how the ketogenic diet works. Some investigators I know have hypothesized that the induction of a low pH in the brain may be the beneficial effect. In other words, hydrogen ion per se is what is being generated in the brain and it is a local acidemia of sorts that is depressing seizure activity. I don't think that is probably likely but perhaps something a perturbation in the cellular redox potential yielding a more favorable state under the circumstance might be the biochemical basis, but to my knowledge no one really understands yet the metabolism which is responsible.

Dr. Bier: I originally wanted to ask you about the MRI studies in PKU but your response to Dr. Walker's question generated two comments. First it is important when we talk about knockout mice that are so popular today to point out that the human knockouts came first, allowing us to start thinking about how to deal with single gene defects. This is something which is frequently completely lost to our molecular colleagues. Second I was surprised that you didn't talk about the differences between the galactose-1-phosphate transferase knockout mouse and the phenotype of human galactosemia.

Dr. Berry: That is actually the worst thing that has happened in the galactosemia field: the mouse doesn't get sick. In fact when I present a knockout mouse to the interns and residents, and I don't tell them the nature of the organism, just give them the values for red blood cell, galactose-1-phosphate levels and the levels of galactose in blood and urine, they think it is a sick baby, but the mouse doesn't get sick. This is a great example of a situation in which there may be one gene product that makes the difference in the mouse not getting sick and the human getting sick. There are so many comparable biochemical abnormalities in the mouse that it makes one think that there is one thing that is protective, and in fact it may not even have anything to do with the galactose-metabolizing pathway, perhaps it is a sensor that recognizes elevated galactose-1-phosphate, and acts to recruit an apoptosis pathway. We really are completely in the dark about that.

Dr. Walker: Dr. Bier and I are always going back and forth between animal models, in vitro studies and human models. I didn't mean to imply that using animal models is going to be the panacea, but over the years having repeatedly heard about metabolic diseases, it seems to me that many of the questions originally asked have still not been answered. I was just suggesting another approach to try to determine the mechanism.

Dr. Berry: Going back to what Dr. German said before about carnitine therapy; there is a great need in the nutrition community to focus on these problems of reduced substrate levels, in this instance carnitine deficiency, and does it really matter for that particular patient. If the valine level in blood should normally be between 120 and 250 µmol/l and it is 90, does that matter for that patient? If there are enough perturbations like that in a particular patient then they may be impacting on their clinical condition. On the other hand, perhaps the carnitine level in skeletal muscle can be as low as 40% of normal and still can be normal because there is so much excess of carnitine that it doesn't matter. We think it is deficient but really it is not of clinical importance.

Dr. Rinaldo: Actually the levels of carnitine in muscle can get as low as 5% of normal and still have a normal function. Yes of course we have animal models, but sometimes a mouse reproduces the human phenotype, and galactosemia is certainly not the only one with such an uninformative outcome. We also see models in which the phenotype is far more severe than the corresponding human disease, and years of work and hundred of thousands of dollars are wasted because no living thing can be found in which to test your hypothesis. In the end, the sad thing is that when the time comes to test therapy, to test treatments, people skip mouse models and go straight back to the human model. This is certainly the case for fatty acid oxidation disorders. We have animal models that are really very close, sometimes just like the human disease, and yet every time a new therapy comes up they are just not used. It is a sad reality that people get funding and do so-called research in generating these models but when the time comes to do something with it, it is no longer fashionable.

Dr. Lau: I would like to revisit the issue on the varying severity of PKU and maple syrup urine disease in different patients. This seems to be common with a lot of monogenic diseases. We like to say they are modifier genes, but are they really there? The example that I am most familiar with is sickle cell anemia. Even though we have known the mutation for a long time yet each patient has very different spectrum of complications. We are beginning to unravel that a little bit, for example we know a little bit about some patients having persistent fetal hemoglobulin synthesis which may help to ameliorate these symptoms. How solid is the evidence in PKU or other inborn errors of metabolism that the severity is genetically regulated?

Dr. Berry: We don't know. The effects could be environmental or could also be induced by a gene perturbation, and a gene perturbation could even impact on development, not necessarily in postnatal life. We try to think mechanistically about the pathophysiology and what would make sense. Using proton NMR spectroscopy to demonstrate that the brain phenylalanine levels in vivo are elevated to the same extent in the patient who is spared CNS disease and has marked hyperphenylalaninemia is a very reasonable thing to do. In this instance the difficulty has been with using the NMR because of the lack of sensitivity, and its utility has not been demonstrated. I think a transporter abnormality makes the most sense for PKU and with association and relevant polymorphism in the genome in the people who are spared. We need to look for plausible things that are logical and follow metabolism principles. The fact is there is nothing there to show a cause and effect relationship at this point in time.

Dr. Lau: If you look at members of the affected families, is there evidence that this level of severity also runs through the families?

Dr. Berry: Yes, there are a few instances where there have been differential effects within a family; it has been very confusing. Again whether that is environment or genetics, including modifier genes is not known, it is complex. Many people who have some interest in the inborn errors probably don't appreciate how the Mendelian defects don't always hold up as would be expected or how they were originally described in the text books. They are not always simple Mendelian disorders, it is just that most of the time 80–90% of the patients behave like they are.

Dr. Koletzko: You have given us very impressive examples on how restrictive diets and inborn errors can lead to short- and medium-term effects and metabolic profiles and clinical outcomes such as isoleucine deficiency. We now are confronted with subjects who have been on these diets for 4 decades, after screening started in the 1960s. Some of these subjects follow strict diets, but many of them are not under good medical control. Isn't that a tremendous opportunity and almost an obligation for us to look at these long-term effects in much more detail?

Dr. Berry: It is actually very sad that with regard to metabolic diseases the adult world of medicine has not been ready to accept metabolic patients. A few centers have really been doing a fantastic job of trying to set up clinics, but this has not been worldwide and at least in the United States there has not been a tremendous amount of support for this. In the next session Dr. Rinaldo will talk about the success of newborn screening, which is so tremendously important. One of the places where we have really failed with newborn screening is in adults with PKU and some other disorders who now don't have medical coverage for their disorders. Coverage can always be found for them, and in fact the Department of Health and Human Services won't allow a patient like this not to be treated properly. The trouble is identifying and getting them to fit in the system. But the other big problem is to get newborn screening done properly which needs good clinical research follow-up to identify what the natural history is because we just don't know that. Take Lowe's disease, for example, an X-linked disorder involving an enzyme defect in phospholipid metabolism, these patients present with slow development early on and congenital cataracts. Later in life many of these patients cannot walk; in addition to corticospinal tract involvement they have what looks like a terrible deforming osteoarthritis that no one even thought about in the first decade of life. Much of this is not well recognized unless you happen to be very interested in this particular disease. This has not been well studied and not been well characterized unfortunately a lot because of funding problems, and not allowing good natural history or impact of therapy studies to be carried on for 2, 3 decades and more.

Dr. Walker: I am not that familiar with metabolic diseases but I am familiar with genetic diseases affecting the gastrointestinal tract and liver. I was thinking of cystic fibrosis where there is a defect in an enzyme and various forms of that defect, and that seems to be related to the phenotypic expression of disease. Does that same phenomenon occur in metabolic diseases or is it just a pure decrease due to a specific enzyme itself?

Dr. Berry: It does occur in the inborn errors, but I believe with the enzyme deficiency states it is less apt to show itself than with integral membrane proteins and proteins that are part of multiprotein complexes. The typical story with the enzymopathies is that of a gene defect associated with a termination codon involving the aminoterminal region. This usually results in a severe state with no enzyme activity because of no protein. So these are general rules with regard to inborn errors. I believe that with the complex protein assemblies linked to an integral membrane protein, very often unique phenotypes can be seen depending on the location or nature of the mutation. A great example of that is the RET proto-oncogene, where in the broader biochemical genetic world, one mutation can lead to Hirschsprung's disease but another mutation can lead to an always-on oncogenic state later on in life, namely medullary carninoma of the thyroid. Where abnormalities are found that don't make sense or are not readily predictable is where an amino acid alteration is seen in a particular domain and where there is the opportunity for another protein to interact in an aberrant protein–protein complex so that novel disease states can emerge.

Bier DM, German JB, Lönnerdal B (eds): Personalized Nutrition for the Diverse Needs of Infants and Children.
Nestlé Nutr Workshop Ser Pediatr Program, vol 62, pp 81–96,
Nestec Ltd., Vevey/S. Karger AG, Basel, © 2008.

Newborn Screening of Metabolic Disorders: Recent Progress and Future Developments

Piero Rinaldo, James S. Lim, Silvia Tortorelli, Dimitar Gavrilov, Dietrich Matern

Biochemical Genetics Laboratory, Division of Laboratory Genetics, Department of
Laboratory Medicine and Pathology, Mayo Clinic College of Medicine, Rochester, MN, USA

Abstract

Tandem mass spectrometry has been the main driver behind a significant expansion
in newborn screening programs. The ability to detect more than 40 conditions by a single
test underscores the need to better understand the clinical and laboratory characteristics
of the conditions being tested, and the complexity of pattern recognition and differential
diagnoses of one or more elevated markers. The panel of conditions recommended by the
American College of Medical Genetics, including 20 primary conditions and 22 secondary
targets that are detectable by tandem mass spectrometry has been adopted as the standard of care in the vast majority of US states. The evolution of newborn screening is far
from being idle as a large number of infectious, genetic, and metabolic conditions are currently under investigation at variable stages of test development and clinical validation. In
the US, a formal process with oversight by the Advisory Committee on Heritable
Disorders and Genetic Diseases in Newborns and Children has been established for nomination and evidence-based review of new candidate conditions. If approved, these conditions could be added to the uniform panel and consequently pave the way to large scale
implementation.

After a period of significant changes and at times controversy, the expansion of newborn screening programs in the United States [1], and in other
countries as well [2], is reaching a higher level of consensus. This process has
been pushed forward by the task of implementing tandem mass spectrometry
(MS/MS) as a single-test platform for the simultaneous detection of over 40
inborn errors of amino acid, fatty acid, and organic acid metabolism [3] by
amino acid and acylcarnitine profiling of neonatal dried blood spots [4, 5].

Critical evidence in support of this expansion came from a report released by an expert panel assembled by the American College of Medical Genetics (ACMG) [6, 7]. This report described the evidence-review process applied to identify a panel of 29 conditions, 20 of them screened for by MS/MS analysis, which is commonly referred to as the 'uniform panel'. An additional 25 conditions, 22 of them also detected by MS/MS, were recommended in a cohort of secondary targets. Table 1 shows a list of these 42 conditions, the number of US states currently screening for each of them, and highlights the need for differential diagnosis due to pervasive overlap of informative markers between primary and secondary targets.

To date (July 2007), screening by MS/MS is provided by 48 of 51 US states (including the District of Columbia), a proportion that translates into approximately 98% of the total number of births per year [8]. However, the extent of implementation of the full panel remains variable (fig. 1), ranging between 5 and 100% (5 states) with an overall average of 75%. Although the uniform panel (20 conditions) has been implemented by a majority of states (38 of 51), only six are pursuing the whole set of secondary targets [8]. The inclusion of the secondary targets has been controversial because in most cases their natural history is poorly understood [9]. However, a defining characteristic of a multiplex platform like MS/MS is the need to perform an extensive post-analytical interpretation and differential diagnosis for most of the metabolites detectable in the amino acid and acylcarnitine profiles [4, 10]. If conditions were to be removed from the list of secondary targets on the sole basis of not requiring a differential diagnosis from a primary condition, only argininemia and 2,4-dienoyl-CoA reductase deficiency would be candidates for exclusion from the panel [10, 11]. Limited appreciation of this reality may lead to unfortunate yet fully avoidable situations, for example the reporting of concurrent diagnoses in a patient with a complex biochemical phenotype, or the assumption that a nominal mass represents only one of several possible isobaric compounds [12, 13]. Moreover, advocates of testing by multiple reaction monitoring rather than the full scan mode, for the purpose of avoiding 'undesirable' findings, apparently fail to recognize the number of potentially misleading findings [14, 15] which can only be recognized properly when the full profile is evaluated.

The impact of a deliberate exclusion of informative markers could be as high as missing approximately 10% of all cases who could be detected if the uniform panel was universally implemented (fig. 2). This estimate is extrapolated from an analysis of: (a) current state panels [1, 8]; (b) incidence data from multiple sources [11, 16–20], and (c) an empirical yet data-driven estimate of correction factors for ethnic variability selected as follows: Caucasians >75% of births; Hispanic >40%; African-American >40%, and Asian/Pacific >50% (2004 ethnic distribution from http://www2.uthscsa.edu/nnsis/). These modifiers are used to define ethnically adjusted rates of detection for conditions with emerging evidence of broad, racially defined incidence rates (table 1), beyond the well-known clustering of specific conditions

Table 1. Inborn errors of metabolism included in the ACMG recommended panels of primary and secondary targets [6]

Group	Condition (inborn errors of amino acid, fatty acid, and organic acid metabolism)[1]	ACMG code[1]	ACMG panel[2]	US states screening for this condition [8]	Interpretation requires differential diagnosis	Primary conditions with same marker(s)	Secondary conditions with same markers	Differences in US incidence on the basis of ethnic distribution	Detection rate in Minnesota (July 2004–July 2007; n = 289,292)
AA	Argininosuccinic acidemia	ASA	UP	45	Yes	CIT	CIT II	1:200,000	1:144,646
AA	Citrullinemia	CIT	UP	45	Yes	ASA	CIT II	1:200,000	None detected
AA	Homocystinuria (CBS deficiency)	HCY	UP	47	Yes	–	MET	1:250,000	1:289,292
AA	Maple syrup (urine) disease	MSUD	UP	47	–	–	–	1:250,000 Asian/Pacific >50% 1:30,000	1:289,292
AA	Phenylketonuria	PKU	UP	51	Yes	–	H-PHE BIOPT (BS) (REG)	1:20,000 Caucasians >75% 1:15,000 Hispanics >40% 1:30,000 Asian/Pacific >50% 1:50,000	1:15,226
AA	Tyrosinemia type I	TYR I	UP	39	Yes	–	TYR II TYR III	1:500,000	None detected
AA	Argininemia	ARG	ST	34	–	–	–	1:250,000	None detected

Table 1. (continued)

Group	Condition (inborn errors of amino acid, fatty acid, and organic acid metabolism)[1]	ACMG code[1]	ACMG panel[2]	US states screening for this condition [8]	Interpretation requires differential diagnosis	Primary conditions with same marker(s)	Secondary conditions with same markers	Differences in US incidence on the basis of ethnic distribution	Detection rate in Minnesota (July 2004 July 2007; n = 289,292)
AA	Hyper-phenyl-alaninemia	H-PHE	ST	51	Yes	PKU	H-PHE BIOPT (BS) (REG)	1:30,000 Caucasians >75% 1:25,000 Hispanics >40% 1:30,000 Asian/Pacific >50% 1:80,000	1:26,299
AA	Citrullinemia type II	CIT II	ST	40	Yes	ASA CIT	CIT II PC	1:200,000	1:144,646
AA	Defects of biopterin cofactor biosynthesis	BIOPT (BS)	ST	22	Yes	PKU	H-PHE BIOPT (REG)	1:500,000	None detected
AA	Disorders of biopterin cofactor regeneration	BIOPT (REG)	ST	22	Yes	PKU	H-PHE BIOPT (BS)	1:250,000	None detected
AA	Hyper-methioninemia	MET	ST	40	Yes	HCY	–	1:200,000	1:144,646
AA	Tyrosinemia type II	TYR II	ST	39	Yes	TYR I	TYR III	1:500,000	None detected

AA	Tyrosinemia type III	TYR III	ST	32	Yes	TYR I	TYR II	1:250,000	None detected
FAO	Carnitine uptake defect	CUD	UP	43	Yes	GA I (mat) 3MCC (mat)	—	1:50,000	1:144,646 1:22,253 (maternal)
FAO	Long-chain 3-OH acyl-CoA dehydrogenase deficiency	LCHAD	UP	45	Yes	TFP	—	1:50,000	1:57,858 (combined with TFP)
FAO	Medium-chain acyl-CoA dehydrogenase deficiency	MCAD	UP	47	Yes	—	GA2 MCKAT	1:15,000 Caucasians >75% 1:12,000 Hispanics >40% 1:21,000 African-Americans >40% 1:30,000 Asian/Pacific >50% 1:50,000	1:11,572
FAO	Trifunctional protein deficiency	TFP	UP	45	Yes	LCHAD	—	1:100,000	See LCHAD
FAO	Very long-chain acyl-CoA dehydrogenase deficiency	VLCAD	UP	45	Yes	—	GA2	1:75,000	1:144,646
FAO	Dienoyl reductase deficiency	DE-RED	ST	15	—	—	—	1:2,000,000	None detected

Table 1. (continued)

Group	Condition (inborn errors of amino acid, fatty acid, and organic acid metabolism)[1]	ACMG code[1]	ACMG panel[2]	US states screening for this condition [8]	Interpretation requires differential diagnosis	Primary conditions with same marker(s)	Secondary conditions with same markers	Differences in US incidence on the basis of ethnic distribution	Detection rate in Minnesota (July 2004–July 2007; n = 289,292)
FAO	Carnitine palmitoyl-transferase Ia deficiency (L)	CPT Ia	ST	35	–	–	–	1:300,000 Alaska 1:1,000	None detected
FAO	Carnitine palmitoyl-transferase II deficiency	CPT II	ST	42	Yes	–	CACT	1:250,000	1:289,292
FAO	Glutaric acidemia type II	GA2	ST	41	Yes	MCAD GA I IVA	SCAD IBG	1:250,000	1:289,292
FAO	Medium/short-chain 3-OH acyl-CoA dehydrogenase deficiency	M/SCHAD	ST	18	–	–	–	1:2,000,000	None detected
FAO	Medium-chain ketoacyl-CoA dehydrogenase deficiency	MCKAT	ST	19	Yes	MCAD GA2	–	1:2,000,000	None detected

FAO	Short-chain acyl-CoA dehydrogenase deficiency	SCAD	ST	38	Yes			1:50,000	1:28,929
FAO	Carnitine/acyl-carnitine translocase deficiency	CACT	ST	41	Yes	CPT II		1:300,000	None detected
OA	3-Methyl-crotonyl-CoA carboxylase deficiency	3MCC	UP	44	Yes	2M3HBA 3MGA	MCD HMG BKT	1:50,000	1:36,162 1:57,858 (maternal)
OA	3-Hydroxy 3-methylglutaric aciduria	HMG	UP	44	Yes	2M3HBA 3MGA	3MCC MCD BKT	1:250,000	None detected
OA	β-Ketothiolase deficiency	BKT	UP	44	Yes	2M3HBA 3MGA	3MCC MCD HMG	1:300,000	None detected
OA	Glutaric acidemia type I	GA I	UP	45	Yes	GA2	–	1:100,000	1:289,292
OA	Isovaleric acidemia	IVA	UP	45	Yes	2MBG GA2	–	1:75,000	1:48,215
OA	Methylmalonic acidemia (A,B)	Cbl A,B	UP	45	Yes	Cbl CD	MUT PA	1:100,000	See MUT
OA	Methylmalonic acidemia (Mut)	MUT	UP	45	Yes	Cbl CD	Cbl AB PA	1:100,000	1:36,162 (combined with Cbl A,B)
OA	Multiple carboxylase deficiency	MCD	UP	43	Yes	2M3HBA 3MGA	3MCC HMG BKT	1:250,000	None detected

Table 1. (continued)

Group	Condition (inborn errors of amino acid, fatty acid, and organic acid metabolism)[1]	ACMG code[1]	ACMG panel[2]	US states screening for this condition [8]	Interpretation requires differential diagnosis	Primary conditions with same marker(s)	Secondary conditions with same markers	Differences in US incidence on the basis of ethnic distribution	Detection rate in Minnesota (July 2004 July 2007; n = 289,292)
OA	Propionic acidemia	PA	UP	45	Yes	MUT Cbl AB	Cbl CD	1:150,000	None detected
OA	2-Methyl-3-hydroxybutyric aciduria	2M3HBA	ST	29	Yes	3MCC MCD HMG BKT	3MGA	1:1,000,000	None detected
OA	2-Methylbutyryl-CoA dehydrogenase deficiency	2MBG	ST	36	Yes	IVA	GA2	1:500,000 Hmong >0.5% 1:15,000	1:12,054
OA	3-Methyl-glutaconic aciduria	3MGA	ST	35	Yes	3MCC MCD HMG BKT	2M3HBA	1:200,000	1:96,431
OA	Isobutyryl-CoA dehydrogenase deficiency	IBG	ST	35	Yes	–	GA2 SCAD	1:100,000	1:57,858
OA	Malonic aciduria	MAL	ST	25	–	–		1:500,000	1:289,292
OA	Methylmalonic acidemia (Cbl C,D)	Cbl C,D	ST	40	Yes	MUT Cbl AB PA	–	1:100,000 Hispanics >40% 1:50,000	1:72,323

[1]Nomenclature and abbreviations from Watson et al. [6; table 1, pp 5S–6S].
[2]From Watson et al. [6; tables 7 and 8, pp 37S–38S]. UP = Uniform panel (primary targets); ST = secondary targets.

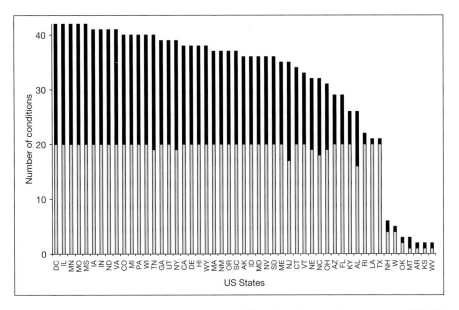

Fig. 1. Number of primary targets (out of 20; □) and secondary targets (22; ■) screened for by US newborn screening programs (MS/MS only). Data from the National Newborn Screening and Genetics Resource Center [8], accessed June 23, 2007.

in small enclaves [21, 22]. This approach, of course, is based on the assumption of mutual compensation when applied across more than four million births in the US. Under these circumstances, a nationwide implementation of the recommended panel of 42 conditions could lead to the identification of approximately 1,600–1,700 cases per year. To date, however, the partial implementation of the ACMG panel implies that more than 180 cases could remain undetected and/or unreported. More than 50 of them would be affected with one of the primary targets, and half of them carry a risk of sudden and unexpected death [3]. In view of available evidence on the high rate of lethality at the first episode of metabolic decompensation, which could be as high as 30–50% in certain disorders of fatty acid oxidation, even under the most conservative scenario as many as ten infants born in the United States this year are at risk of dying because they are affected with a treatable condition not yet included in a state newborn screening panel.

As mentioned above, most of the secondary targets are part of the differential diagnosis of one or more conditions in the core panel. Furthermore, it has become increasingly apparent that there are additional conditions potentially detectable by analysis of the same amino acid and acylcarnitine markers

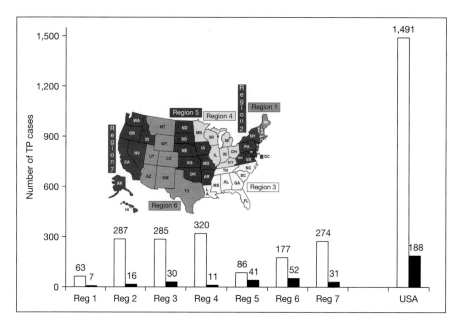

Fig. 2. Estimates of the number of true positive (TP) cases identifiable (targeted; □) and potentially undetected/unreported (■) by US newborn screening program. States are combined according to the boundaries of current regional collaborative projects (http://www.nccrcg.org).

[23–25]. This observation suggests a need in the near future to update the list of secondary targets, and possibly upgrade a few of the existing ones to a status of primary target on the basis of new evidence obtained after the implementation of expanded screening by MS/MS [26]. Table 2 summarizes these emerging conditions, their respective informative markers, and the number of cases known to us as a result of data collection in the context of a collaborative project which has grown to include 82 laboratories worldwide (see www.region4genetics.org).

Although much progress has taken place recently, a large number of other conditions are still actively being considered for future expansion of newborn screening programs. Table 3 is a representative, but likely incomplete, list of conditions currently being considered. Analytical development of screening tests and clinical validation through prospective pilot studies for many of them are in progress. For example, our laboratory is actively involved in three projects, namely screening for lysosomal storage diseases [27, 28], Wilson disease [29], and X-linked adrenoleukodystrophy [30].

Table 2. Additional conditions detectable by amino acid and acylcarnitine analysis of dried blood spots by MS/MS (not included in the ACMG uniform panel)

Condition	Code	Marker	Differential diagnosis	Cases detected by NBS[1]
Ethylmalonic encephalopathy [5]	EE	C4 C5	SCAD IBG GA2	7
Pyruvate carboxylase deficiency [23]	PC	CIT	CIT-I CIT-II ASA	2
Formiminoglutamic academia	FIGLU	Figlu (m/z 287)	SCAD IBG EE	>10
SUCLA2 deficiency [24]	SUCLA2	C3 C4DC	MUT Cbl AB Cbl CD	–
Methylene tetrahydrofolate reductase deficiency	MTHFR	MET (low)	Cbl E Cbl G	1
Defect of cobalamin metabolism	Cbl E	MET (low)	MTHFR Cbl G	–
Defect of cobalamin metabolism	Cbl G	MET (low)	MTHFR Cbl E	–

From the true positive database of the Regional Collaborative project 'Laboratory quality improvement of newborn screening by tandem mass spectrometry', http://www.region4genetics/org. Accessed July 31, 2007.

In anticipation of the outcome of several ongoing projects, the Secretary Advisory Committee on Heritable Disorders and Genetic Diseases in Newborn and Children (ACHDGDNC; http://mchb.hrsa.gov/programs/genetics/committee/) has developed a process for the nomination of conditions to be considered for inclusion in the uniform panel, which is based on sequential stages of administrative review, committee approval to proceed, and appointment of an evidence review group (ERG). The charge of the ERG is to assess all available evidence and make recommendations back to ACHDGDNC. In case of a positive outcome, a recommendation could be made to add the approved condition to the uniform panel [31]. However, it is likely that a vigorous, iterative process will first take place to address gaps in the understanding of the natural history of the condition, and the availability of clinical validation data, which must include a prospective pilot study and modality, efficacy, and availability of treatment options. More information on the nomination process, which was launched on June 22, 2007, can be found at the website listed above. Based on anecdotal information, it appears more than likely that several conditions will be nominated formally in the near future, with a review process taking place between 2008 and 2009.

Table 3. Conditions under active investigation toward the development and validation of a high throughput method targeting population screening (listed in alphabetical order)

Creatine metabolism (disorders of)
Duchenne muscular dystrophy
Familial hypercholesterolemia
Fragile X syndrome
Glucose-6-phosphate dehydrogenase (G6PD) deficiency
Infectious diseases
 HIV
 Toxoplasmosis
 Cytomegalovirus (CMV)
Lysosomal storage diseases (partial list)
 Fabry disease
 Gaucher disease
 Krabbe disease
 Metachromatic leukodystrophy (MLD)
 MPS I, II, IV
 Niemann Pick disease type A,B
 Pompe disease
Severe combined immunodeficiency (SCID)
Smith-Lemli-Opitz syndrome (and possibly other disorders of sterol metabolism)
Spinal muscular atrophy (SMA)
Wilson disease
X-linked adrenoleukodystrophy (X-ALD)

References

1 Therrell BL, Adams J: Newborn screening in North America. J Inherit Metab Dis 2007;30:447–465.
2 Bodamer OA, Hoffmann GF, Lindner M: Expanded newborn screening in Europe 2007. J Inherit Metab Dis 2007;30:439–444.
3 Rinaldo P, Hahn SH, Matern D: Inborn errors of amino acid, organic acid, and fatty acid metabolism; in Burtis CA, Ashwood ER, Bruns DE (eds): Tietz Textbook of Clinical Chemistry and Molecular Diagnostics, ed 4. Philadelphia, Saunders, 2005, pp 2207–2247.
4 Chace DH, Kalas TA, Naylor EW: Use of tandem mass spectrometry for multianalyte screening of dried blood specimens from newborns. Clin Chem 2003;49:1797–1817.
5 Rinaldo P, Tortorelli S, Matern M: Recent developments and new applications of tandem mass spectrometry in newborn screening. Curr Opin Pediatr 2004;16:427–432.
6 Watson MS, Mann MY, Lloyd-Puryear MA, Rinaldo P, Howell RR (eds): Newborn screening: toward a uniform screening panel and system (executive summary). Genet Med 2006;8(suppl):1S–11S.
7 Watson MS, Lloyd-Puryear MA, Mann MY, Rinaldo P, Howell RR (eds): Newborn screening: toward a uniform screening panel and system (main report). Genet Med 2006;8(suppl):12S–252S.
8 National Newborn Screening and Genetics Resource Center: US National Newborn Screening Information System. http://genes-r-us.uthscsa.edu. Accessed June 14, 2007.
9 Pollitt RJ: Introducing new screens: why are we all doing different things? J Inherit Metab Dis 2007;30:423–429.
10 Sweetman L, Millington DS, Therrell BL, et al: Naming and counting disorders (conditions) included in newborn screening panels. Pediatrics 2006;117:S308–S314.

11 Rinaldo P, Zafari S, Tortorelli S, Matern D: Making the case for objective performance metrics in newborn screening by tandem mass spectrometry. Ment Retard Dev Disabil Res Rev 2006;12:255–261.

12 Abdenur JE, Chamoles NA, Guinle AE, et al: Diagnosis of isovaleric acidaemia by tandem mass spectrometry: false positive result due to pivaloylcarnitine in a newborn screening programme. J Inherit Metab Dis 1998;21:624–630.

13 Oglesbee D, He M, Majumder N, et al: Development of a newborn screening follow-up algorithm for the diagnosis of isobutyryl-CoA dehydrogenase deficiency. Genet Med 2007;9: 108–116.

14 Vianey-Saban C, Boyer S, Levrat V, et al: Interference of cefotaxime in plasma acylcarnitine profile mimicking an increase of 3-hydroxypalmitoleylcarnitine (C16:1-OH) using butyl esters. J Inherit Metab Dis 2004;27(suppl 1):94.

15 Magera MJ, Tortorelli S, Hahn SH, et al: Dextrose – An Artifact Detectable by Newborn Screening as a Butylated Acylcarnitine. Portland, Association of Public Health Laboratories, Newborn Screening and Genetic Testing Symposium, 2005, p 67.

16 Zytkovicz TH, Fitzgerald EF, Marsden D, et al: Tandem mass spectrometric analysis for amino, organic, and fatty acid disorders in newborn dried blood spots: a two-year summary from the New England Newborn Screening Program. Clin Chem 2001;47:1945–1955.

17 Schulze A, Lindner M, Kohlmuller D, et al: Expanded newborn screening for inborn errors of metabolism by electrospray ionization-tandem mass spectrometry: results, outcome, and implications. Pediatrics 2003;111:1399–1406.

18 Wilcken B, Wiley V, Hammond J, et al: Screening newborns for inborn errors of metabolism by tandem mass spectrometry. N Engl J Med 2003;348:2304–2312.

19 Hoffmann GF, von Kries R, Klose D, et al: Frequencies of inherited organic acidurias and disorders of mitochondrial fatty acid transport and oxidation in Germany. Eur J Pediatr 2004;163:76–80.

20 Frazier DM, Millington DS, McCandless SE, et al: The tandem mass spectrometry newborn screening experience in North Carolina: 1997–2005. J Inherit Metab Dis 2006;29:76–85.

21 Matern D, He M, Berry SA, et al: Prospective diagnosis of 2-methylbutyryl-CoA dehydrogenase deficiency in the Hmong population by newborn screening using tandem mass spectrometry. Pediatrics 2003;112:74–78.

22 Alaska Division of Public Health: CPT-1 Deficiency. Available at http://www.hss.state.ak.us/dph/wcfh/metabolic/downloads/cpt1_brochure.pdf

23 Merinero B, Perez-Cerda C, Ruiz Sala P, et al: Persistent increase of plasma butyryl/isobutyrylcarnitine concentrations as marker of SCAD defect and ethylmalonic encephalopathy. J Inherit Metab Dis 2006;29:685.

24 Garcia-Cazorla A, Rabier D, Touati G, et al: Pyruvate carboxylase deficiency: metabolic characteristics and new neurological aspects. Ann Neurol 2006;59:121–127.

25 Carrozzo R, Dionisi-Vici C, Steuerwald U, et al: SUCLA2 mutations are associated with mild methylmalonic aciduria, Leigh-like encephalomyopathy, dystonia and deafness. Brain 2007;130:862–874.

26 Lorey F, Enns G, Cederbaum S, et al: Should Cobalamin C (Cbl C) be a core target? Evidence for increased prevalence, detection, and effectiveness of treatment intervention in California newborn screening. Proc 2007 Newborn Screening and Genetic Testing Symp. Minneapolis, Association of Public Health Laboratories, 2007, p 36. http://www.aphl.org.

27 Meikle PJ, Grasby DJ, Dean CJ, et al: Newborn screening for lysosomal storage disorders. Mol Genet Metab 2006;88:307–314.

28 Gelb MH, Turecek F, Scott CR, Chamoles NA: Direct multiplex assay of enzymes in dried blood spots by tandem mass spectrometry for the newborn screening of lysosomal storage disorders. J Inherit Metab Dis 2006;29:397–404.

29 Kroll CA, Ferber MJ, Dawson BD, et al: Retrospective determination of ceruloplasmin in newborn screening blood spots of patients with Wilson disease. Mol Genet Metab 2006;89:134–138.

30 Hubbard WC, Moser AB, Tortorelli S, et al: Combined liquid chromatography-tandem mass spectrometry as an analytical method for high throughput screening for X-linked adrenoleukodystrophy and other peroxisomal disorders: preliminary findings. Mol Genet Metab 2006;89:185–187.

31 Watson MS: Current status of newborn screening: decision-making about the conditions to include in screening programs. Ment Retard Dev Disabil Res Rev 2006;12:230–235.

Discussion

Dr. Koletzko: Tandem screening was introduced in Bavaria in January 1999 and we are just as enthusiastic and consider this a quantum leap in the early detection of disease, not only because we have a larger number of diagnoses. It is also important in that the diagnosis has become far more precise and there are much fewer false-positive results. With respect to newborn screening I really wonder whether the motto the bigger the better is always true; whether the longer list is always the better list. The longer list obviously is of greater advantage if we talk about research applications. It is also of greater advantage if we try to diagnose symptomatic patients, then the more we can detect will give us a greater likelihood of making a diagnosis. But from the European perspective screening is really a public health concept that should be offered to all newborns in a nation regardless of where they are born. Then there is not only the question of benefit, there is also the question of harm and not to do harm will be the guiding principle. From that point of view in our country we feel that analytical methodology is only one part of the concept. In addition to a good analytical tool, it is very important that a tracking system is established to monitor and find those who have not been screened, and also to make sure that those who have been screened and have a positive result are really followed up. Experience has shown that without a tracking system a lot of problems occur. The other concern is that one would not want to introduce detection of disorders where there is no true benefit for the child. For example organic acidemias; the link has been made between the biochemical abnormality and 3-methylcrotonyl-CoA carboxylase (3MCC) deficiency. In the literature there are a number of symptomatic patients with that biochemical abnormality, but the experience of the last 8 years has shown that most children affected by 3MCC deficiency in the newborn screening don't have any disease. So there is no benefit from screening for this deficiency. The same is true with newborn screening for hypercholesterolemia, there is really no benefit. Obviously, yes, we want to detect those with primary genetic hypercholesterolemia but when is the right time? Is newborn screening really the right time or is it the right time when you can't intervene?. If you make a diagnosis and cannot offer anything to the family in terms of treatment for a newborn, then I think the adverse effects need to be considered. Adrenoleukodystrophy is the same, it can be diagnosed, and there may be some benefit from prenatal diagnosis in a sibling, but there is no agreement that treatment is really beneficial. This needs to be looked at more closely and I could not agree with you more in terms of research or evaluation that the list should be enlarged, but in terms of implementation of public health service, that needs to be thoroughly discussed.

Dr. Rinaldo: The point is actually not about 3MCC, it is about the same marker being diagnostic for six different conditions. The diagnoses of HMG-CoA lyase deficiency or β-ketothiolase or 3-methylglutaconic aciduria must be clearer. We can have long discussions about the fact that it goes back to the environment and the modifiers; I have seen comatose patients with 3MCC. There is beautiful paper in the *American Journal of Human Genetics*, well-presented data, and yet not a single word about the differential diagnosis of 3MCC, and that is a problem. The point is what about those patients. To say that there are adverse effects is highly questionable. In fact it is mostly anecdotal based on a single case; so we really have to keep things in a perspective. 3MCC could be asymptomatic for a long time, in fact maternal cases have been diagnosed. Yet under the right circumstances it could even be a life-threatening disease. We just don't know what makes the difference between the two scenarios. The same goes for excluding propionic acidemia and methylmalonic acidemia, conditions that nobody should doubt, as presented earlier by Dr. Berry, because they can cause life-threatening episodes and serious damage and pancreatitis. To deny a patient the best possible chance of being treated in the best possible way is just against every fiber of my body and everything I believe in. The point is a public policy cannot be generalized so that it compromises the chances of individual patients to be treated in the best possible way. It is not a decision for politicians or policy makers, it is a decision for the individual families and their physician. What is best; we need the information; we need to know.

Dr. Lagercrantz: Why do people still continue to collect blood from the heel of babies? In Sweden we take a venous sample; it is much less painful and you can get much more blood [1].

Dr. Rinaldo: An excellent point and there is really no good reason to continue to do it this way.

Dr. Strandvik: I want to support what Dr. Koletzko said. As a clinician I have seen dramatic pathology in the relation between mother and child when a diagnosis is made very early or if formation is obtained about something which sometimes won't result in a clinical disease for many years. In these cases, many parents become hesitant to bond to the child because they are afraid of losing it. The first period in a small infant's life is extremely important for this bonding [2]. When you show such a high percentage of positive results with this enormous tandem spectrometry, indicating a lot of diseases, do you give psychological support for all this or how do you handle it?

Dr. Rinaldo: It really should be mentioned that human screening is not a test, it is a system that includes various components such as evaluation and follow-up and support. It is interesting though that although we seem to be so focused on the potential negative consequences of a diagnosis of a known condition, nobody really talks about the real problem: false-positives. The acceptability of screening could be greatly improved if we reduced the false-positives. That is why in our collaborative project we have performance metrics and we say that if a program has a false-positive regulator of more than 0.3% by tandem mass spectrometry then there is a problem, and yet there are programs with a false-positive rate of 1–2%. That is really why we are teaching pediatricians to start asking tough questions because it is probably not helpful to know what the sensitivity or the specificity of a system is overall. If you ask what the positive predictive value is, I can probably answer that mine is 47% over 4 years, meaning that 1 in every 2 that I report as abnormal is real. In most cases the false-positive predictive value will be a single digit, meaning that for every 1 shown positive there will be 20 false-positives. With a low positive predictive value, a lot of downstream problems and issues are actually being created with acceptance of testing and disattached parents. Waisbren et al. [3] have published a beautiful paper showing the number of hospitalizations, visits to the emergency room and all sorts of problems in families of children who are false-positive. So the point is, bigger might not be better if it isn't handled well. If it is done well, if the performance metrics are kept in check, then it is very powerful. There will always be exceptions; there will always be situations where people may object. Do you want to know at birth about the risk of heart disease; do you want to know at birth that your teenage child will be in a wheelchair; it is an incredibly tough question. Again the hope is that if you pick them up early, there will be a better outcome, and there is only one way to find out.

Dr. Berry: Actually we need to think about this in a different way, some more to immunization, especially if other genetic diseases are screened for in the future. From a public health point of view, it is just may be economically so much more advantageous to screen in the newborn period for adult-onset diseases and multifactorial complex genetic diseases that it overweighs any ideas to the contrary. It may be necessary for countries to come to grips with the idea that newborn screening to identify disorders that aren't present in newborn period may be better for the common good; that actually a greater number of individuals may be helped while, at the same time, there are psychological problems that occur to a minority. Perhaps it is just only financially feasible to do this in the newborn period, and so some difficult decisions might need to be made in the future.

Dr. Rinaldo: I could not agree more. In fact I hope I didn't give anybody the impression that all this is black and white and clear cut, it is incredibly complex. But you are right, even Minnesota will screen 75,000 babies, 99.5% coming from 118 birthing places, so the collection is centralized. The moment you lose the opportunity to do something in an existing system that is really focused on a relatively small number of sites where the specimens are procured, and you start going to the individual doctors' offices then you start going into the tens of thousands. The old systems, especially when it comes to fairness and universality, are almost impossible to comply with. That is actually a very good point, for the greater good the newborn screening card has a massive potential. Under certain circumstances, in some cases, that again could have perceived negative consequences, but the greater of good would be well served.

References

1 Larsson BA, Tannfeldt G, Lagercrantz H, Olsson GL: Venipuncture is more effective and less painful than heel lancing for blood tests in neonates. Pediatrics 1998;101:882–886.
2 Klaus MH, Kennell JH: Bonding: The Beginnings of Parent–Infant Attachment. St Louis, Mosby, 1983.
3 Waisbren SE, Albers S, Amato S, et al: Effect of expanded newborn screening for biochemical genetic disorders on child outcomes and parental stress. JAMA 2003;290:2564–2572.

Bier DM, German JB, Lönnerdal B (eds): Personalized Nutrition for the Diverse Needs of Infants and Children.
Nestlé Nutr Workshop Ser Pediatr Program, vol 62, pp 97–110,
Nestec Ltd., Vevey/S. Karger AG, Basel, © 2008.

The Phenotype of Human Obesity: The Scope of the Problem

Dennis M. Bier

USDA/ARS Children's Nutrition Research Center,
Baylor College of Medicine, Houston, TX, USA

Abstract

The prevention and treatment of childhood obesity have proven to be extremely difficult problems. Since the equation for maintaining energy balance is an extremely simple one, having only two terms, 'energy in' and 'energy out', the difficulties encountered in its application for obesity management are not immediately obvious. Among the problems that make practical application of the energy balance equation more difficult than expected are: (1) the precise feedback control system that is designed to maintain weight within a given range; (2) the aggressive resistance of the system to attempts to exceed its boundaries; (3) inaccurate assessment of energy intake in practice; (4) the dominant role of genes in determining body weight; (5) the polygenic nature of obesity and the fact that any single gene accounts for a small fraction of the genetic variation in weight; (6) underestimation of the genetic contribution to the current 'epidemic' of obesity; (7) the fact that 'modifiable' risk factors may be less modifiable than expected; (8) appreciation that family role modeling may be less influential than anticipated, and (9) the realization that our knowledge about the development of physical activity behaviors in childhood is extremely limited.

Introduction

Obesity is the most prevalent form of malnutrition in the developed world. At first glance, one might imagine that obesity should be a relatively simple condition to correct. After all, the energy balance equation has only two terms. Thus:

Dietary energy intake − Energy expended in activity = Body fat stored

In theory, then, one has merely to reduce the amount of energy consumed in food and/or increase the amount of energy expended in daily activities and the problem is solved. Moreover, the tool necessary to measure the primary endpoint variable, body weight, is simple, readily available, and easy to interpret – namely a reliable scale. Likewise simple, readily available and easy to interpret are the tools necessary to measure the secondary endpoint variable, body fat distribution. These are a tape measure and mirror for assessing body fat distribution. Nevertheless, both treating established obesity and preventing the development of obesity have proven almost intractable in practice. Why is this so? The answer is not simple. If it were, we would not be in this predicament. The plausible, proximate explanations lie in the fact that there are significant problems that confound a straightforward application of the energy balance equation.

Problem No. 1

Man has evolved an exquisitely sensitive and precise feedback control system to maintain body weight within a genetically set range [1–8]. Because an effective body mass is critical to survival, during the course of human evolution, man has developed an exquisitely sensitive and precise system for assessing the status of body energy intake and fuel stores [1–5] and for maintaining body weight within a relatively narrow range [6–8]. It is now abundantly clear that both gut and adipose tissue are in constant communication with the brain via the hormones cholecystokinin, ghrelin, glucagon-like peptide-1, peptide YY, enterostatin, bombesin, oxyntomodulin, secreted by the gut, insulin release by the pancreas and leptin released by adipocytes. Insulin and leptin signal the magnitude of fat stores and leptin inhibits neural pathways that stimulate food intake while promoting pathways that reduce feeding [6–8]. Ghrelin stimulates appetite, while the remaining hormones provide satiety signals [1–5]. Correspondingly, the brain responds with the appropriate efferent hormonal signals that regulate food intake and energy expenditure [6–8]. Thus, neuropeptide-Y and Agouti-related peptide stimulate eating while the pro-opiomelanocortin-derived peptides α- and β-melanocortin-stimulating hormones reduce eating [6–8]. When one attempts to reduce body weight, there is increased secretion of ghrelin, neuropeptide-Y and Agouti-related peptides, accompanied by a decreased release of leptin, insulin, and pro-opiomelanocortin. Further, sympathetic nervous system tone decreases and less thyroxine is converted to triiodothyronine, the active thyroid hormone [6, 7]. The net result of these changes is that energy expenditure declines [6, 7]. That this resistance is operative and effective in man has been amply demonstrated by rigorous clinical investigation. Leibel et al. [7] demonstrated that a weight reduction of 10% was accompanied by a decrease in total daily energy expenditure in the order of 6–8 kcal/kg of fat-free mass.

Problem No. 2

The system conspires against our attempts to exceed its boundaries. While it is well known that obesity results in peripheral resistance to the actions of insulin, it is less well appreciated that the hypothalamus in obese individuals also develops a resistance to the actions of leptin. While it is not entirely clear whether the leptin resistance develops in cells that respond directly to leptin itself or in cells that are further 'downstream' of leptin's proximate action, the overall result is that leptin's role in reducing food intake is blunted [8].

In consort then, the overall effects of Problem No. 1 and Problem No. 2 are to increase the difficulty of losing weight since there is an effective 'hormonal resistance' to attempts to diminish body mass by reducing energy expenditure and by reducing the break on satiation [6–8]. In clinical practice, the net result is that the involuntary, long-term, biological regulatory system outlasts the voluntary, short-term response system of human compliance and perseverance.

Problem No. 3

We do not have practice tools that will let us know confidently which term in the energy balance equation is the culprit in any individual circumstance. The long-established tools of direct and indirect calorimetry, including the doubly labeled water method, are extremely accurate and very precise by any usual standard of methods applied to human physiology. Thus energy expenditure can be measured to a precision of about ±2–5% [9, 10]. However, a long-term, daily energy excess of 2–5% is greater than that necessity to result in a significant degree of obesity.

Tools to measure energy intake, on the other hand, are notoriously inaccurate. Trabulsi and Schoeller [11] compared multiple conventional approaches to assessing dietary intake in humans with unbiased estimates of actual intake derived from simultaneous measurement of total daily energy expenditure using doubly labeled water. Conventional methods of dietary assessment regularly and significantly underestimated actual energy intake by about −20% on average [11]. In the context of maintaining energy balance, an inaccuracy of 20% is a truly gargantuan amount. In practical terms, this means that, except under conditions of gross over-consumption, dietary intake data are not sensitive enough to permit confident conclusions about the role of modest increments in energy intake as a contributing factor in the development and/or maintenance of obesity in individuals.

Problem No. 4

Our genes account for a greater fraction of the variance in body weight than all other physiological, biochemical, and behavioral variables combined. Body weight is largely determined by genetics. Long-term

Table 1. Human obesity gene map

1 The Y chromosome is the only chromosome without a putative obesity locus
2 More than 250 quantitative trait loci for body weight have been identified in more than 60 genome-wide scans
The *FTO* gene has been the most consistently observed gene associated with the common form of human obesity
3 More than 125 candidate obesity genes have been identified
More than 20 of these are supported by findings from 5 or more separate studies
4 Fifty obesity-related syndromes have been mapped
Causal or candidate genes have been identified in most of these syndromes
5 More than 175 cases of human obesity have been shown to be due to more than 70 single mutations in 11 genes (monogenic obesity)
The vast majority of these are mutations in the melanocortin-4 receptor gene, accounting for the obesity observed in approximately 90% of the people who have been found to have monogenic causes of obesity

Adapted from Rankinen et al. [16].

and well-established studies carried out in many thousands of twin pairs have confirmed that genes are responsible for 50–90% of the variance in BMI [12]. Consensus overall estimates derived from such twin studies estimate that about two thirds to three quarters of the variance in BMI distribution in populations is the result of genetics. Likewise, genes are a major contributor to body fat mass, fat distribution, energy intake, and responses to alterations in energy intake and diet composition [13–15].

Problem No. 5

The common form of human obesity is a polygenic disorder in which many genes contribute to the body weight phenotype and each gene contributes only a small fraction of the variance. Table 1 shows the status of the human obesity gene map at the end of 2005 [16]. All chromosomes but the Y chromosome house genes with loci that contribute to body weight. In syndromes that have obesity as part of their phenotypes, more than 50 loci have been mapped and causal or candidate genes have been identified in most of these [16]. However, as a rule, the identified genes have not provided a mechanism for the development of obesity.

For the forms of obesity commonly present in the general population, more than 250 quantitative trait loci have been identified in more than 60 genome-wide scans (table 1). From such scans, genetic variants in the *FTO* gene have now been most consistently identified as the most important contributors to common obesity phenotypes [17–20]. Individuals with at-risk

FTO haplotypes 'yield a proportion of attributable risk of 22% for common obesity' [18], weigh 'about 3 kg more' [19], have a '1.67-fold increased odds of obesity' [19] and are, 'on average, 1.0–3.0 BMI units heavier' [17] than those who do not have the at-risk haplotypes.

More than 70 mutations in eleven genes have now been identified as monogenic causes of human obesity [16] (table 1). As opposed to the case of the genes in obesity syndromes, the genes identified as monogenic causes of obesity do provide clear mechanisms for the obesity phenotype. The majority of these genes account for only a very few obese individuals [21, 22]. One, however, represents a significant contributor to human obesity. Loss of function mutations in the melanocortin-4 receptor gene have been identified in 2–5% of individuals with childhood onset obesity [23–25].

Nonetheless, the majority of the other candidate genes [16] have not been demonstrated to contribute individually to a significant fraction of the variation observed in body weight. Thus, for example, Masud et al. [26] reported a meta-analysis of the relationship of PPARγ polymorphisms and BMI in more than 19,000 individuals, showing that the polymorphism effect size was less than one BMI unit. Similarly, a meta-analysis of the association of β3-adrenergic receptor gene polymorphisms with BMI in more than 6,000 persons demonstrated a gene variant effect on BMI of only 0.3 BMI units [27].

Problem No. 6

The common refrain that genes are not contributing to the current obesity 'epidemic' is oversimplified. Because the prevalence of obesity has more than doubled over the last several decades and because gene variations due to environmental evolutionary pressures do not occur on this time scale, genetic contributions to the current problem are often dismissed. This is not an entirely defensible position. First, Helmchen and Henderson [28] presented evidence that the increase in population BMI actually began more than a century ago. The prevalence of obesity in the early 1880s in 40- to 59-year-old adults was less than 2%. At the end of the 19th century, the prevalence was nearly 5% [28]. Thus, like the doubling of obesity prevalence that has taken place in the final two decades of the 20th century, there was also a doubling of the prevalence of obesity in the last two decades of the 19th century. However, since the absolute prevalence was low a century ago, there was little notice and less public health concern. Nonetheless, a century is still a trivial time period on the evolutionary scale required for changes in the DNA of the population.

In order to further appreciate why an individual's genotype remains an important consideration in the modern obesity 'epidemic', it is first necessary to understand that the term 'heritable' defines the proportion of the total phenotype variance in a trait that is caused by genes. The twin studies discussed above demonstrate that the majority of the shape of the bell-shaped distribution of BMI is due to genes within the population. In an environment where there is little food and where a significant amount of energy must be expended to obtain the food (human hunter-gatherer prehistory, for instance), the shapes of the 'genetic' body weight distribution curve and of the phenotypic 'actual' body weight distribution curve are the same, but the observed phenotypic distribution itself is shifted to the left (thinner). Conversely, in an environment such as that which exists in developed countries today, where food is available in excess and physical activity is minimized, the shape of the 'genetic' body weight distribution curve has not changed from that found in prehistoric times. However, the 'actual' observed phenotypic distribution of body weight has shifted to the right (fatter). In other words, genes have not changed and still account for the majority of the distribution variance, but the measured body weights themselves have moved into the obese range. Support for this right-shifting position comes from established population measurements in the United States demonstrating that children who are at the upper end of the body weight distribution curve are becoming fat faster than those in the middle of the distribution [29].

An additional reason not to 'count out' a genetic contribution to the current obesity 'epidemic' is the fact that while genes themselves may not have changed, the distribution of gene frequencies within the population may have been altered by influences such as assortative mating due, for instance, to obese individuals being more likely to marry other obese individuals or, conversely, to thin people being less likely to marry obese people. Redden and Allison [30] demonstrated that this is not a trivial consideration in altering the prevalence of obesity across several generations of matings. Likewise, Speakman et al. [31] demonstrated convincingly that assortative mating exists for obesity by directly determining adiposity using DXA. Moreover, social ties may contribute to this phenomenon because obesity has been shown clearly to spread within social networks [32, 33].

Problem No. 7

The traditional therapeutic paradigm that tends to minimize 'non-modifiable' risk factors and focus on 'modifiable' risk factors may be flawed by the fact that many 'modifiable' risk factors may not be so modifiable after all. Most conventional approaches to obesity treatment tend to minimize the 'non-modifiable' risk factors such as genes, gender and age, while focusing on 'modifiable' risk factors such as eating habits and physical activity behaviors. In this context, considerable discussion has focused on the environmental factors [34] and on societal policies and processes [35] that might be modifiable and alter the development, progression, or treatment of obesity. In pediatrics, particular attention is paid to early infancy where common logic has it that, since children who gain weight rapidly in early infancy are more likely to be obese later, we can successfully prevent obesity by intervening during this 'modifiable' window of opportunity by, among other measures, altering dietary intake and fostering healthful dietary eating behaviors.

Nonetheless, this window of opportunity may be less modifiable than anticipated. The genetic contribution to rapid growth during the first 2 years of life is substantially more than is commonly appreciated [36]. Heritability is by far the principal determinant of weight from birth to 3 years of age and is the major contributor to the change in body weight Z score from birth to 6 months of age, from birth to 12 months of age and from birth to 24 months of age [36]. Moreover, we are beginning to identify the genes responsible for rapid weight gain in childhood [18, 19, 37].

Likewise, childhood eating behaviors might not be as modifiable as commonly proposed. Thus, for example, Fisher et al. [38] recently demonstrated significant heritability contributions to eating behaviors in overweight Hispanic children and a genome-wide scan has identified a significant genetic linkage with the appetite-stimulating hormone, ghrelin [39]. Additionally, animal studies have shown that leptin signaling during the developmental period in which hypothalamic feeding circuits are 'hard wired' in mice permanently alters these circuits in adult mice [40, 41]. Likewise, oral leptin availability during lactation in rats can prevent the development of adult obesity when the animals are fed high-fat diets [42]. If similar phenomena exist in human infants, once CNS appetite and satiety circuits are 'hard wired' during early infant and childhood development, they may be effectively 'immune' to behavioral modification in later childhood and adolescence. Some evidence that eating behaviors are developed very early comes from studies showing that children as young as 2–3 years of age, like adults, already over-consume food when presented with large portion sizes and that these actions lead to excess energy consumption [43, 44].

Problem No. 8

Modeling the family environment may not be as effective as commonly believed. There is no question that parents influence the eating behaviors of their children [45]. However, the net effects of such influences on the eating behaviors of the child are complex and influenced by parenting styles [45, 46]. Although the family environment is commonly viewed as a shared environment for the family's children, individual children often are subject to different (non-shared) aspects of this environment. Keller et al. [46] have shown that 'whether or not maternal feeding practices are shared or non-shared components of the home environment depends on the specific feeding domain being measured'. This is particularly important since 'behavioral genetic studies … suggesting that the environmental experiences that make children vary in weight status are primarily those that *differ* among children in the same family' [46]. Thus, in this context, weight concerns, restrictive feeding practices and pressures to eat were unshared environmental factors among the children who 'shared' the overall family environments in the study by Keller et al. [46]. More than a decade ago, Klesges et al. [47] demonstrated the limited parental influences on food selection in children. In this study, 4- to 7-year-old children, who were well aware of their mother's categories of 'non-nutritious' foods, nonetheless voluntarily chose such foods for lunch, unless they knew that they would be monitored by their parent [47]. In other words, the daily parental influence over the child's eating habits during the entire early phase of the child's life was essentially ineffectual when the child was left to his or her own devices. Parental preferences had no fundamental influence on the child's own desired eating preference, other than they were altered by possible punitive consequences.

Problem No. 9

We know virtually nothing about the developmental aspects of the energy expenditure term of the balance equation in very young children. Nor do we confidently know whether most aspects of childhood physical activity behaviors have really changed during the decades of the obesity epidemic. Very little is known about how children develop physical activity behaviors. Essentially all the studies of childhood physical activity have been conducted in school-aged children. Nonetheless, one study of 4- to 10-year-old monozygotic and dizygotic twin pairs has suggested that genetic variability does not explain the observed familial resemblance in physical activity behaviors [48]. This resemblance, rather, is explained principally by the environmental factors shared within the family [48]. Recently, Sturm [49, 50] reviewed the secular changes in childhood physical activity behaviors that took place over the last two decades of the 20th century in America, coincident with the development of the obesity 'epidemic'. The results were surprising. He found that children's free time had declined substantially 'because of increased time away from home, primarily in school, daycare, and after-school programs' [49]. Additionally, childhood 'participation in organized activities (including sports) has increased', while time for unstructured play correspondingly decreased [49]. Further, time spent watching television actually declined at the start of the obesity 'epidemic', but time spent in transportation increased [49]. Finally, there were not indications that increased homework has led to less available free time [49]. Overall, the changes found in children's physical activity over the last two decades have been smaller than generally believed.

Conclusion

Despite the deceptive simplicity of the energy balance equation, its practical application in the prevention and/or treatment of childhood obesity is not a simple issue at all.

References

1 Korner J, Leibel RL: To eat or not to eat – how the gut talks to the brain. N Engl J Med 2003; 349:926–928.
2 Woods SC: Signals that influence food intake and body weight. Physiol Behav 2005;86: 709–716.
3 Wren AM, Bloom SR: Gut hormones and appetite control. Gastroenterology 2007;132: 2116–2130.
4 Murphy KG, Bloom SR: Gut hormones and the regulation of energy homeostasis. Nature 2006;444:854–859.
5 Coll AP, Farooqi S, O'Rahilly S: The hormonal control of food intake. Cell 2007;129:251–262.
6 Rosenbaum M, Leibel RL, Hirsch J: Obesity. N Engl J Med 2007;337:396–407.
7 Leibel RL, Rosenbaum M, Hirsch J: Changes in energy expenditure resulting from altered body weight. N Engl J Med 1995;332:621–628.
8 Friedman JM: Modern science versus the stigma of obesity. Nat Med 2004;10:563–569.
9 Moon JK, Vohra FA, Omar S, et al: Closed-loop control of carbon dioxide concentration and pressure improves response of room respiration calorimeters. J Nutr 1995;125:220–228.
10 Trabulsi J, Troiano RP, Subar Af, et al: Precision of the doubly labeled water method in a large-scale application: evaluation of a streamlined-dosing protocol in the Observing Protein and Energy Nutrition (OPEN) study. Eur J Clin Nutr 2003;57:1370–1377.
11 Trabulsi J, Schoeller DA: Evaluation of dietary assessment instruments against doubly labeled water, a biomarker of habitual energy intake. Am J Physiol Endocrinol Metab 2001;281: E891–E899.
12 Maes HH, Neale MC, Eaves LJ: Genetic and environmental factors in relative body weight and human adiposity. Behav Genet 1997;27:325–351.
13 Faith MS, Pietrobelli A, Nuñez C, et al: Evidence for independent genetic influences on fat mass and body mass index in a pediatric twin sample. Pediatrics 1999;104:61–67.
14 Faith MS, Rha SS, Neale MC, et al: Evidence for genetic influences on human energy intake: Results from a twin study using measured observations. Behav Genet 1999;29:145–154.
15 Pérusse L, Bouchard C: Gene-diet interactions in obesity. Am J Clin Nutr 2000;72: 1285S–1290S.
16 Rankinen T, Zuberi A, Chagnon YC, et al: The human obesity gene map: the 2005 update. Obesity 2006;14:529–644.
17 Scuteri A, Sanna S, Wei-Min C, et al: Genome-wide association scan shows genetic variants in the *FTO* gene are associated with obesity-related traits. PLoS Genet 2007;3:e115.
18 Dina C, Meyre D, Gallina S, et al: Variation in *FTO* contributes to childhood obesity and severe adult obesity. Nat Genet 2007;39:724–726.
19 Frayling TM, Timpson NJ, Weedon MN, et al: A common variant in the *FTO* gene is associated with body mass index and predisposes to childhood and adult obesity. Science 2007;316: 889–894.
20 Field SF, Howson JMM, Walker NM, et al: Analysis of the obesity gene *FTO* in 14,803 type 1 diabetes cases and controls. Diabetologia 2007;50:2218–2220.
21 Farooqi IS, O'Rahilly S: Genetics of obesity in humans. Endocr Rev 2006;27:710–718.
22 Farooqi IS, O'Rahilly S: Monogenic obesity in humans. Annu Rev Med 2005;56:443–458.
23 Vaisse C, Clement K, Durand E, et al: Melanocortin-4 receptor mutations are a frequent and heterogeneous cause of morbid obesity. J Clin Invest 2000;106:253–262.
24 Farooqi IS, Keogh JM, Yeo GSH, et al: Clinical spectrum of obesity and mutations in the melanocortin 4 receptor gene. N Engl J Med 2003;348:1085–1095.

25 Hinney A, Hohmann S, Geller F: Melanocortin-4 receptor gene: case-control study and transmission disequilibrium test confirm that functionally relevant mutations are compatible with a major gene effect for extreme obesity. J Clin Endocrinol Metab 2003;88:4258–4267.
26 Masud S, Ye S: Effect of the peroxisome proliferator activated receptor-γ gene Pro12Ala variant on body mass index: a meta-analysis. J Med Genet 2003;40:773–780.
27 Kurokawa N, Nakai K, Kameo S, et al: Association of BMI with the β3-adrenergic receptor gene polymorphism in Japanese: meta-analysis. Obesity Res 2001;9:741–745.
28 Helmchen LA, Henderson RM: Changes in the distribution of body mass index of white US men, 1890–2000. Ann Hum Biol 2004;31:174–181.
29 Troiano RP, Flegal KM: Overweight children and adolescents: description, epidemiology, and demographics. Pediatrics 1998;101:497–504.
30 Redden DT, Allison DB: The effect of assortative mating upon genetic association studies: spurious associations and population substructure in the absence of admixture. Behav Genet 2006;36:678–686.
31 Speakman JR, Diafarian K, Stewart J, et al: Assortative mating for obesity. Am J Clin Nutr 2007;86:316–323.
32 Jacobson P, Torgerson JS, Sjöström L, et al: Spouse resemblance in body mass index: effects on adult obesity prevalence in the offspring generation. Am J Epidemiol 2007;165:101–108.
33 Christakis NA, Fowler JH: The spread of obesity in a large social network over 32 years. N Engl J Med 2007;357:370–379.
34 Keith SW, Redden DT, Katzmarzyk PT, et al: Putative contributors to the secular increase in obesity: exploring the roads less traveled. Int J Obes 2006;30:1585–1594.
35 World Health Organization: Obesity: preventing and managing the global epidemic. Report of a WHO consultation. World Health Organ Tech Rep Ser 2000;894:i–xii, 1–253.
36 Demerath EW, Choh AC, Czerwinski SA, et al: Genetic and environmental influences on infant weight and weight change: the Fels Longitudinal Study. Am J Hum Biol 2007;19:692–702.
37 Cai G, Cole SA, Haack K, et al: Bivariate linkage confirms genetic contribution to fetal origins of childhood growth and cardiovascular disease risk in Hispanic children. Hum Genet 2007;121:737–744.
38 Fisher JO, Cai G, Jaramillo SJ, et al: Heritability of hyperphagic eating behavior and appetite-related hormones among Hispanic children. Obesity 2007;15:1484–1495.
39 Voruganti VS, Goring JJ, Diego VP, et al: Genome-wide scan for serum ghrelin detects linkage on chromosome 1p36 in Hispanic children: results from the Viva La Familia study. Pediatr Res 2007;62:445–450.
40 Bouret SG, Simerly RB: Developmental programming of hypothalamic feeding circuits. Clin Genet 2006;70:295–301.
41 Bouret SG, Simerly RB: Minireview: leptin and development of hypothalamic feeding circuits. Endocrinology 2004;145:2621–2626.
42 Picó C, Oliver P, Sánchez J, et al: The intake of physiological doses of leptin during lactation in rats prevents obesity in later life. Int J Obes 2007;31:1199–1209.
43 Fisher JO: Effects of age on children's intake of large and self-selected food portions. Obesity 2007;15:403–412.
44 Fisher JO, Liu Y, Birch LL, et al: Effects of portion size and energy density on young children's intake at a meal. Am J Clin Nutr 2007;86:174–179.
45 Savage JS, Fisher JO, Birch LL: Parental influences on eating behavior: conception to adolescence. J Law Med Ethics 2007;35:22–34.
46 Keller KL, Pietrobelli A, Johnson SL, et al: Maternal restriction of children's eating and encouragements to ear as the 'non-shared environment': a pilot study using the child feeding questionnaire. Int J Obes 2006;30:1670–1675.
47 Klesges RC, Stein RJ, Eck LH, et al: Parental influence on food selection in young children and its relationships to childhood obesity. Am J Clin Nutr 1991;53:859–864.
48 Franks PW, Ravussin E, Hanson RL: Habitual physical activity in children: the role of genes and the environment. Am J Clin Nutr 2005;82:901–908.
49 Sturm R: Childhood obesity – what we can learn from existing data on societal trends, part 1. Prev Chronic Dis 2005;2:A12.
50 Sturm R: Childhood obesity – what we can learn from existing data on societal trends, part 2. Prev Chronic Dis 2005;2:A20.

Discussion

Dr. Lagercrantz: This was very interesting but you didn't mention anything about the effect of breastfeeding. I would think that breastfeeding would be good for the babies. The paradox is that the prevalence of breastfeeding in France is very low and the prevalence of obesity is also low.

Dr. Bier: The data on breastfeeding with regard to obesity are very mixed and even those where the effects on the whole are put together only account for a small percent of the variance, but it is not the principal issue. One of the reasons why breastfeeding may be protective has primarily to do with the issue of infants controlling their own appetite, not with putting the extra half ounce in the bottle. The infant stops feeding, falls asleep at the breast, and finally the mother stops feeding. This may be an issue; there are people who believe it may have to do with the different flavors that babies are exposed to in breast milk, etc., but again the data are very noisy. If you look at the standard errors in some of the meta-analyses they are very large, and some total differences are relatively small. It is really hard to do those kinds of cross-cultural comparisons because there are too many other variables.

Dr. Szajewska: I have a question regarding a study published in *Nature*[1]. Could you comment on this study with regard to microbiota and obesity?

Dr. Bier: I think these are very intriguing observations. As we know in other context, they tell us that the gut microbiota talk to the systemic system, and that tells us that they may have effects in a way that we never understood before. I am particularly interested in this from a developmental perspective because I think it is entirely possible that we have a microbiota system that is influencing developmental genes or developmental progression in the enterocyte, for example perhaps in the intestinal lymphatic system or germ-free mice, in signals that go systemically to alter the pathways of fat oxidation in a permanent way if they are in the proper developmental window. This is one of the most interesting things that people should be pursuing from a very hard science point of view. I also think it would be extremely interesting to apply non-culture techniques to the earliest times in infancy when colonization takes place.

Dr. Strandvik: There is one problem which I would like to hear your opinion on. By advising very low fat intake, the consumption of carbohydrate beverages has increased. Could that trigger insulin which then induces the consumption of large food portions? Another thing which has been discussed is that fat consumption has not decreased but it also has not increased. What has happened in the last decades is that due to our restriction of saturated fat we advise a lot of n-6 fatty acids which are adipogenic. I wonder especially about fast foods where there are a lot of items fried with vegetable oils containing high amounts of n-6. Could that be one part of the epidemic? We also have to realize that corn is being exchanged for other seeds in the world, replacing the more original kind of feeding. What is your opinion about the hypothesis that the increase in n-6 fatty acids worldwide might contribute to the obesity epidemic [2]?

Dr. Bier: There have been a very significant number of highly controlled clinical research center studies which have unequivocally shown that a calorie is calorie, either in weight maintenance or weight reduction. If you look at the curves or the numbers, when the macronutrient content of the diet was surreptitiously changed, it didn't make any difference, it was an energy issue. Now when it comes to whether or not there are certain things that people are consuming more of many people argue that, for example, soft drinks are contributing to extra calories, and they are. But remember when diet records and surveys are done, how precise and accurate can they be? When it comes to these kinds of data, it is much easier to identify a can of soft drink in a diet survey than it is the hidden fat in a pastry or something else. So part of the reason why some of these things may drop out may have nothing to do with the fact that it is a soft drink, it may have to do with the fact that the variance is less in that particular measurement. When we talk about things like soft drinks, they are not energy-dense compared to fat. Whether it is an excess of calories by carbohydrates or an excess of calories by fat, people are eating too much. I am not familiar with the other parts of the world, but for years national survey data have been collected in the United States, and they tell us that people are doubling the prevalence of obesity without eating anymore. Now if you believe this, we are at a standstill somewhere; it just doesn't happen.

Dr. Strandvik: We investigated healthy 4-year-olds and the results showed that the children who ate more fat were slimmer than those who ate less fat and also had a higher carbohydrate intake. But one point which was very interesting was that the overweight and obese also had less n-3 fatty acids in the diet [3]. So what is happening is the ratio between n-6 and n-3 fatty acids has changed a lot. Although I agree with you that these big portions contribute to obesity, the kind of fat has a different impact on gene expression and this factor might be of importance in this change in quality of fat.

Dr. Bier: Very extensive studies have been done in rodents, and others have tried to reproduce them in human infants but were unable to show any difference in energy expenditure or growth depending on those fats. When I look at the sum total of the metabolic data on obesity over several decades, where people have tried every possible macronutrient permutation, my impression is that a calorie is a calorie, and it certainly doesn't make such a dramatic difference to account for the nature of the vast difference on obesity that we have. That is my belief.

Dr. Walker: What generally happens in the United States when we see an overweight child is that the parents are both also overweight or obese. If you go to China where one sees increasing numbers of children who are overweight, their parents are not obese. How do you explain that phenomenon in a single generation?

Dr. Bier: Because they are giving their children the food they would have eaten had they had the opportunity. People become obese by sitting around and doing nothing. It is actually really hard to become that obese unless you are overeating. So more calories are going in than the energy is being expended.

Dr. Walker: That is my point. It is not a pure genetic phenomenon; it appears also to be an environmental phenomenon.

Dr. Bier: The distribution of the curve is set by the genes. I don't know if any of you have ever participated or tried to do overfeeding experiments. Ethan Sims in the United States started these in the 1960s in prisoners who were fed Swanson TV dinners. He discovered, as have various people since then, that when you try to overfeed people there are some whose weight changes 1 g for every calorie, 4 g for 4 calories they receive, and other people who burn this off because suddenly their metabolic rate changes dramatically. This is a wide variance and it is set by the genes. This is also going to be true in some Chinese children who are going to get fatter and others who are going to deal with it well. It moves the distribution of the curve, and where they are is set by the genes.

Dr. Gluckman: The difficulty is the use of the word heritability, which is not necessarily the same thing as genes. There are many aspects of heritability other than genes: there is the environmental component; there is the epigenetic component which can be either direct or indirect through re-creation of the developmental niche which triggers the change in the next generation. We have to be very careful just to be certain of what we are talking about. For instance, looking at the transgenerational correlations in birth size and birth weight, the work of the Aberdeen study [4] highlights the other ways in which this can occur rather than necessarily just being a genetic explanation for heritability. But putting that aside, the conclusions are still the same that in fact these things occur very early on. Certainly in our experiments in animals and, in fact, the clinical data show that many children are getting visceral obesity from birth. Other studies very clearly show that hardwiring and changes in appetite regulation are there before any other phenotypic changes; so that is happening very early in life. The basic point we are making is that if the cycle is going to be broken, then yes we have got to deal with the macroenvironment because ultimately, whatever your hardwired physiology is, it is the environment you live in which either leads to you manifesting disease or not. If we are going to tackle this we have to think about the early developmental origins for how we can actually intervene if it is not genetic, otherwise the only way to intervene is to try to reprogram or re-hardwire, or we have to think of the thing we can't do which is persuade people to eat less and exercise more. Just on the side, there is extensive animal or comparative biology literature on organisms in the gastrointestinal tract causing epigenetic changes in physiology. What is your opinion on this interest in the macronutrient balance in terms of appetite regulation, namely that the change in the protein to carbohydrate lipid ratios may play a role in determining when satiety occurs?

Dr. Bier: The last one first, again the literature is very noisy on this but I think it is plausible, just like the change in the different kinds of fats. One can show that these different mechanisms exist but trying to show what fraction they contribute to human obesity is very difficult because these things contribute a small fraction of the variance and showing it in some systematic way requires huge numbers of people, it is just very hard to do. The heritability, gene factor, I completely agree with you that there are some parts of the environment that are extremely difficult to tease out from the genes and some studies suffer from that more than others. In most cases the heritability estimates of factors relative to body weight are so high that even if they go down 10% on this basis, they still account for the majority of the distribution. It is an important point and I agree entirely that this heritable environmental factor is perhaps setting the development of programming that permanently keeps the memory.

Dr. Netrebenko: Several studies have been done on infant nutrition, some in United States by Stettler et al. [5] and others, showing that high weight gain during the first 4 or 6 months results in obesity at 7 years. I wonder what kind of nutrient could cause obesity if the children only receive it during the first 4 months of life?

Dr. Bier: This is again highly controversial. I have a very fundamental feeling about early weight gain as we have been unable to change the trajectory of weight gain in any group in a systematic way. The earlier a person starts to get fat, the fatter they will be at the end, regardless of what happens in between, because nothing that physicians or parents or anybody has done has been able to change that trajectory. If for example a child at that age has the right genes for catch-up growth plus has been overfed, then he starts getting fatter earlier, and that by the way has some other effect on hardwiring appetite and satiety centers; they end up being fat later. We just don't know, but what is clear is that this is something that starts early. Early development actually starts with the mother and if we are going to be effective we have to be a generation ahead, and in fact for girls, we have to be two generations ahead to really change this.

Dr. Koletzko: This issue of early weight gain as a predictor of later overweight and obesity has been looked at in a large number of studies, far more than 20 now and 3 meta-analyses. All have described that rapid weight gain in early life, not only in the first 4 months but in infancy and early childhood, is associated with a 2- to 3-fold higher risk of overweight in school age children and beyond. This somehow matches the observation that in populations of breastfed infants there is a slightly but significantly lower risk of later overweight and obesity. It is plausible that breastfeeding in fact might protect by the lesser weight gain in the population at the end of the first year. Your question then is, is that something that one can modify or is it all predetermined by genetics or other intrauterine or whatever factors? A randomized intervention study was performed in five countries in a European childhood and obesity project where healthy term infants of normal birth weight were randomized to two different infant formulas and follow-on formulas with lower and higher protein, based on the hypothesis that this difference between breastfed and formula-fed infants might be due to the higher nitrogen intake with infant formula leading to higher levels of branched chain amino acids which then would be expected to have higher levels of insulin IGF-I. The total cohort consisted of about 1,000 children, of which roughly 300 were breastfed for 4 months and 700 were randomized to the two different formulas. The infants have now all reached the age of 2 years. It was found that with the lower protein intake the growth curves, the weight gain, weight for height and BMI matched that of the breastfed population or the WHO growth standard, whereas with the higher protein intake there was significantly higher weight for height and BMI from the age of 6 months onwards and the relative difference was maintained until the age of 2 years, even though the intervention was stopped at 12 months. So it appears that modification of micronutrient supply can actually influence weight gain in infancy and early childhood, even though obviously we would like to understand more about the underlying mechanism.

Dr. Bier: Any blinded randomized studies that give a clue to what may affect this trajectory are important. In this field there have been thousands of studies of all kinds and until the results are reproduced or confirmed, it remains a nice hypothesis. All of us are looking for anything that will help us change this trajectory, and then finding the mechanism for one and also putting it into practice are important.

Dr. Walker: I think from the studies that have been done to get people to stop smoking, the conclusion is that preventing them from starting to smoke is much more effective than trying to get them to stop smoking. I believe that gives more credence to approaching obesity by trying to prevent it from occurring and, as Dr. Gluckman and others have said, start very early. It is an important issue. One of the problems, at least in the United States, is the data that you just presented are virtually unknown by practicing pediatricians. They don't really follow the babies that closely and they are not aware of how important weight gain is initially in the long-term effect on overweight. What we have to do is translate observations and make recommendations to those who actually see overweight children who are continuing to gain excessively.

Dr. Bier: The problems that we have in trying to set the child's weight gain trajectory are firstly that we are not very good at how to do this, and secondly we have no idea what the down side risks might be. It is a research field and the kind of studies that Dr. Koletzko talked about are necessary to understand even what the limits are for any individual child.

References

1 Turnbaugh PJ, Ley RE, Mahowald MA, et al: An obesity-associated gut microbiome with increased capacity for energy harvest. Nature 2006;444:1027–1031.
2 Ailhaud G, Massiera F, Weill P, et al: Temporal changes in dietary fats: role of n-6 polyunsaturated fatty acids in excessive adipose tissue development and relationship to obesity. Prog Lipid Res 2006;45:203–236.
3 Garemo M, Lenner RA, Strandvik B: Swedish pre-school children eat too much junk food and sucrose. Acta Paediatr 2007;96:266–272.
4 Batty GD, Morton SM, Campbell D, et al: The Aberdeen Children of the 1950s cohort study: background, methods and follow-up information on a new resource for the study of life course and intergenerational influences on health. Paediatr Perinat Epidemiol 2004;18:221–239.
5 Stettler N, Zemel BS, Kumanyika S, Stallings VA: Infant weight gain and childhood overweight status in a multicenter, cohort study. Pediatrics 2002;109:194–199.

Bier DM, German JB, Lönnerdal B (eds): Personalized Nutrition for the Diverse Needs of Infants and Children.
Nestlé Nutr Workshop Ser Pediatr Program, vol 62, pp 111–125,
Nestec Ltd., Vevey/S. Karger AG, Basel, © 2008.

Intestinal Immune Health

Michelle E. Conroy, W. Allan Walker

Mucosal Immunology and Developmental Gastroenterology Laboratories,
Massachusetts General Hospital for Children, Department of Pediatrics,
Harvard Medical School, Boston, MA, USA

Abstract

The fetal intestinal immune system is structurally intact from a very early gestational age. At birth, the neonate is challenged with an extraordinary and variable bacterial challenge. This mucosal and bacterial interface is the site of critical symbiotic and potentially pathogenic interactions. Neonatal inflammatory reactions are often exaggerated, creating a situation in a newly colonized gut whereby homeostasis must be actively achieved. Fortunately, the neonate is armed with a multitude of protective mechanisms by which to ensure a productive microbiota in the setting of an intact mucosal surface. The intestinal epithelium orchestrates complex interactions and signaling through a variety of intrinsic and extrinsic stimuli. Chief among these is the immunomodulatory capacity of breast milk which is increasingly implicated in the achievement of intestinal and immunologic health via a multitude of mechanisms. Additionally, developmental expression of enzymes, pattern recognition, downstream signaling and dendritic cell interaction all contribute to intestinal homeostasis. Current research is uncovering the molecular mechanisms behind many of these mechanisms. These strategies lend insight into the establishment of tolerance so critical to neonatal health. In a clinic context of increasing food allergy and inflammatory bowel disease, elucidating this machinery is increasingly pertinent. Future research should explore these molecular interactions more closely for their potential therapeutic applications.

Introduction

Fetal development and the transition from the womb imply an elegant anatomic and physiologic preparation for drastic changes in environment and exposure. The immune system of the neonate requires both instant readiness in the event of perinatal infection but also education about its new surroundings. As a result, the infant is in the unique immune circumstance of readied ignorance. The intestinal mucosa can be likened to the neonate itself. Initially sterile and then rapidly exposed to a completely novel environment, this single epithelial layer must quickly and effectively learn and react. But the larger challenge in this mucosal context lies in the challenge of how to reap the benefits of the vast luminal bacterial world while minimizing harm to the mucosa and the host at large. Therefore, the infant's immune system must quickly establish a fine balance between Th1 and Th2 responses. Excess of either is well known to lead to either inflammatory diseases such as inflammatory bowel disease or atopic diseases, respectively. The kinetics of the immune system are being elucidated with inspiring rapidity. This review will incorporate both well-established and recent data to present an abbreviated depiction of fetal and neonatal mucosal immune development and some of the potential molecular mechanics driving gut homeostasis.

Fetal Immune Structure and Function in the Gut

Throughout gestation, the fetus undergoes predictably timed assembly of and protection by various immune system components and surrogates. In fact, the basic template of the mucosal immune system is established very early. Specifically, the intestinal villi are first observed at about 10 weeks and the crypts/stem cells at 10–11 weeks. Groupings of lymphocytes resembling Peyer's patches are observable by about 100 days of gestation. These areas further develop into increasingly organized areas of B cell follicles and T cell zones by 130–140 days [1]. B cells within these lymphoid collections are sIgM+, SIgD+, and CD5+ with only occasional IgA+ and IgG+ cells. This exception continues through birth when the lamina propria remains devoid of these same immunoglobulin-specific cells. There are MHC-II-positive cells in this space, but the definitive cell type has not been defined [2]. It is also important to note the absence of germinal centers and, hence, B-cell proliferation throughout fetal life. It is also noteworthy that the intestine's ability to produce IgA in either fetal life or early infancy is virtually nonexistent. As such, the basic components for mucosal immune function are present quite early in gestation. This is essentially the same for the systemic immune system, the development of which occurs in parallel with the mucosal system [for review see, 3].

Though maternal immunoglobulin dominates fetal and neonatal immunity, the fetus is capable of generating IgM and IgG. This occurs in the spleen and peaks at approximately 17 weeks of gestation. Despite this, immunoglobulin levels are low at birth and are virtually all maternal in origin [3]. Passive transfer of maternal antibody begins at approximately week 16 of gestation. The initial ratio of fetal to maternal immunoglobulin is quite low, but a subsequent increased concentration of immunoglobulins results in near maternal levels by the third trimester. Therefore the majority of transfer occurs late in gestation. Immunoglobulin receptors have been demonstrated on placental tissue through radiolabeling. Studies of mRNA transcripts have demonstrated variable expression of the three different FcγR reflecting consistent expression of FcγRI and FcγRIII, but variable expression of FcγRIIb, which increases significantly in the second and third trimesters [4]. Notably, the FcγRIIb is typically not expressed on any adult endothelial surfaces other than the placenta. Recently, it has been shown that FcγRIIb associates with a novel IgG-containing intracellular organelle within placental epithelial cells. This may likely be a mechanism by which the fetus specifically accumulates maternal IgG, particularly given the temporal correlation between increased fetal immunoglobulin levels and expression of this particular receptor [5]. The fetus is thus protected passively via this transfer of maternal immunoglobulin.

While the fetal immune system has traditionally been regarded as quiescent, it is clear that it can mount adaptive, inflammatory immune responses. As an example, Hermann et al. [6] demonstrated impressive, oligoclonal T-cell expansion in the cord blood of newborns who had been congenitally infected with *Trypanosoma cruzi*. This expansion was accompanied by the expression of effector molecules including IFNγ and TNFα indicating competence of these T cells. A similar capability has been noted in response to other infectious agents, which has raised questions regarding the resting state of the fetal immune system. It has previously been demonstrated in vitro that immature human enterocytes demonstrate exaggerated IL-8 secretion via IL-1β and TNFα stimulation [7]. Therefore, mediators must exist that dampen this fetal tendency toward overt inflammatory responses. A regulatory safety net is implicated to protect the fetus and neonate from this immune reactivity. CD4+CD25+ T cells have been detected in fetal tissue at 13 weeks gestational age which occurs in tandem with other T-cell migration from the thymus. These regulatory cells were stable in number throughout gestation and birth. This is in contrast to other T cells which demonstrate variable levels and maturation evidenced through analysis of surface markers [8]. A recent study demonstrated a large population of CD4+CD25+ T cells present in cord blood and fetal mesenteric lymph nodes at higher levels than in adults. Subsequent removal of these cells from fetal mediastinal lymph node culture resulted in significant T-cell proliferation and IFNγ production. This cellular expansion and IFN production did not occur in adult tissue culture upon the removal of regulatory cells [9]. This striking difference between fetal and adult tissue highlights the critical importance of regulatory activity in establishing peripheral tolerance in the fetus.

Thus, as the neonate readies for birth and entrance into the contaminated world, the issue of potentially excessive inflammatory responses becomes critical. Clearly the fetal to neonatal transition must include means through which this inflammatory default must be mitigated. Much work has been done to understand the mechanisms behind this process which leads ultimately to the enigma of oral tolerance.

The Variable Inoculation of Birth

The amniotic environment is a sterile one that protects the developing fetus from infection. As a result, the fetus is presumably 'sterile' prior to birth. However, birth itself results in a massive introduction of bacteria, regardless of the mode of delivery. Significant differences exist in the microbial exposure and resultant colonization in babies born by cesarean section (CS) versus vaginal delivery (VD). Infants born vaginally acquire maternal resident vaginal and colonic microbes. The sterile conditions of surgical birth necessarily predict that environment will make a larger contribution to the babies born by CS. When fecal microbial content was evaluated from 3 days of age to 6 months of age, there were marked differences in VD versus CS infants. Most notably, there was no colonization with *Bacteroides fragilis* in the CS group before 2 months of age. By 6 months, the bacteroides colonization rate was half that of infants born by VD. Additionally, VD infants had greater colonization with lactobacillus and bifidobacter, whereas the CS infants were more colonized with clostridium. All of these results were significant [10]. This variance in mode of delivery and resultant colonization has clinical implications. CS has been cited as a risk factor for allergic disease. Specifically, CS has been associated with an increased risk of allergic rhinoconjunctivitis and asthma [11]. It has also been implicated as a risk factor for infantile diarrhea and IgE responses to food antigen including egg [12]. Therefore, even these initial bacterial interactions with the neonatal epithelium have lasting impact and effects. This bacterial proximity reinforces the intensive need for protection from the neonate's tendency toward inflammatory reactions. Almost right away, there is another microbial onslaught via feeding. The ability to tolerate intake of novel dietary antigen is one of the major immunologic tasks of the neonate. While the mechanisms are far from understood, it is clear that the neonate is assisted via the interaction of the gut epithelium, commensal bacteria, and human milk. Inappropriate function at any of these interfaces may lead to inflammation or allergy. It is a great, delicate task of balance and resultant homeostasis.

The Feeding Frenzy

It is intuitive that feeding influences the microbial flora and antigenic stimulation of the developing intestine. The aforementioned initial colonization via birth is rapidly altered by the introduction of feeding. One study of 40 infants from days 3–21 of life demonstrated marked variability in colonization between breast- and bottle-fed infants. In this study, which confirms others, bifidobacter becomes the dominant bacteria by 1 week of age in breastfed infants. Bottle-fed infants show a much more diverse flora with a predominance of bacteroides [13]. Bottle-fed infants continue to show more diverse

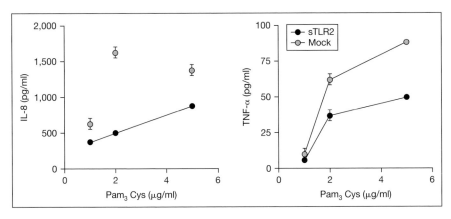

Fig. 1. sTLR2 inhibits cell activation. IL-8 and TNF-α production by Mono Mac-6 cells (5×10^4) cultured in the presence of sTLR2. From LeBouder et al. [16].

and potentially pathogenic flora including clostridia throughout the first months of life. Thus, breastfed babies support more 'beneficial' microbial colonization. The mechanisms by which this occurs elucidates the protective nature of human milk. In a broad sense, human milk serves to 'quiet' the hyperactive inflammatory response of the neonate. There are multiple milk components that appear responsible for this modulation of neonatal inflammation. Human milk concentrations of TGFβ were shown to decrease TNFα-induced IL-8 secretion in vitro. This reduction was shown to be more dramatic in fetal intestinal epithelial cells than in more mature cells [14]. Soluble Toll-like receptor-2 (TLR2) is present in human milk as well as plasma [15]. It appears to be another mechanism through which excess inflammation may be avoided (fig. 1). Human milk also contains soluble CD14 (sCD14), a co-receptor for TLR4 recognition of LPS. Intestinal epithelial cell responses via TLR4 are dependent on the presence of sCD14. But other currently unknown milk components are responsible for enhancing cellular responsiveness to stimulation via TLR4. This milk factor likely assists the neonatal gut in its response to gram-negative organisms [16]. Human milk contains carbohydrates that are unique and reach the distal gut of the neonate structurally intact. This ultimately encourages synergistic microbial colonization which results in inhibition of harmful inhabitants [17]. It is therefore clear that the epithelial layer of the gut interacts with microbes and milk (human or artificial) products to establish protection and immune modulation for the neonate. These interactions, when appropriate, begin to create a process in which tolerance can be established. While the exact mechanisms of this are unknown, multiple epithelially based processes are being discovered that provide clues.

Barrier Function

As the infant is bombarded with billions of bacteria that are of variable potential pathogenicity, the epithelium must provide effective barrier protection. It has help from other mucosal cells including the antimicrobial proteins of Paneth cells and the mucous of goblet cells. There are also tight junctions between the epithelial cells, but these are not impenetrable as dendritic cells traverse through as do pathogenic bacteria. It turns out that the TLRs expressed on intestinal epithelia contribute to protecting the intact barrier. In MyD88−/− animals morbidity and mortality after administration of an epithelial toxic substance were marked and significant. The animals exhibited colonic bleeding and anemia which likely led to their increased mortality. Intact TLRs prevented this extensive epithelial damage, likely by the induction of pathways yielding protective and reparative factors such as IL-6 and heat-shock proteins [18]. The pattern recognition of colonized bacteria, then, likely assists the epithelium in maintaining a constitutive barrier to invasion. With one cell layer constituting such a critical separation, reparation via commensal stimulation is an efficient example of coexistence.

Another study also implicates TLRs and NFκB in the maintenance of epithelial integrity. NEMO knockout mice were shown to exhibit chronic intestinal inflammation. These mice also had decreased production of antimicrobial peptides and increased TNF-induced epithelial apoptosis. As a result, not only is chronic inflammation induced, but epithelial integrity is compromised leading to bacterial translocation and an additional stimulus for inflammation. Notably, mice bred to lack both NEMO and MyD88 did not exhibit this pathology. This clearly implicates the central role of epithelial TLRs in signal transduction leading to the eventual inflammatory state in the absence of these modifiers [19]. The neonatal gut barrier, then, is reliant on epithelial–bacterial interaction to maintain a strong barrier against invasive organisms.

Changing the Locks

From the moment of impact, initial bacterial docking, the epithelium has devised ways of regulating the colonization of the gut. Bacteria utilize cell surface glycoconjugates as receptors for epithelial adherence. In rodents, this is apparently under both regional and developmental regulation resulting in variability of terminal epithelial glycosylation by age and anatomical location [20]. This specifically relates to activity of sialyl- and fucosyltransferases which have predictable activity based on age and weaning. Most notably, germ-free animals do not appear to express these enzymes variably, regardless of age or weaning [21]. With the introduction of colonizing organisms, however, the germ-free animals express increased fucosyltransferase similar to their conventional counterparts (fig. 2). This relationship between bacterial

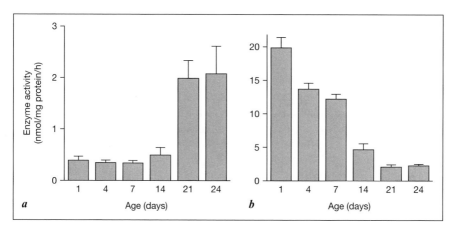

Fig. 2. Developmental regulation of fucosyltransferase (*a*) and sialytransferase (*b*) as a function of postpartum age in the newborn mouse ileum. From Dai et al. [20].

presence and epithelium function points again to the critical importance of proper initial and maintained colonization. A step further in logic suggests that alternative bacterial presence will result in a varied epithelial surface response. In turn, this may encourage less symbiotic and more pathogenic bacterial effect in the gut. This bacterial and epithelial interaction is compelling. Because of its circular nature, it again reinforces the pertinence of proper initial colonization.

The Dynamic Duo

The polarity of the epithelial layer creates the consummate separation of self and non-self. Various recent studies are elucidating the elegance of this proximity in bridging that discrepancy and allowing non-inflammatory coexistence. It seems increasingly clear that dendritic cells and epithelial cells are partners in the game of gut homeostasis. Rimoldi et al. [22] demonstrated that human gut dendritic cells show a bias toward the Th2 response, which seems logical given the proximity of microbes and the need to avoid chronic inflammation. But their studies implicated the epithelium in the generation of this tendency. Epithelial cells release thymic stromal lymphopoietin (TSLP) which influences dendritic cell maturation and leads to T-cell encouragement in the Th2 direction. TSLP is a product of NFκB transcription, the downstream effect of TLR stimulation by bacteria [22]. However, and perhaps more compelling within the same study, is that invasive bacteria reaching the basolateral side of the epithelial layer can induce TSLP production. When this occurs, local TSLP levels are greatly increased as compared to levels in the noninvasive scenario. In this TSLP flood, dendritic cells regain the ability to release IL-12 and a Th1 response is elicited. The study included evidence that epithelial cells constitutively express TSLP but only when co-cultured with bacteria. This study gives evidence of another mechanism through which neonatal excessive inflammation is reigned via interactions between commensal bacteria, epithelium and downstream immune cells.

Other TLR intermediaries are also implicated in the task of inflammation modulation. Zaph et al. [23] showed that removal of epithelial Ikk, part of the TLR→NFκB pathway, resulted in an intensive inflammatory response in animal models. Ikk would normally activate NFκB with resultant downstream gene expression including TSLP which, as mentioned previously, yields a Th2 response. In the setting of a parasitic infection in Ikk-deficient animals, there was extensive damage via Th1 and Th17 responses, but no evidence of a protective Th2 response [23]. Interestingly, it is also the case that IkB is developmentally regulated. In immature intestinal epithelial cells, IkB levels were notably lower in immature cells. This was coincident with increased levels of IL-8 expression via bacterial component stimulation [24]. Taken together, these results point to another mechanism by which neonates tend toward inflammation. They also lift up the critical balance between and among immune cells at the gut interface (fig. 3).

But dendritic cells are hardly passive bystanders. As mentioned above, they can push through the epithelial barrier to sample bacterial antigen and induce the maturation of T cells via antigen presentation and cytokine milieu. However, like the epithelial cells, these cells extract advantage out of another kind of restriction. Specifically, dendritic cells take bacteria from the lumen only so far as the mesenteric lymph nodes. Here B- and T-cell stimulation and maturation can occur with subsequent re-homing to the gut. The systemic immune system is taken out of the commensal equation, thus compromising another example of protective sequestration within the mucosal immune system [25]. It is also worth wondering if regulatory T-cell presence in these same lymph nodes assists the infant early on in providing extra prophylaxis against a systemic immune response.

Hanging in the Balance

The variable colonization of the neonatal gut has immune responses that hinge directly on the specificity of the predominant organism. While correlations between clinical manifestations and colonization have been made, the molecular basis of these phenotypes is being elucidated. Recently, Mazmanian et al. [26] identified a unique surface polysaccharide of *B. fragilis* that induces CD4+ T-cell proliferation via novel carbohydrate MHC-II presentation by dendritic cells. Apparently the polysaccharide induces dendritic cell

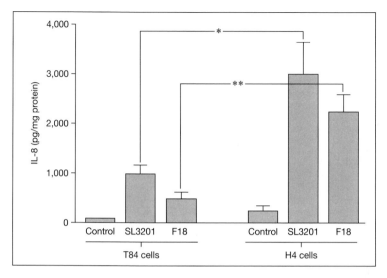

Fig. 3. Fetal H4 cells secrete significantly more IL-8 in response to the pathogenic *Salmonella* strain SL3201 and the commensal *E. coli* strain F18 than do adult T84 cells. Asterisks denote significance at p < 0.05 for the comparison of the values indicated by the brackets. From Claud et al. [24].

maturity in order to allow for T-cell reactivity. Dendritic cells subsequently produced IL-12 which led to an increase in T-cell-generated IFNγ, the characteristic Th1 cytokine. Concurrent experiments demonstrated that CD4+ cells from germ-free mice overproduce IL-4, the cytokine associated with Th2 responses [26]. These results clearly demonstrate the potential balance achieved via competing results of epithelial responses to the gut microenvironment. It also begins to establish a molecular link to clinical observations. Recall that neonates born via CS have both decreased bacteroides colonization and increased allergic risk.

In keeping with the molecular theme of balance, two lactobacillus strains were shown to prime dendritic cells to yield regulatory T cells. These particular strains have surface glycosylation patterns that render them recognizable by DC-SIGN, a C-type lectin on the dendritic cell surface. It appears that this interaction nudges the dendritic cell toward the regulatory pathway. This effect was optimized at a bacterium to dendritic cell ratio of 1:1. A predominance of bacteria interestingly did not induce a regulatory effect. The authors speculate that this may be adaptive in the setting of bacterial overload or infection when a regulatory response would be inappropriate [27]. Again, the critical intersection of neonatal gut colonization and the interaction with epithelial and dendritic cells has another molecular manifestation. Both of these examples, while different, demonstrate the necessary underlying machinery the neonate utilizes to assimilate the benefits of the bacterial onslaught at birth.

Conclusion

The fetus transitions through birth to infancy with an immune system that is readied but necessarily harnessed through regulatory mechanisms. The enormous transition from sterility to non-inflammatory colonization requires intricate adaptive responses. This is accomplished through various specific and nonspecific means, but the epithelial layer is central to the infant's ability to be colonized without harm. These interactions are central to both the immediate need to avoid infection and the long-term goal of tolerance. Recent studies have elucidated the molecular basis of the epithelial ability to provide barrier function, a non-inflammatory resting state, and protection against invasive organisms. The neonate is further assisted by the powerful exogenous immune influence via human milk. Not only does it allow proper colonization, but human milk clearly modulates neonatal excessive inflammation. Future research should be focused on better understanding the Ikk, DC-SIGN, and both the directly immune and non-immune functions of TLRs. Given the intestinal epithelial layer's open access to the environment, it seems clear that clinical intervention at this locus is inevitable. Taken in context with the widespread clinical issues of childhood allergy and inflammatory bowel disease, the gut mucosa becomes even more pertinent. The infant's acquisition of both local and systemic tolerance is complex with the reward of immunologic pearls awaiting discovery.

References

1 Spencer J, Macdonald T, Finn T, et al: Development of Peyer's patches in human fetal terminal ileum. Clin Exp Immunol 1986;64:536–543.
2 MacDonald TT, Weinel A, Spencer J: HLA-DR expression in human fetal intestinal epithelium. Gut 1988;29:1342–1348.
3 Holt PG, Jones CA: The development of the immune system during pregnancy and early life. Allergy 2000;55:688–697.
4 Koyama M, Saji F, Kameda T, et al: Differential mRNA expression of three distinct classes of Fc gamma receptors at the feto-maternal interface. J Reprod Immunol 1991;20:103–113.
5 Mishima T, Kurasawa G, Ishikiawa G, et al: Epithelial expression of Fc gamma receptor IIb in the full-term human placenta. Placenta 2007;28:170–174.
6 Hermann E, Truyens C, Alonso-Vega C, et al: Human fetuses are able to mount adult-like CD8 T cell responses. Immunobiology 2002;100:2153–2158.
7 Nanthakumar NN, Fusunyan RD, Sanderson I, et al: Inflammation in the developing human intestine: a possible pathophysiologic contribution in necrotizing enterocolitis. Proc Natl Acad Sci USA 2000;97:6043–6048.
8 Darasse-Jeze G, Marodon G, Salomon B, et al: Ontogeny of CD4+CD25+ regulatory/suppressor T cells in human fetuses. Immunobiology 2005;105:4715–4721.
9 Michaëlsson J, Mold J, McCune J, et al: Regulation of T cell responses in the developing human fetus. J Immunol 2006;176:5741–5748.

10 Grölund MM, Lehtonen OP, Eerola E, et al: Fecal microflora in healthy infants born by different methods of delivery: permanent changes in intestinal flora after cesarean delivery. J Pediatr Gastroenterol Nutr 1999;28:19–25.
11 Renz-Polster H, David MR, Buist AS, et al: Cesarean delivery and the risk of allergic disorders in childhood. Clin Exp Allergy 2005;11:1466–1472.
12 Labereau B, Filipiak-Pitroff B, von Berg A, et al: Cesarean section and gastrointestinal symptoms, atopic dermatitis, and sensitization during the first year of life. Arch Dis Child 2004;89: 993–997.
13 Harmsen HJM, Wildeboer-Veloo ACM, Alida CM, et al: Analysis of intestinal flora development in breast-fed and formula-fed infants by using molecular identification and detection methods. J Pediatr Gastroenterol Nutr 2000;30:61–67.
14 Claud EC, Savidge T, Walker AW: Modulation of human intestinal epithelial cell IL-8 secretion by human milk factors. Pediatr Res 2003;53:419–425.
15 LeBouder E, Rey-Nores JE, Rushmere NK, et al: Soluble forms of Toll-like receptor (TLR) 2 capable of modulating TLR2 signaling are present in human placenta and breast milk. J Immunol 2003;171:6680–6689.
16 LeBouder E, Rey-Nores JE, Raby A-C, et al: Modulation of neonatal microbial recognition: TLR-mediated innate immune responses are specifically and differentially modulated by human milk. J Immunol 2006;176:3742–3752.
17 Macfarlane GT, Macfarlane S: Human colonic microbiota: ecology, physiology, and metabolic potential of intestinal bacteria. Scand J Gastroenterol Suppl 1997;222:3–9.
18 Rakoff-Nahoum S, Paglino J, Eslami-Verzaneh F, et al: Recognition of commensal microflora by Toll-like receptors is required for intestinal homeostasis. Cell 2004;118:229–241.
19 Nenci A, Becker C, Wullaert A, et al: Epithelial NEMO links innate immunity to chronic intestinal inflammation. Nature 2007;446:557–561.
20 Dai D, Nanthakumar NN, Newburg D, et al: The role of indigenous microflora in the development of murine intestinal fucosyl- and sialyltransferases. Am J Physiol Gastrointest Liver Physiol 2002;282:480–490.
21 Nanthakumar NN, Dai D, Newburg D, et al: The role of indigenous microflora in the development of murine intestinal fucosyl- and sialyltransferases. FASEB J 2003;17:44–46.
22 Rimoldi M, Chieppa M, Salucci V, et al: Intestinal immune homeostasis is regulated by crosstalk between epithelial cells and dendritic cells. Nat Immunol 2005;6:507–514.
23 Zaph C, Troy A, Taylor B, et al: Epithelial-cell-intrinsic IKK-β expression regulates intestinal immune homeostasis. Nature 2007;446:552–556.
24 Claud EC, Lu L, Amon PM, et al: Developmentally regulated IkB expression in intestinal epithelium and susceptibility to flagellin-induced inflammation. Proc Nat Acad Sci USA 2004;101:7404–7408.
25 Macpherson AJ, Uhr T: Induction of protective IgA by intestinal dendritic cells carrying commensal bacteria. Science 2004;303:1662–1665.
26 Mazmanian SK, Liu CH, Tzianabos AO, et al: An immunomodulatory molecule of symbiotic bacteria directs maturing of the host immune system. Cell 2005;122:107–118.
27 Smits HH, Engering A, van der Kleij D, et al: Selective probiotic bacteria induce IL-10-producing regulatory T cells in vitro by modulating dendritic cell function through dendritic cell-specific intracellular adhesion molecule 3-grabbing nonintegrin. J Allergy Clin Immunol 2005;115:126.

Discussion

Dr. Isolauri: Yesterday we talked briefly about bacterial translocation and breast milk bifidobacteria. Now you have nicely summarized the current understanding of mechanisms; how that kind of uptake could take place, and how these bacteria could be coated by IgA. Do we know anything about their fate in the common mucosal immune system after that process?

Dr. Walker: There is a study from Lausanne in *Pediatrics* which suggests that maternal bacteria in a mother's intestine, can be taken up across the intestine, pass through the circulation and move to the breast where they are secreted into the breast milk [1]. I think unfortunately these studies are very early on and I don't know how to interpret them. Your group has made very interesting observations using probiotics in the latter stages of gestation showing a protective effect against allergy [2]. I think that is an area that needs to be explored, particularly in the context of programming within the intrauterine environment.

Dr. Berry: The inborn errors of metabolism sometimes provide great insight into the normal physiology. One of the things that has plagued the metabolic field for years is this mystery of *Escherichia coli* sepsis in babies with hereditary galactosemia. It only occurs in the newborn period, and appears to require exposure of the infants to lactose causing the galactose-1-phosphate levels to rise. Data are continuing to accumulate, suggesting that there is a secondary defect in glycosylation in babies with galactosemia. For example serum transferrin, the majority of molecules circulating in plasma are missing the entire chain so that the n-linked glycan with sialic acid residues is missing and as the babies are taken off lactose the assembly defect gradually disappears. We thought for some time that it was perhaps the mechanism for allowing a greater ability of *E. coli* to transfer from the lumen into the circulation of the baby and produce sepsis. The congenital defects in glycosylation where there are inherited defects in the glycosyltransferase assembling factors exist; they are terrible diseases, but they don't have *E. coli* sepsis as part of their features early on. Later on some of the patients can get protein-losing enteropathies and are susceptible to infection but it is not the *E. coli* galactosemia phenotype. One of the things that has been curious for us over the years is we have had instances in which blood cultures have been done in babies with galactosemia and evidence for *E. coli* antigens was detected in the blood but the cultures were negative, even in the absence of antibiotic exposure. Must the dendritic cell bring in the intact organism like *E. coli* or just parts of it to stimulate the proper immune response?

Dr. Walker: There is a publication by Garcea et al. [3] showing that *Bacteriodes fragilis* has surface PSA on the organism. In this situation dendritic cells take up the entire organism and then the organism is modified and presented to the lymphocyte, but there are also circumstances in which secreted products from bacteria can potentially interact with pattern recognition receptors and produce the same phenomena. Macpherson and Smith [4] have done studies showing the mechanism by which commensal bacteria are taken up across M cells into dendritic cells or by dendritic cells projecting through the epithelium, and these cells are then transported to the mesenteric lymph nodes where they preferentially produce a local immune response but not a systemic response. I can't make further comments beyond those bits of information.

Dr. Prescott: I was very interested in your findings on Toll-like receptor (TLR) regulation, particularly in view of the fact that we recently observed that children who develop allergic disease actually have increased expression of TLR function to, particularly, TLR2, 3 and 4 in the neonatal period, even before significant colonization has taken place. Could you to comment on that, and also on the recent observation that breast milk appears to differentially regulate the expression of TLRs?

Dr. Walker: This is an area that is evolving. We have looked at fetal enterocytes and shown that there is an increased expression of TLR2 and 4 and that this is modulated by inflammatory circumstances. What we think is happening as part of the rationale for having increased inflammation is that immature cells express Toll receptors on the luminal surface, adult enterocytes don't; so you don't get the TLR4-mediated response that you do in the immature cell. We think that it is a maturational process which helps affect the decrease in inflammatory stimuli within the intestine. I can't comment on the allergic versus non-allergic, but I would not be surprised if Toll receptors were involved. The whole field of innate immunity in breast milk is opening up and there are lots of factors in breast milk that we have or have not identified. There is work being done on TLR4, TLR2 as well as CD14, suggesting again that this is something that breast milk produces that can potentially help enhance its immune protection.

Dr. Isolauri: You mentioned that in breast milk there are some other agents that could modify the immune response to microbes. These include fatty acids which actually engage the same TLR CD14.

Dr. Walker: That is a very important observation because initially the feeling was that Toll receptors only interacted with microbial molecular patterns. We know now that there are endogenous ligands including fatty acids. That is also true incidentally in the inflammatory response in obesity.

Dr. Salminen: I would like to focus on your results from probiotics. We know from several studies that probiotics are very strain-specific and you have used the probiotic preparation that was defective in necrotizing enterocolitis (NEC). Are there differences in mechanistic details when different probiotic strains are compared?

Dr. Walker: We took the two strains of probiotics which were used in a clinical study done in Taiwan [5] showing a decrease in NEC in patients at risk, that is 1,500 g and less. We collected the strains that were described from the NIH ATTC bank and grew them in media. Because we were dealing with the xenograph model and the skid mouse, we were worried about putting live strains into the xenograph, so we started by taking media from these cells and fortuitously it had an effect. It represents a response using the same probiotics that were used clinically to prevent NEC. I totally agree with you, you can't equate one probiotic with another because they all have different effects and that is why we specifically used those strains. We are now considering a multicenter trial through the neonatal network in United States, but we are not sure which of those two probiotics is more effective. My bias would be the bifidobacteria but I don't know. We are also not sure as to when probiotics should be introduced in the feeding regimen of a severely premature infant, although hopefully we will soon have some information from your institution where you have had good success in the first introduction of feeding using probiotics.

Dr. Kunz: Like you I am very much in favor of human milk oligosaccharides. However I don't agree in one point. Like many others you compare the prebiotic effect of human milk oligosaccharides with prebiotic oligosaccharides from plants or modified from lactose. If the structures are compared, they are not at all the same, and with regard to the prebiotic effect, it is most likely that human milk oligosaccharides have a prebiotic effect but it is not shown in humans, we only have in vitro data. I agree absolutely that there are very specific effects of human oligosaccharides on bacteria but I am just not sure if we can call it prebiotic effects.

Dr. Walker: It depends on how prebiotics are defined. I define prebiotics as the effect of oligosaccharides on increasing the proliferation of endogenous flora. What I tried to show in this very new observation, in the absence of bacterial flora, this was a cell culture situation, we used the prebiotic to reduce inflammation. To me, at least in the preliminary observation, it appears that this might represent a primary effect as well as a secondary effect of the oligosaccharides in the form of prebiotics. I agree with you, milk oligosaccharides represent about 8% of the total carbohydrates in breast milk and that is an enormous mixture of oligosaccharides, so it is very hard to isolate out from that specific oligosaccharide. I just used as an example some of the commercial oligosaccharides that presumably also exist in breast milk, although you are right, the structure may be different.

Dr. Kunz: May You mentioned the change in sialylation to fucosylation in the early postnatal period. Where does the fucose come from? Is it a self-regulated process of the epithelial cell or does fucose come from breast milk or is it derived from microorganisms?

Dr. Walker: Sonnenburg et al. [6] showed that these organisms can take complex carbohydrates and produce fucose as a substrate for the organism and presumably it is also present in the milieu. Certainly the breast milk or other forms of feeding contain fucose. I don't think the problem is the substrate, it is the enzyme which expresses the fucose and the surface glycolipids and proteins in the glycosylation process. There are some very recent data which suggest that fucose expressed on the Toll receptor is an important determinant in glycosylation and in protection of the gut against inflammatory bowel disease in animal models. It is a very complex process and we have just began to touch the surface of it.

Dr. German: In terms of actually personalizing and bring this in essence to practice, it could be said that if a child is getting antibiotics then that would be a time to selectively avoid novel foods to avoid breaking oral tolerance. Can you imagine a time when we would actually build a tolerogenic cocktail?

Dr. Walker: As we understand more about the process, it is still again studies in progress, I would be inclined to give a child on antibiotics a probiotic because there is pretty good evidence that it protects against some of the complications.

Dr. Savilahti: Thank you for your excellent review and so much information about this development. I would like to discuss the role of prematurity in the genesis of allergic diseases, the data are rather conflicting. We completed a study about 7 years ago in which small premature babies whose birth weight was below 1,500 g were studied and again at the age of 10 years. Their allergy prevalence was one third of the control population, and the same was true for sensitization [7]. We speculated that it is probable that these very premature infants develop tolerance because we also found low levels of IgG and IgA antibodies to food antigens. So under those conditions in which there is increased permeability, there is also a possibility for tolerance development and increased permeability is always detrimental for immunological development [7, 8].

Dr. Walker: Your point is very well taken. It is much more controversial in the premature than it is in babies born by cesarean section and the use of antibiotics. You are absolutely right.

Dr. Savilahti: Another comment I would like to make is about this mechanism of probiotics because in a clinical setting we recently studied both treatment and prevention. We saw that markers of inflammation are activated during treatment. We saw an increase in CRP concentration in the serum of these infants and we also saw an increase in IL-6 concentrations and they correlated with each other [9, 10]. The probiotic was *Lactobacillus* GG, but the same happened with a combination of 4 species which we used in the prevention study [10]. Going to this hygiene hypothesis I presume that you need some kind of inflammation in the intestine.

Dr. Walker: The low grade physiologic inflammation that was discussed. The other point I want to make is I don't think we can extrapolate from the in vitro studies that I presented, other than what we think is the possible mechanism of clinical trials. Nothing substitutes for trying a probiotic in which you think would be effective in the clinical setting in which you think it could be used.

Dr. Björkstén: We have to remember that the story is not about oral tolerance but immune modulation of relevance for respiratory allergies. It is not even about asthma, which is an inflammatory disease, but about IgE regulation and inhalant allergies. You referred to the studies by Sudo. There are actually two aspects on this. One is that gut bacteria are a prerequisite for the induction of oral tolerance. The other is that Sudo showed another type of immune regulation, that is downregulation of specific IgE antibodies by gut microbes. As you know IgE-mediated food allergy is uncommon after the age of 3 years. So I am wondering whether the discussion on mechanisms of oral tolerance has very little to do with atopic disease.

Dr. Walker: Good point. Again I am giving you basic observations that we carried over into the clinical setting. In most instances, for example, my using the term Th1-dominant versus Th2 for allergy versus autoimmune disease, I don't think that holds up in humans. There is lots of evidence that the study done in Africa with schistosomiasis has a protective effect against the expression of allergy, not allergy per se, but allergic symptoms. It is a much more complex process than we think.

Dr. Björkstén: In Africa immune deviation is said to be due to parasites, but we have published almost identical cytokine immune responses in Estonian as compared to Swedish children, and Estonians don't have parasites that influence the IgE antibody formation. I would suggest that it is conceivable that what you see in Africa may not only be due to parasites. They may also have a totally different gut flora. This has not been looked at. As I said we have excluded parasites in Estonia.

Dr. Walker: Another good point. There are lots of clinical questions that need to be resolved. In the interest of time, I was more or less trying to tweak your interest by giving you an overview in a somewhat simplistic fashion.

References

1   Perez PF, Doré J, Leclerc M, et al: Bacterial imprinting of the neonatal immune system: lessons from maternal cells? Pediatrics 2007;119:e724–e732.
2   Rautava S, Kalliomäki M, Isolauri E: Probiotics during pregnancy and breast-feeding might confer immunomodulatory protection against atopic disease in the infant. J Allergy Clin Immunol 2002;109:119–121.
3   Garcea RL, Salunke DM, Caspar DL: Site-directed mutation affecting polyomavirus capsid self-assembly in vitro. Nature 1987;329:86–87.
4   Macpherson AJ, Smith K: Mesenteric lymph nodes at the center of immune anatomy. J Exp Med 2006;203:497–500.
5   Lin HC, Su BH, Chen AC, et al: Oral probiotics reduce the incidence and severity of necrotizing enterocolitis in very low birth weight infants. Pediatrics 2005;115:1–4.
6   Sonnenburg JL, Chen CT, Gordon JI: Genomic and metabolic studies of the impact of probiotics on a model gut symbiont and host. PLoS Biol 2006;4:e413.
7   Siltanen M, Kajosaari M, Pohjavuori M, Savilahti E: Prematurity at birth reduces the long-term risk of atopy. J Allergy Clin Immunol 2001;107:229–234.
8   Siltanen M, Kajosaari M, Savilahti EM, et al: IgG and IgA antibody levels to cow's milk are low at age 10 years in children born preterm. J Allergy Clin Immunol 2002;110:658–663.
9   Viljanen M, Pohjavuori E, Haahtela T, et al: Induction of inflammation as a possible mechanism of probiotic effect in atopic eczema-dermatitis syndrome. J Allergy Clin Immunol 2005;115:1254–1259.
10 Marschan E, Kuitunen M, Kukkonen K, et al: Probiotics in infancy induce protective immune profiles that are characteristic for chronic low-grade inflammation. Clin Exp Allergy 2008; 38:611–618.

Bier DM, German JB, Lönnerdal B (eds): Personalized Nutrition for the Diverse Needs of Infants and Children.
Nestlé Nutr Workshop Ser Pediatr Program, vol 62, pp 127–140,
Nestec Ltd., Vevey/S. Karger AG, Basel, © 2008.

Gut Decontamination with Norfloxacin and Ampicillin Enhances Insulin Sensitivity in Mice

Chieh Jason Chou, Mathieu Membrez, Florence Blancher

Nestlé Research Center, Lausanne, Switzerland

Abstract

Recent data suggest that gut microbiota plays a significant role in fat accumulation. However, it is not clear whether gut microbiota is involved in the pathophysiology of type-2 diabetes. To address this issue, we modulated gut microbiota with two combinations of antibiotics in two different mouse models with insulin resistance. Treatment with norfloxacin and ampicillin for 2 weeks reduced the cecal bacterial DNA below the level of detection in ob/ob, diet-induced obese and insulin resistance (DIO) mice, and significantly improved fasting glycemia and oral glucose tolerance of the treated animals. The enhanced insulin sensitivity was independent of food intake or adiposity because pair-fed ob/ob mice were as glucose intolerant as the untreated ob/ob mice. The reduced liver triglycerides, increased liver glycogen and improved glucose tolerance in the treated mice indicate broad impacts on metabolism by gut decontamination. The treatment with non-absorbable antibiotics polymyxin B and neomycin significantly modified cecal microbiota profile in the DIO mice, and the modified intestinal microbiota was associated with a gradual reduction in glycemia during a washout period. In summary, modulation of gut microbiota ameliorated glucose intolerance in mice and altered the hormonal, inflammatory and metabolic status of the host.

Background

The human digestive tract contains a significant number of microorganisms, bacteria being the most dominant. The composition and functionality of the microbiota in each section of the digestive tract have been an area of active research for many years. Several studies, based on the variations in 16S rRNA gene sequence derived from clone libraries, have made comprehensive surveys on the profile of the microbiota in different parts of the digestive tract. These studies, utilizing culture-independent methods, have revealed unique microbiota profiles in the periodontal pocket [1], the distal esophagus [2], the stomach [3] and the colon [4]. Especially in the gut, microbial communities have been shown to play a critical role in its maturation [5, 6], development of innate immunity [7], production of essential vitamins [8], and the biotransformation of endogenous and exogenous compounds [9].

Recently gut microbiota has been shown to affect fat storage and energy harvesting, which suggests that intestinal microorganisms may play a role in the development of obesity. Bäckhed et al. [10] demonstrated that germ-free mice had defects in storing fat in white adipose tissue and that this was due to higher amounts of circulating lipoprotein lipase inhibitor Fiaf produced by the gut. In support of this, germ-free Fiaf knockout mice gained more weight than their germ-free wild-type littermates when all mice were fed a Western diet, confirming the protective role of Fiaf on body fat accumulation [11]. Also, the composition of cecal microbiota in obese and insulin-resistant ob/ob mice differed from lean controls with a higher ratio of Firmicutes/Bacteroidetes found in the ob/ob mice [12]. Metagenomic analyses revealed that the cecal microbiota in the ob/ob mice was more capable of producing short-chain fatty acids by fermenting dietary fibers. The increased energy harvesting from dietary fibers contributed partly to the excessive weight gain of the ob/ob mice [13]. In humans, the fecal Firmicutes/Bacteroidetes ratio also decreased after obese individuals consumed different low-calorie weight-loss diets, providing an association between gut microbiota profile and weight management [14]. Thus, available evidence suggests that the microbiota could be a contributing factor to obesity.

In both in vitro and in animal models, an increase in proinflammatory cytokines such as TNFα causes tissue insulin resistance [15, 16]. When the systemic inflammation is suppressed by pharmaceutical interventions, the whole body insulin sensitivity is also improved in both mice and humans [17, 18]. However, the source of the low-grade inflammation has not been clearly defined. In type-2 diabetic patients with periodontal problems, treatments with topical antibiotics lower serum TNFα and improve the markers of insulin sensitivity such as HOMA-IR and HbA-1c levels [19]. This finding suggests that reducing local infection can decrease systemic inflammation and enhance whole body insulin sensitivity. Cani et al. [20] showed that subcutaneous infusion of a low dose of lipopolysaccharide (LPS), a component of the gram-negative bacteria cell wall, leads to excessive weight gain and insulin resistance in mice. In the gut, pattern-recognition Toll-like receptors (TLRs) are important for host defense against bacterial infection and the development of innate immunity [21, 22], and TLR4 is responsible for recognizing bacterial LPS. Upon activation of TLR4, NFκB is translocated to the nucleus where it turns on the expression of inflammatory genes such as TNFα and COX2 [23]. Due to the large number of LPS-containing gram-negative bacteria residing in the gut, chronic stimulation of intestinal TLR4 may exacerbate the low-grade inflammation associated with obesity and insulin resistance. To test this hypothesis, we eliminated most members of the gut microbiota in ob/ob and diet-induced obese and insulin resistant (DIO) mice using two different combinations of antibiotics. We postulated that insulin resistance can be reversed by removing or reducing the gut microbiota in the two animal models. Our data demonstrate that gut microbiota modulation improves whole body glucose tolerance and reduces hepatic steatosis, suggesting that controlling gut microbiota could be a novel therapeutic strategy in treating or managing type-2 diabetes.

Efficacy of Gut Decontamination

To test the hypothesis, we decided to use one or a combination of several broad range antibiotics to remove the majority of the gut microbiota in ob/ob mice. Since the outcomes of the study depended very much upon the success of gut decontamination, we first checked the efficacy and specificity of several antibiotics in in vitro screening tests. Fecal samples from ob/ob mice were diluted and plated on different selective media for bifidobacteria, lactobacillus, enterobacteria or bacteroides. Our data showed that norfloxacin was the only antibiotic capable of killing fecal enterobacteria, while ampicillin was the most efficient antibiotic in eliminating bacteroides. For lactobacillus and bifidobacteria, both ampicillin and amoxicillin were equally effective. Based on these results, the combination of norfloxacin and ampicillin, both effective against gram-positive and gram-negative bacteria, was selected for the purpose of gut decontamination.

Consuming high doses of antibiotics can cause gastrointestinal irritation with nausea, vomiting and diarrhea. These symptoms can have a significant impact: short-term on food intake, and long-term on body weight and the state of insulin sensitivity of the mice. To minimize these undesirable side effects and to determine the most efficient dose of the antibiotic combination, we performed a dose-response study using different concentrations of the norfloxacin and ampicillin combination in ob/ob mice. At the end of the treatment period, cecal samples were collected and cultured in aerobic and anaerobic conditions. A treatment with norfloxacin and ampicillin at 1 g/l in drinking water achieved the highest level of suppression in the number of cecal aerobic and anaerobic bacteria population in ob/ob mice. With this dose, there was no significant difference in body weight (48.6 ± 1.0 vs. 47.6 ± 1.3 g) but a 17% reduction in food intake did occur (67.1 ± 3.86 g in control vs. 55.4 ± 2.86 g in the 1-g/l group) during the 2-week antibiotic treatment period.

Body Weight and Body Fat Are Affected by Food Intake but Not by Gut Decontamination

Based on the notable reduction in food intake during the dose-response experiment, we designed a pair-feeding study to control for potential impacts

Table 1. Body weight and body composition of ob/ob mice treated with antibiotics

	Control	Nor + Amp	Pair-fed
Body weight, g	47.8 ± 0.9	47.2 ± 0.6	46.1 ± 0.9
Total fat pad weight, g	5.95 ± 0.18[b]	5.43 ± 0.11[a]	5.46 ± 0.11[a]
Gut weight, g	4.03 ± 0.13[b]	6.00 ± 0.05[a]	3.59 ± 0.13[b]

Body weights, total fat pad weights and the gut weights were obtained at sacrifice after overnight fasting. Total fat pad includes epididymal, retroperitoneal and mesenteric fat pads. The gut weight includes the weight of the whole digestive tract from the stomach to the anus. Nor + Amp = Norfloxacin and ampicillin. Data are median ± rob SEM (n = 12). Different letters represent statistical significance: $p < 0.05$ using Kruskal-Wallis test followed by Wilcoxon test.

of reduced food intake caused by the antibiotic treatment. As observed in the previous experiment, the treated and the control ob/ob mice had comparable weights. However, both groups tended to weigh more than the pair-fed mice (table 1). The weight of epididymal, retroperitoneal and mesenteric fat pads was similar in the treated and pair-fed mice, and both groups tended to have a lower total fat pad weight than the control group (table 1). This result suggests that the amount of food ingested, rather than gut decontamination, determined the fat mass of the ob/ob mice. Thus, gut decontamination did not affect nutrient digestion and absorption in the ob/ob mice. The reason for the higher body weight and lower fat mass in the treated group was due to the weight of the gut, especially cecum weight. As shown in table 1, the gut weight of treated mice was about 2 g heavier than the control and the pair-fed groups, which is approximately equal to the difference observed in body weight between the treated and the pair-fed animals. In spite of the enlarged cecum, the cecal microbiota was strongly suppressed by gut decontamination. We assessed the profile of the cecal microbiota populations by denatured gradient gel electrophoresis based on the unique DNA sequences of 16S rRNA in bacteria. Unlike the control and pair-fed groups, we were unable to obtain a sufficient amount of DNA to perform denatured gradient gel electrophoresis in cecal samples collected from the treated mice. Despite the 17% food restriction, pair-feeding did not alter the profile of gut microbiota.

Gut Decontamination Improved Oral Glucose Tolerance of ob/ob Mice

Before the overnight fasted ob/ob mice were challenged with an oral glucose tolerance test (OGTT), gut decontaminated ob/ob mice demonstrated completely normalized basal glucose concentrations table 2. The treated mice

Table 2. Plasma and liver parameters in the ob/ob mice in the fasting and non-fasting states

	Fasting state			Non-fasting state	
	control	Nor + Amp	pair-fed	control	Nor + Amp
Blood glucose, mg/dl	156.3 ± 17.9^b	97.5 ± 13.2^a	181 ± 14.8^b	165.3 ± 20.7^b	101.6 ± 7.3^a
Plasma insulin, ng/ml	$3.27 \pm 0.39^{a,b}$	2.07 ± 0.44^a	3.25 ± 0.47^b	23.6 ± 5.1^b	13.9 ± 3.9^a
Liver glycogen, mg/g liver	3.72 ± 1.42	3.88 ± 1.02	1.92 ± 1.38	37.51 ± 6.14^a	58.88 ± 4.58^b
Liver triglycerides, μg/g liver	200.8 ± 15.3^b	159.6 ± 14.7^a	$182.6 \pm 21.4^{a,b}$	159.2 ± 5.3^b	122.8 ± 4.1^a

Samples were collected either after 15-hour fasting or in the morning. Liver samples were collected at sacrifice. Data are median ± rob SEM (n = 12 for data in the fasting state; n = 6 for data in the non-fasting state). Different letters represent statistical significance: $p < 0.05$ using Kruskal-Wallis test followed by Wilcoxon test.

also had much improved oral glucose tolerance with a smaller area under the glucose curve (AUC) during the OGTT (fig. 1a, b). Basal plasma insulin concentrations and insulin responses during the OGTT were also reduced in the treated group (fig. 1c). Despite consuming less food and weighing less than the control group, the pair-fed ob/ob mice were as glucose intolerant as the control mice. In contrast to germ-free mice that have a reduced expression of intestinal SGLT-1 [5], the expression of SGLT-1 in the jejunum was not affected by gut decontamination suggesting that the improved oral glucose tolerance was not due to a defect in glucose absorption. In addition, non-fasting blood glucose concentrations in the treated ob/ob mice were also significantly lower than both the control and pair-fed groups (table 2). Together with improved glucose tolerance, lower glucose and insulin concentrations, our data suggest that removing gut microbiota with norfloxacin and ampicillin significantly enhanced insulin sensitivity in ob/ob mice.

Gut Microbiota Modulation Improved Glucose and Lipid Metabolism in the Liver

Liver glycogen is often lower in patients with type-2 diabetes, and restoration of liver glycogen storage is associated with increased hepatic insulin

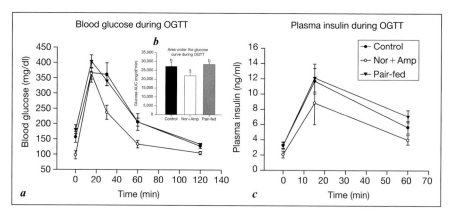

Fig. 1. Results of blood glucose (*a*), area under the glucose curve (*b*) and plasma insulin concentrations (*c*) levels from oral glucose tolerance tests in ob/ob mice. All mice were fasted overnight (15 h) before the OGTT. Data are median ± rob SEM (n = 12). Kruskal-Wallis test followed by Wilcoxon tests for pair-wise comparisons were applied. Statistical significance: p < 0.05.

sensitivity [24]. Indeed, in the non-fasting state, the control ob/ob mice had less liver glycogen than mice treated with antibiotics (table 2). As expected, all groups showed depleted liver glycogen after an overnight fast. In the state of hepatic insulin resistance, insulin is unable to suppress gluconeogenesis in the liver. Thus, we examined whether gut microbiota modulation had a direct effect on the expression of genes involved in gluconeogenesis. In the liver of antibiotic-treated ob/ob mice, the expression of glucose-6-phosphatase was significantly lower than that in the control group, which provides supportive evidence for the normalized blood glucose concentrations and elevated liver glycogen storage observed in ob/ob mice treated with norfloxacin and ampicillin.

The amount of liver triglycerides is also positively associated with insulin resistance. In the untreated ob/ob mice, a high amount of fat can be seen, whereas gut microbiota modulation considerably reduced the amount of micro- and macrovesicular steatosis in hepatocytes. Pair-feeding did not significantly change liver steatosis in ob/ob mice. Table 2 illustrates the quantification of liver triglyceride levels in both the non-fasting and fasting states. In the gut-decontaminated group, there was a significant reduction in hepatic fatty acid synthase and acetyl CoA carboxylase-1 mRNA levels in the non-fasting state, suggesting that reduced lipogenesis possibly contributed to the lower level of liver triglycerides observed in the gut-decontaminated ob/ob mice.

Table 3. Plasma parameters of ob/ob mice treated with norfloxacin and ampicillin

	Control	Nor + Amp	Pair-fed
LPS, EU/ml	24.74 ± 2.67[b]	16.93 ± 1.73[a]	28.20 ± 4.25[b]
Adiponectin, μg/ml	15.79 ± 0.57[b]	18.23 ± 0.78[a]	15.93 ± 1.12[a, b]
ALT activity, U/l	194.2 ± 36.3[b]	116.6 ± 16.9[a]	163.5 ± 23.6[a, b]

Plasma samples were collected after 15-hour fasting. Data are median ± rob SEM (n = 12). Different letters represent statistical significance: $p < 0.05$ using Kruskal-Wallis test followed by Wilcoxon test.

Gut Microbiota Modulation Suppressed Intestinal Immune Responses

Some of the interactions between gut microbiota and host tissues rely on the activation of TLRs. For example, bacterial lipopeptide in gram-positive bacteria and LPS in gram-negative bacteria can be recognized by TLR2 and TLR4, respectively [25]. Activation of TLR4 particularly leads to the activation of NFκB and inflammatory pathways including expression of TNFα [26]. Since a significant reduction in total cecal bacteria and Enterobacteria was observed after treatment with norfloxacin and ampicillin, the question was asked whether inflammatory responses in the gut were also reduced. First, the expression of genes involved in the TLR4-signaling pathway in the jejunum was examined. Gut microbiota modulation did not alter the expression of TLR4, CD14, or MyD88. As predicted, the TNFα mRNA concentration in the jejunum was reduced in the ob/ob mice treated with norfloxacin and ampicillin.

Gut Microbiota Modulation Reduced Plasma Endotoxemia

LPSs from gram-negative bacteria in the gut have been shown to play an important role in the development of insulin resistance [20] and non-alcoholic fatty liver disease [27]. To examine whether the plasma endotoxin level was associated with improved insulin sensitivity in the gut microbiota-modulation group, we measured plasma LPS concentrations in all groups, and found that plasma LPS levels were reduced by 32% in the antibiotic-treated ob/ob mice (table 3). The counts of cecal Enterobacteria, one of the sources of LPS, were also reduced by 5 logs after antibiotic treatment. In addition, plasma adiponectin concentrations were 14% higher in the treated ob/ob mice than the control mice (table 3). Reduced plasma LPS and increased adiponectin levels support the results of improved oral glucose tolerance and liver metabolism in ob/ob mice that received gut decontamination. To rule out the possibility that antibiotics caused toxic side effects to the liver, we measured plasma alanine transaminase (ALT) activity. As shown in table 3, plasma ALT activity was markedly reduced after gut microbiota modulation suggesting that it improved liver functions in ob/ob mice.

Gut Microbiota Modulation Improved Glucose Tolerance in Diet-Induced Obese Mice

To further demonstrate the beneficial effect of gut microbiota removal on insulin sensitivity in mice, we treated DIO mice with two combinations of antibiotics: (1) polymyxin B and neomycin, and (2) norfloxacin and ampicillin. Polymyxin B and neomycin were selected because of their low oral bioavailability, which allowed us to directly examine the role of gut microbiota in the regulation of glucose tolerance in animals. In contrast to the previous observations using the combination of norfloxacin and ampicillin, the combination of polymyxin B (0.5 g/l) and neomycin (1.0 g/l) only resulted in gut microbiota modulation. We treated DIO mice with polymyxin B and neomycin and examined whether the alternative profile of gut microbiota by a 'milder' antibiotic combination can improve the regulation of blood glucose. In addition, using the DIO rather than ob/ob mouse model allowed us to validate the beneficial effects of gut decontamination by norfloxacin and ampicillin. After 10 weeks of high-fat diet feeding, DIO mice were treated with a placebo control, the combination of polymyxin B and neomycin, or the combination of norfloxacin and ampicillin for 2 weeks. At the end of the antibiotic treatment period, half of the mice in each group were sacrificed, and the remaining mice entered a 4-week washout by removing antibiotics from their drinking water. Similar to the results found in the previous experiment with ob/ob mice, blood glucose concentrations in the norfloxacin- and ampicillin-treated DIO mice were markedly reduced (table 4), indicating the robust effect of gut decontamination. In contrast, the blood glucose concentrations in DIO mice treated with polymyxin B and neomycin were not different from the mice in the control group. Surprisingly, during the washout period, mice previously treated with polymyxin B and neomycin showed a continuous reduction in blood glucose concentration whereas the blood glucose concentrations of the norfloxacin- and ampicillin-treated mice remained at the same level as at the end of antibiotic treatment (table 4). The effect of washout on the blood glucose concentration was not due to food intake or body weight as mice in all groups consumed a similar amount of food and gained a similar amount of weight. The microbiota profile, however, was very different among all groups. At the end of the 2-week antibiotic treatment period, polymyxin B and neomycin significantly altered the cecal microbiota profile, and norfloxacin

Table 4. Blood glucose concentrations of DIO mice treated with different antibiotic combinations

	Blood glucose, mg/dl		
	baseline	after treatment	after washout
Control	159.6 ± 5.3	164.9 ± 8.1^b	161.3 ± 4.1^b
Poly + Neo	170.4 ± 4.2	156.8 ± 3.8^b	145.6 ± 3.0^a
Nor + Amp	168.5 ± 4.5	139.4 ± 1.7^a	140.2 ± 3.3^a

Blood and plasma samples were collected after 6-hour food deprivation in the light cycle. Poly + Neo = Polymyxin B and neomycin; Nor + Amp = norfloxacin and ampicillin. Data are median $\pm$ rob SEM (n = 12). Different letters represent statistical significance: $p < 0.05$ in each period using Kruskal-Wallis test followed by Wilcoxon test.

and ampicillin drastically reduced the cecal bacterial DNA concentrations below the limit of detection. After the 4-week washout period, the pattern of cecal microbiota was similar to that observed at the end of antibiotic treatments, regardless of the combination of antibiotics. Our data demonstrate that a drastic reduction in gut decontamination by norfloxacin and ampicillin rapidly reduced the blood glucose concentrations in DIO mice, and a milder gut microbiota modulation by polymyxin B and neomycin gradually ameliorated the hyperglycemia of DIO mice.

Conclusions

Gut decontamination with norfloxacin and ampicillin reversed the insulin resistance characteristic of ob/ob mice via multiple pathways (fig. 2). Gut microbiota modulation with polymyxin B and neomycin altered the gut microbiota composition and then reduced fasting glycemia further, supporting the importance of interactions between intestinal bacteria and the host in the regulation of glycemic control in mice. Although the mechanisms of how gut microbiota influence host physiology are still unknown, it is plausible that bacterial-induced inflammatory responses in the gut play a significant role. Since low-grade systemic inflammation is observed in the insulin-resistant state, the presence of certain gut bacteria might exacerbate the inflammatory responses and insulin resistance. Our data indicate that gut microbiota affected insulin resistance independent of obesity, since the mice treated with antibiotics were more insulin-sensitive and yet had similar adiposity to those of the pair-fed mice. Our results support the idea that modulating gut microbiota plays a vital role in whole body insulin sensitivity. However, more work has to be done in order to prove that gut microbiota modulation is an effective therapeutic strategy to treat or manage type-2 diabetes.

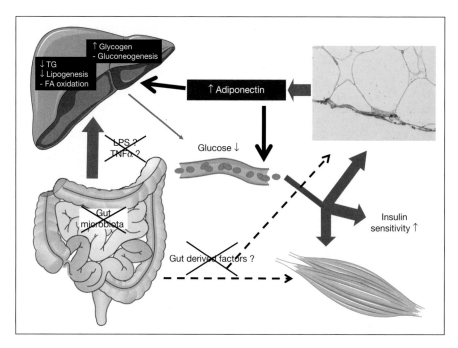

Fig. 2. Gut microbiota modulation improved whole body glucose tolerance by reducing the population of gut microbiota and suppressing gut microbiota originated factors including TNFα and LPS. The liver responded to the changes by increasing glycogen storage and decreasing triglyceride accumulation. Elevated adiponectin levels further enhanced insulin sensitivity. Together, a reduced low-grade systemic inflammation was likely the cause of enhanced insulin sensitivity by gut microbiota modulation.

References

1   Paster BJ, Boches SK, Galvin JL, et al: Bacterial diversity in human subgingical plaque. J Bacteriol 2001;183:3770–3783.
2   Pei Z, Bini EJ, Yang L, et al: Bacterial biota in the human distal esophagus. Proc Natl Acad Sci USA 2004;101:4250–4255.
3   Bik EM, Eckburg PB, Gill SR, et al: Molecular analysis of the bacterial microbiota in the human stomach. Proc Natl Acad Sci USA 2006;103:732–737.
4   Eckburg PB, Bik EM, Bernstein CN, et al: Diversity of the human intestinal microbial flora. Science 2005;308:1635–1638.
5   Hooper LV, Wong MH, Thelin A, et al: Molecular analysis of commensal host-microbial relationships in the intestine. Science 2001;291:881–884.
6   Stappenbeck TS, Hooper LV, Gordon JI: Developmental regulation of intestinal angiogenesis by indigenous microbes via Paneth cells. Proc Natl Acad Sci USA 2002;99:15451–15455.
7   Mazmanian SK, Liu CH, Tzianabos AO, Kasper DL: An immunomodulatory molecule of symbiotic bacteria directs maturation of the host immune system. Cell 2005;122:107–118.
8   Hill MJ: Intestinal flora and endogenous vitamin synthesis. Eur J Cancer Prev 1997;6(suppl 1): S43–S45.
9   Blaut M, Clavel T: Metabolic diversity of the intestinal microbiota: implications for health and disease. J Nutr 2007;137:751S–755S.

10 Bäckhed F, Ding H, Wang T, et al: The gut microbiota as an environmental factor that regulates fat storage. Proc Natl Acad Sci USA 2004;101:15718–15723.
11 Bäckhed F, Manchester JK, Semenkovich CF, Gordon JI: Mechanisms underlying the resistance to diet-induced obesity in germ-free mice. Proc Natl Acad Sci USA 2007;104:979–984.
12 Ley RE, Bäckhed F, Turnbaugh P, et al: Obesity alters gut microbial ecology. Proc Natl Acad Sci USA 2005;102:11070–11075.
13 Turnbaugh PJ, Ley RE, Mahowald MA, et al: An obesity-associated gut microbiome with increased capacity for energy harvest. Nature 2006;444:1027–1031.
14 Ley RE, Turnbaugh PJ, Klein S, Gordon JI: Microbial ecology: human gut microbes associated with obesity. Nature 2006;444:1022–1023.
15 Hotamisligil GS, Peraldi P, Budavari A, et al: IRS-1-mediated inhibition of insulin receptor tyrosine kinase activity in TNF-alpha- and obesity-induced insulin resistance. Science 1996;271:665–668.
16 Hotamisligil GS, Budavari A, Murray D, Spiegelman BM: Reduced tyrosin kinase activity of the insulin receptor in obesity-diabetes. Central role of tumor necrosis factor-alpha. J Clin Invest 1994;94:1543–1549.
17 Yuan M, Konstantopoulos N, Lee J, et al: Reversal of obesity- and diet-induced insulin resistance with salicylates or targeted disruption of Ikkbeta. Science 2001;293:1673–1677.
18 Hundal RS, Petersen KF, Mayerson AB, et al: Mechanism by which high-dose aspirin improves glucose metabolism in type 2 diabetes. J Clin Invest 2002;109:1321–1326.
19 Iwamoto Y, Nishimura F, Nakagawa M, et al: The effect of antimicrobial periodontal treatment on circulating tumor necrosis factor-alpha and glycated hemoglobin level in patients with type 2 diabetes. J Periodontol 2001;72:774–778.
20 Cani PD, Amar J, Iglesias MA, et al: Metabolic endotoxemia initiates obesity and insulin resistance. Diabetes 2007;56:1761–1772.
21 Rakoff-Nahoum S, Paglino J, Eslami-Varzaneh F, et al: Recognition of commensal microflora by toll-like receptors is required for intestinal homeostasis. Cell 2004;118:229–241.
22 Medzhitov R: Toll-like receptors and innate immunity. Nat Rev Immunol 2001;1:135–145.
23 Fukata M, Chen A, Klepper A, et al: Cox-2 is regulated by Toll-like receptor-4 (TLR4) signaling: role in proliferation and apoptosis in the intestine. Gastroenterology 2006;131:862–877.
24 Magnusson I, Rothman DL, Katz LD, et al: Increased rate of gluconeogenesis in type II diabetes mellitus. A 13C nuclear magnetic resonance study. J Clin Invest 1992;90:1323–1327.
25 Abreu MT, Fukata M, Arditi M: TLR signaling in the gut in health and disease. J Immunol 2005;174:4453–4460.
26 Cario E: Bacterial interactions with cells of the intestinal mucosa: Toll-like receptors and NOD2. Gut 2005;54:1182–1193.
27 Solga SF, Diehl AM: Non-alcoholic fatty liver disease: lumen-liver interactions and possible role for probiotics. J Hepatol 2003;38:681–687.

Discussion

Dr. Bier: I would just like to view the persistence of the gut bacteria in a somewhat different way, and it goes back to discussions we have had about the fetal origins of disease for some years, that is how does the adult organ or cell know what it ate as a fetus or a young child. We have talked about changes in developmental programming, now we have hardwiring, we have talked about clonal selection, etc. Another way of maintaining memory is the introduction and persistence of bacteria that are sending signals and talking. So this is just perhaps another memory phenomenon working to the gut bacteria and I think it is very exciting.

Dr. Chou: Of course this could be true. In our study after we modulate the flora and do the washout, the flora maintains the same pattern in support of your hypothesis. But the question is, after we change the pattern of the flora, can the body relearn new things? So we refresh the memory by exposing it to new environmental stimulation.

Dr. Bier: Of course that is another question: can we change something that has happened. At least some of the implications of the work in humans is that the gut microbiota patterns are different among people but remarkably stable within the people. If that is the case, in a sense this is personalized gut memory being carried in the microflora. The issue was always that cells turnover in a matter of days and a person lives 50 years, so how is this memory being maintained? The gut microbiota can be turning over all the time, but if they are remaining approximately the same species over time, they are carrying the same memory. I just think we are opening up areas of really interesting kinds of research.

Dr. Chou: It is an interesting idea to find associations between the colonization of gut microbiota in an infant and certain physiological outcomes in adult life. Another thing that I would like to emphasize: not only is the diversity of gut microbiota important, the functionality of gut microbiota is as well. New technology, such as metagenomic analysis, would help us to gain more insight into the metabolic pathways of gut microbiota. The activity of gut microbiota could contribute to the tissue memory of humans.

Dr. Walker: I have a question about microbiota in the context of before and after the ob/ob mice developed excessive weight and fat distribution. Is the flora different? Theoretically once flora is formed because of genetic implications and environmental factors, it remains fairly stable during the entire lifetime. The question is does the development of obesity and excessive deposition of fat influence a change in the existing flora or does that flora exist prior to their developing the obese state?

Dr. Chou: That is a great question, and I have the same question regarding the data published by Turnbaugh et al. [1]. I think in that study the different composition of the gut microbiota found in ob/ob mice was due to excessive food intake rather than obesity. Ob/ob mice eat about 6 g/day in our study, which is twice as much as a regular wild-type animal consumes daily. When imaging gut microbiota in ob/ob mice, you also have to deal with an excessive amount of dietary fiber and other nutrients. So is the response of the gut microbiota in ob/ob mice a result of genetic predisposition (leptin deficiency) or just excessive food intake?

Dr. Salminen: In your mouse experiment you showed that 40 days after withdrawal from antibiotic treatment the blood glucose levels were still quite significantly low. Do you also have gut microbiota data for that point? How quickly does this change return to the baseline you started from? In germ-free mice or in mice treated with antibiotics cecal enlargement is always observed. Is it perhaps an adaptive physiological mechanism, or is it actually the consequence of the changes in nutrient absorption?

Dr. Chou: Regarding your first question whether the difference in gut microbiota profile remained after 4 weeks of washout, the answer is yes. To be honest we were surprised by the results because we thought the composition of the gut microbiota would quickly return to baseline. And to answer your second question about cecal enlargement, I think some data have shown that if some dietary ingredients such as chlorides are introduced to germ-free mice, the size of the cecum is reduced [2]. So the size of the cecum is a result of physiological adaptation to the germ-free state.

Dr. Saavedra: This is a great and probably the most provocative presentation yet in terms of all the things we probably need to learn regarding those relationships between bacteria and humans. First just a comment: I think this may have something to do with the concept that Peter Gluckman was mentioning earlier yesterday with regard to a relative mismatch. Yesterday we were talking of this mismatch relative to an energy rich world: Can this mismatch be relative to the hypobacterial world that we live in today compared to what we were before? The reason for this question is that the secular trends in increasing autoimmune disease and obesity are so similar that they could almost be superimposed one over the other. Could the bacterial changes in our diet and environment be related to both autoimmune disease and obesity? My question goes to the other concept that we were talking about yesterday relative to the differences between flora in the cecum and colon versus flora in the small bowel. There are a number of very nice experiments showing that the cytokine response pattern of the same bacteria orally ingested in the small bowel is very different from the cytokine response when you expose the colon to those bacteria. Can you comment on that?

Dr. Chou: We looked at the gene expressions in the inflammatory pathway in the small intestine. The TLR2 TLR4 expressions were not changed in the jejunum of the antibiotic-treated ob/ob mice. The intestinal TNFα mRNA level was slightly reduced in the treated mice. Also the flora in the small intestine could not only trigger different inflammatory responses but could also directly compete with the nutrient absorption in the host. The result published by Dumas et al. [3] supports the argument that gut microbiota is able to alter nutrient bioavailability and eventually affect the metabolic phenotypes of mice. So there are quite a few hypotheses ongoing that we are very interested in but we don't have any results.

Dr. Berry: Concerning the lipotoxicity hypothesis in type-2 diabetes or specifically the toxicity of free fatty acids; did you actually measure the plasma concentration of short-chain fatty acids? Did they change during the course of antibiotic exposure?

Dr. Chou: We did not measure the concentration of short-chain fatty acids but we did measure the typical long-chain fatty acids which were not different in the treated ob/ob mice.

Dr. Berry: They are not reduced. You probably have to use a different technique to measure the head space chromatography. Is that something you are planning to do?

Dr. Chou: Yes, we are working with another group in NRC, and we are trying to use metabonomic technology, a proton NMR, to find out the profile of lipids in the liver and plasma.

Dr. Berry: Do you think that the amount of short-chain fatty acids that is being produced could significantly impact plasma levels? I am interested in the short-chain fatty acids as a fuel versus the signaling agents that could produce insulin desensitivity.

Dr. Chou: I talked to a colleague who did a stable isotope tracer study in humans. Short-chain fatty acids, like acetate, contributed about 7% of the whole body energy supply, and 40% of those short-chain fatty acids come from fermentation in the gut [4]. When the calculation is done, about 2.8% of the whole body energy source comes from the acetate produced in the gut. Assuming that an adult consumes 2,400 kcal/day, the contribution of energy from the fermentation in the gut is less than 70 kcal. Given a generous reduction of short-chain fatty acid production by 50% due to the different gut microbiota composition, we are talking about a less than 40 cal/day difference. Does that really mean it will cause obesity? That is questionable.

Dr. Berry: Has anyone infused the short-chain fatty acids to try to induce a state of glucose intolerance in these experimental mice?

Dr. Chou: In the past I did long-chain fatty acid infusion causing insulin resistance, but I have never done a short-chain fatty acid infusion because it is known that long-chain fatty acids induce insulin resistance. But I am not sure about short-chain fatty acid.

Dr. Bier: I don't think acetate is 40% of the energy of the organism. We don't work on acetate, we work on acetyl-CoA. There may be some acetate coming into the gut bacteria, I am just not sure of that. It is a little bit awkward to know what it means when you say acetate is responsible for 40% of the energy because the acetyl moiety comes through oxidation of fat, but it is not really acetate.

Dr. Chou: Actually the study looked at acetate and acetyl-CoA together as a total pool level of acetate. Also the energy contribution of total acetate is 7%, not 40%. 40% of the total acetate pool comes from the gut. So it is a very small amount.

Dr. Bier: Given that this is almost certainly an exploding field, and entirely new methods are being introduced into a field where there are a lot of old methods, and where there are people reporting things in different ways, etc., is there any effort through, for example, Nestlé or Danone or some international organizations to set the rules about how we are going to describe the organisms, the amounts, etc., so that we are all comparing the same things when the studies start being published?

Dr. Chou: I had the same problem when I tried to summarize the literature results; a lot of them cannot be used because of the way the data were presented. I think it requires collaborative efforts from everybody here to promote this idea.

Dr. Bier: The issue of probiotic becomes a problem in a journal unless it is described. I think that the field needs a set of rules and standardization. If it were done with some of the international microbiology societies and the industry or whatever, and a set of rules and descriptions were produced of what actually enhances the publication issues, then I think several journals might be interested in publishing that kind of document or using it as the standard for reporting of things that have to go into those journals. So it seems to me that the time has come to think about these things.

Dr. Salminen: We have discussed a lot about the strain-specific properties of probiotics. It is really our duty and that of any respectable scientific journal to clearly identify the strains used, and use the international culture collection reference numbers and have the strains accessible to researchers. This is the only way that we can actually promote reliable science in probiotics. The same applies in a different way to prebiotics, to actually describe and identify clearly what kind of component is being used.

Dr. Bier: I agree with that, but it seems to me that more is involved: the method, for example, which one, what are the quantities involved, etc. We heard percent colonization yesterday but what fraction of the total of the bacteria; what are the numbers that we need to know to compare studies? I honestly don't know all of them, but having a group who is knowledgeable to set the rules would be very helpful. This is going to grow extraordinarily in the next decades.

Dr. Chou: There is also the issue of how to assess the gut microbiota. Currently several techniques for the assessment of gut microbiota are being developed, such as microarray-based analyses, cloned library sequencing and quantitative PCR. Each technique has its pros and cons. The results will be much clearer after a comparative study using different technologies has been done. Then we can decide on the best technology to go forward.

References

1   Turnbaugh PJ, Ley RE, Mahowald MA, et al: An obesity-associated gut microbiome with increased capacity for energy harvest. Nature 2006;444:1027–1031.
2   Asano T: Modification of cecal size in germfree rats by long-term feeding of anion exchange resin. Am J Physiol 1969;217:911–918.
3   Dumas ME, Barton RH, Toye A, et al: Metabolic profiling reveals a contribution of gut microbiota to fatty liver phenotype in insulin-resistant mice. Proc Natl Acad Sci USA 2006;103: 12511–12516.
4   Pouteau E, Nguyen P, Ballèvre O, Krempf M: Production rates and metabolism of short-chain fatty acids in the colon and whole body using stable isotopes. Proc Nutr Soc 2003;62:87–93.

Bier DM, German JB, Lönnerdal B (eds): Personalized Nutrition for the Diverse Needs of Infants and Children.
Nestlé Nutr Workshop Ser Pediatr Program, vol 62, pp 141–155,
Nestec Ltd., Vevey/S. Karger AG, Basel, © 2008.

Individual Epigenetic Variation: When, Why, and So What?

Marcus V. Gomes, Robert A. Waterland

Departments of Pediatrics and Molecular and Human Genetics, Baylor College of Medicine,
USDA Children's Nutrition Research Center, Houston, TX, USA

Abstract

Epigenetics provides a potential explanation for how environmental factors modify the risk for common diseases among individuals. Interindividual variation in DNA methylation and epigenetic regulation has been reported at specific genomic regions including transposable elements, genomically imprinted genes and the 'inactive' X chromosomes in females. We currently have a very poor understanding of the factors that contribute to interindividual epigenetic variation. In particular, it is important to understand when during the life cycle epigenetic variation arises, why epigenetic regulation varies among individuals, and whether epigenetic interindividuality affects susceptibility to diet-related chronic disease. In this review we will summarize current progress toward answering these questions.

Introduction

In recent decades many people have changed their lifestyles and nutritional habits in the interest of personal health. Whereas general nutrition recommendations like eating a varied diet and maintaining a healthy weight are probably universally beneficial, there is growing interest in tailoring nutrition recommendations to match individual metabolic characteristics. The nascent field of nutrigenomics is based on the assertion that responses to nutrition are dependent on each individual's genotype [1]. Herein we propose that epigenetic interindividuality should also be considered. Just as genetic variation affects nutrient metabolism, so too can epigenetic variation, and recent studies have documented myriad epigenetic differences among individuals. Important questions, however, remain unanswered: When during the life cycle does epigenetic variation arise? What are the factors that contribute to interindividual epigenetic variation? Does epigenetic interindividuality affect susceptibility to diet-related chronic disease? In this review we will summarize current progress toward answering these questions.

Epigenetic Gene Regulation

Epigenetics is the study of mitotically heritable changes in gene expression potential that occur without changing the DNA sequence [2]. Epigenetic regulation enables the developmental acquisition and lifelong maintenance of tissue-specific gene expression, despite continuous cellular turnover and DNA replication. Epigenetic mechanisms include methylation of CpG dinucleotides in DNA, autoregulatory DNA-binding proteins, and various modifications to the histone proteins that package DNA in nuclear chromatin [3].

DNA methylation of cytosine residues within CpG dinucleotides is one of the best characterized epigenetic modifications. DNA methylation is the most stable epigenetic mark, and is often correlated with transcriptional activity [2]. Histone modifications have attracted increasing attention as important epigenetic marks. Their dynamic nature, however, coupled with the lack of a known mechanism for their perpetuation through mitosis, have recently led some leaders in the field to question whether histone modifications are truly epigenetic [4]. A relatively underexplored field is the role of autoregulatory DNA-binding proteins in the maintenance of epigenotype. For these reasons, the bulk of this review focuses on DNA methylation.

DNA methylation is critical for the regulation of embryonic development, cellular differentiation, X chromosome inactivation in females, suppression of transposable elements, and genomic imprinting [2]. The methylation pattern in a specific genomic locus affects gene transcription via direct or indirect interaction with DNA-binding proteins.

Interindividual Variation in Epigenotype

In addition to genotypic variation, epigenetic differences can contribute to stable phenotypic differences among individuals, such as metabolic variation, susceptibility to chronic disease, etc. [5]. Further, the incomplete penetrance of susceptibility genes and variation in phenotype (severity of disease) in genetically predisposed individuals may in part be explained by differences in epigenetic regulation [5]. We currently have a very poor understanding of the factors that contribute to interindividual epigenetic variation. Nonetheless, recent studies have documented substantial interindividual epigenetic variation in humans.

Dramatic interindividual variation in DNA methylation has been reported at specific transposable elements, viral-derived elements scattered throughout the genome [6]. This variation is not inconsequential; transposons, which comprise roughly 45% of the genome, are found in about 4% of human genes [7]. *Alu* elements are short retrotranposons present at over a million copies in the human genome. Investigating the CpG methylation of 19 specific members of *Alu* sub-families in human DNA isolated from whole blood, Sandovici et al. [8] found significant interindividual variation in the level of methylation among 48 three-generation families. Interindividual epigenetic variation at *Alu* elements in the human genome was later confirmed in an epigenomic analysis [9].

Animal models corroborate that specific transposable elements potentiate interindividual epigenetic differences among mammals. Two of the best characterized examples are the agouti viable yellow (A^{vy}) and the axin fused ($Axin^{Fu}$) mice. The murine A^{vy} mutation resulted from transposition of an IAP retrotransposon upstream of the *agouti* gene, which normally regulates the production of yellow pigment in fur. The IAP contains a promoter that drives ectopic agouti expression and variation in CpG methylation of the A^{vy} IAP, causing dramatic variation in coat color and other phenotypes among genetically identical A^{vy}/a mice [10]. Similarly, the $Axin^{Fu}$ mutation resulted from transposition of an IAP into intron 6 of the *Axin* gene, which normally regulates anterior-posterior axial patterning during development. The $Axin^{Fu}$ IAP induces a downstream cryptic promoter which drives the expression of a biologically active 3′ truncated transcript of *Axin*, causing a kinky tail phenotype [11]. Hypermethylation at $Axin^{Fu}$ silences expression from the cryptic promoter, preventing tail kinks.

These vividly illustrative mouse models show that even among genetically identical individuals, dramatic variation in phenotype can occur due to epigenetic variation at specific transposable elements. Rakyan et al. [12] proposed the term 'metastable epialleles' to describe genomic regions at which epigenotype is established probabilistically during development but then maintained stably throughout life. We envision that metastable epialleles likely exist in the human genome, affecting individual susceptibility not to yellow coats or kinky tails, but rather to various chronic diseases.

The human epigenome project is an effort to identify, catalog and interpret genome-wide DNA methylation profiles of all human genes in all major tissues [13]. The pilot project analyzed CpG methylation across the entire human major histocompatibility locus on chromosome 6 in several human tissues from different individuals. Over 100 gene regions displayed a difference of greater than 50% between the lowest and highest methylation values in different individuals [13]. For example, both the *CYP21A2* gene and the gene encoding tumor necrosis factor showed marked interindividual variation (fig. 1). Following up on the success of the human epigenome pilot project, a larger study profiled methylation across most of human chromosomes 6, 20, and 22 [14]. Unfortunately, however, DNA from multiple individuals was pooled for each 'sample' characterized in that study, preventing the analysis of interindividual epigenetic variation.

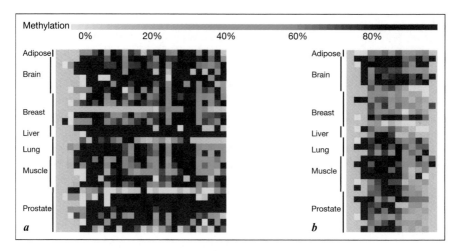

Fig. 1. Interindividual variation in DNA methylation in two human genes. Each column represents a CpG site, and each row a different individual. Colors represent percent methylation and gray boxes indicate missing data. **a** 27 CpG sites within the *CYP21A2* gene. **b** 13 CpG sites within the *tumor necrosis factor* gene. Reprinted from Rakyan et al. [13], with permission.

Interindividual variation in humans has also been found at genomically imprinted genes. Genomic imprinting is an epigenetic phenomenon whereby certain genes are expressed preferentially from either the maternally or paternally inherited allele [15]. At the 11p15.5 human chromosome region, methylation at the paternally inherited allele of the H19 differentially methylated region (H19DMR) contributes to the regulation of monoallelic expression of both the *insulin-like growth factor-2* (*IGF2*) and *H19* genes. Variation of both allelic expression of *IGF2* and methylation at the *H19* DMR has been reported. For example, multiple studies on distinct human populations [16, 17] have found appreciable bi-allelic expression of *IGF2* in about 10% of normal adults. Importantly, this *IGF2* 'loss of imprinting' appears to increase susceptibility to colon cancer [17].

Interindividual variation in humans has also been reported in the epigenetic control of X inactivation [18]. Within each cell, most genes on one of each woman's two X chromosomes are silenced to achieve dosage compensation. However, about 10% of X-linked genes show variable patterns of inactivation and are expressed to different extents from the 'inactive' X chromosome (fig. 2) comprising an additional source of epigenetic heterogeneity specific to females [18].

Studies on monozygous (MZ) twins provide knowledge about both the occurrence and biological consequences of epigenetic variation. Although MZ

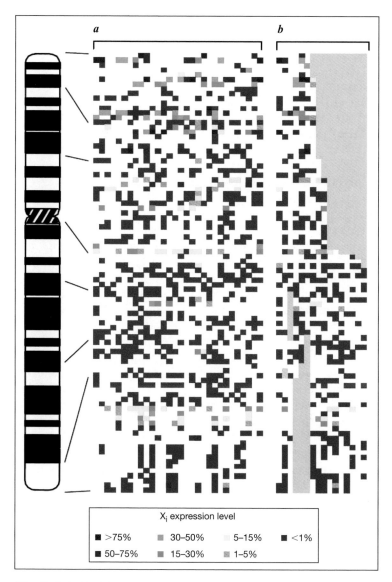

Fig. 2. Individual heterogeneity in gene expression from the 'inactive' X chromosome (X_i) in primary human fibroblasts from normal X_i chromosomes (***a***) and from structurally abnormal X_i chromosomes (***b***). Each column represents a different individual, and each row a different gene. Approximate correspondence to chromosome location is indicated. Colors reflect X_i expression levels and grey boxes (***b***) indicate absent portions of the X chromosome due to deletions or translocations. Clearly, specific X-lined genes show extensive interindividual variation in expression from X_i. Reprinted from Carrel and Willard [18], with permission.

twins are genetically identical, they are often discordant for various diseases such as schizophrenia and bipolar disorder [5]. Interindividual variation in epigenetic marks is a potential candidate to explain the discordances among MZ twins [5]. For example, in MZ twin pairs discordant for Beckwith-Wiedemann syndrome (BWS), a congenital disorder caused by abnormal imprinting at the 11p15.5 chromosomal region, Weksberg et al. [19] showed that only the affected members display abnormal methylation of KvDMR, the CpG island upstream of the imprinted *KCNQ1OT1* gene.

When Do Epigenetic Differences among Individuals Arise?

During embryogenesis, epigenetic reprogramming results in the establishment of diverse patterns of gene expression that characterize the differentiated state of diverse cell and tissue types [20]. Increasingly, data are indicating that this epigenetic reprogramming is not limited to early embryonic development, but continues throughout fetal development and even into early postnatal life. Given that developmental establishment of epigenotype can be influenced by environmental stimuli such as nutrition [21], it is important to determine the critical developmental periods when interindividual variation in epigenetic regulation is first established in humans.

In an extensive epigenomic analysis of MZ twins, Fraga et al. [9] concluded that epigenetic differences among MZ twins are not present during the early years of life, but rather arise in older MZ twins, related to environmental differences and epigenetic changes accumulated with aging. This conclusion, however, was based upon only two pairs of 3-year-old twins! A recent study [14] involving methylation analysis at human chromosomes 6, 20 and 22 in several tissues from two age groups of healthy individuals (one group having a mean age of 26 years and the second 68 years) did not find a significant overall effect of age, in apparent contradiction to the conclusion of Fraga et al. [9].

The data from Weksberg et al. [19] showing divergent methylation patterns at *KCNQ1OT1* in MZ twins discordant for BWS clearly indicates that interindividual epigenetic variation can be established very early in embryonic development. Similarly, Oates et al. [22] reported that discordances for methylation pattern at the promoter region of the *AXIN1* gene are associated with discordances for caudal duplication anomalies in MZ twins aged 7 months.

Data from mouse models indicate that methylation profiles are dynamic and vary during prenatal and/or postnatal life. For example, Weaver et al. [23] documented remarkable developmental changes in methylation at specific CpG sites in the glucocorticoid receptor promoter in the rat hippocampus, during the first few days of postnatal life. Moreover, the level of maternal caregiving during this period permanently changed offspring physiology and behavior by affecting this developmental process.

In addition to the prenatal and early postnatal periods, changes in DNA methylation at specific loci do correlate with age. For example, in human colonic mucosa, aberrant hypermethylation of the estrogen receptor gene increases linearly with age [24]. Analogously, in a study of nutritional effects on epigenetic changes in the post-weaning period, it was shown that developmental changes in allelic methylation at the mouse *Igf2* DMR2 in kidney continue into adulthood [25].

Overall, the data indicate that epigenetic differences among individuals can arise at diverse periods throughout life. Unlike the gradual changes that accumulate with aging, the rapid changes in epigenetic regulation that occur during prenatal and early postnatal development present brief periods during which nutrition and other environmental exposures may wield relatively powerful influence.

What Are the Sources of Interindividual Epigenetic Variation?

Potential sources of interindividual epigenetic variation include environmental factors, genetic inheritance, epigenetic inheritance, and stochastic (random) variation [26].

Among environmental factors, nutrition has been shown to affect the development of epigenotype. The source of one carbon units for biological methylation reactions is S-adenosylmethionine. S-Adenosylmethionine levels are dependent on diet since mammals cannot synthesize sources of one-carbon units such as methionine and choline, or critical cofactors for methyl metabolism such as folic acid and vitamin B_{12}. An unbalance (excess or deficiency) of these critical nutrients may alter the supply of methyl groups [21].

The first direct evidence that maternal nutrition can affect offspring epigenotype was obtained by studies in mouse models. Nutritionally induced changes in the coat color of A^{vy}/a mice were demonstrated to be consequent to an increased methylation at the A^{vy} locus [27]. Additionally, dietary methyl donor deficiency during the post-weaning period causes persistent changes in the allelic expression of *Igf2* in mice [25], showing that the influence of nutrition on epigenetic development is not limited to the prenatal period.

The artificial environment to which the early embryo is exposed during in vitro fertilization might also result in epigenetic defects, and genomically imprinted genes might be especially susceptible [28]. Indeed, a recent study [29] showed aberrant DNA methylation and histone modifications at the *Igf2/H19* imprinted domain in embryonic stem cells derived from in vitro fertilization. The association between assisted reproductive technologies and imprinting alterations in humans provides a foreboding corroboration of the results from mouse studies. Epidemiological studies show a 4- to 9-fold increased risk for BWS in children conceived by assisted reproductive technologies compared to those naturally conceived [30].

Alcohol consumption may also induce epigenetic alterations. Alcohol has an antagonistic effect on folate methyl group metabolism and can negatively affect folate levels, and the folate perturbation affects DNA methylation and DNA synthesis. It was shown in rats that chronic alcohol consumption induces hypomethylation in genomic DNA [31].

Genetic variation among individuals can also contribute to epigenetic variation. Recently, Heijmans et al. [32] investigated the relative contribution of heritable influences versus environmental and stochastic factors in determining DNA methylation at the *IGF2/H19* imprinted domain in 196 adolescent and 176 middle-aged twins. By assessing epigenetic similarity among MZ and dizygotic twin pairs, they estimated heritability of *H19* and *IGF2* methylation. Their data indicate that heritable processes explain most of the variation in epigenotype at the imprinted locus [32]. Polymorphisms in genes affecting one carbon metabolism may influence the establishment of methylation marks and the individual predisposition to epigenetic diseases. Methylenetetrahydrofolate reductase (MTHFR) reduces 5,10-methylenetetrahydrofolate (methylene-THF) to 5-methyl-THF, a fungible methyl donor. A common polymorphism (C677T) in the *MTHFR* gene reduces enzyme activity and is associated with DNA hypomethylation [33].

Lastly, although it has long been assumed that the epigenetic slate is wiped clean in the embryo shortly after fertilization [34], transgenerational inheritance of epigenetic marks does sometimes occur in mammals [35]. Recent studies have suggested epigenetic inheritance of germline epimutation at the promoter region of the DNA repair genes *MLH1* and *MSH2* in individuals with a familial history of cancer [36, 37]. This is an extremely difficult area of study in humans, however, as it may be impossible to distinguish epigenetic inheritance from transgenerational recapitulation of epigenotype associated with genetic inheritance [38].

In addition to environment, genetic and epigenetic inheritance, stochastic processes clearly contribute to individual variation in epigenotype [26]. The many diverse sources of interindividual epigenetic variation will complicate studies aimed at understanding the role of diet in determining epigenotype.

So What? Epigenetics and Human Disease

It is clear that epigenetic dysregulation causes developmental diseases and cancer [39]. The role of epigenetics in the pathogenesis of chronic diet-related diseases such as obesity, cardiovascular disease, and type-2 diabetes, although of major interest [26], is not yet clear. Any disease that can have a genetic basis, however, can equally likely have an epigenetic basis. Studies are currently underway to elucidate epigenetic mechanisms that contribute to the pathogenesis of common diseases, both in animal models and in human studies, for example in MZ twins.

Conclusion

Consideration of interindividual epigenetic variation adds an entirely new level of complexity to the field of nutrigenomics. Whereas genetic variation can influence nutritional requirements, epigenetic variation can both influence nutritional requirements and be induced by nutritional stimuli during critical developmental periods. Moreover, the interaction between epigenetics and nutrition is likely to be affected by genetics. If, as anticipated, epigenetic variation plays an important role in the pathogenesis of diet-related chronic diseases, 'personalized nutrition' may merit especially important consideration during the prenatal and early postnatal periods when nutrition can wield a lasting impact on epigenotype.

Acknowledgements

R.A.W. is supported by NIH grant 5K01DK070007, research grant No. 5-FY05–47 from the March of Dimes Birth Defects Foundation, and USDA CRIS No. 6250–51000–049.

References

1 Stover PJ, Garza C: Nutrition and developmental biology – implications for public health. Nutr Rev 2006;64:S60–S91.
2 Jaenisch R, Bird A: Epigenetic regulation of gene expression: how the genome integrates intrinsic and environmental signals. Nat Genet 2003;33(suppl):245–254.
3 Lande-Diner L, Cedar H: Silence of the genes – mechanisms of long-term repression. Nat Rev Genet 2005;6:648–654.
4 Kouzarides T: Chromatin modifications and their function. Cell 2007;128:693–705.
5 Wong AH, Gottesman II, Petronis A: Phenotypic differences in genetically identical organisms: the epigenetic perspective. Hum Mol Genet 2005;14(Spec No 1):R11–R18.
6 Slotkin RK, Martienssen R: Transposable elements and the epigenetic regulation of the genome. Nat Rev Genet 2007;8:272–285.
7 Nekrutenko A, Li WH: Transposable elements are found in a large number of human protein-coding genes. Trends Genet 2001;17:619–621.
8 Sandovici I, Kassovska-Bratinova S, Loredo-Osti JC, et al: Interindividual variability and parent of origin DNA methylation differences at specific human Alu elements. Hum Mol Genet 2005;14:2135–2143.
9 Fraga MF, Ballestar E, Paz MF, et al: Epigenetic differences arise during the lifetime of monozygotic twins. Proc Natl Acad Sci USA 2005;102:10604–10609.
10 Morgan HD, Sutherland HG, Martin DI, Whitelaw E: Epigenetic inheritance at the agouti locus in the mouse. Nat Genet 1999;23:314–318.
11 Vasicek TJ, Zeng L, Guan XJ, et al: Two dominant mutations in the mouse fused gene are the result of transposon insertions. Genetics 1997;147:777–786.
12 Rakyan VK, Blewitt ME, Druker R, et al: Metastable epialleles in mammals. Trends Genet 2002;18:348–351.
13 Rakyan VK, Hildmann T, Novik KL, et al: DNA methylation profiling of the human major histocompatibility complex: a pilot study for the human epigenome project. PLoS Biol 2004;2: e405.

14 Eckhardt F, Lewin J, Cortese R, et al: DNA methylation profiling of human chromosomes 6, 20 and 22. Nat Genet 2006;38:1378–1385.

15 Reik W, Walter J: Genomic imprinting: parental influence on the genome. Nat Rev Genet 2001;2:21–32.

16 Sakatani T, Wei M, Katoh M, et al: Epigenetic heterogeneity at imprinted loci in normal populations. Biochem Biophys Res Commun 2001;283:1124–1130.

17 Cui H, Cruz-Correa M, Giardiello FM, et al: Loss of IGF2 imprinting: a potential marker of colorectal cancer risk. Science 2003;299:1753–1755.

18 Carrel L, Willard HF: X-inactivation profile reveals extensive variability in X-linked gene expression in females. Nature 2005;434:400–404.

19 Weksberg R, Smith AC, Squire J, Sadowski P: Beckwith-Wiedemann syndrome demonstrates a role for epigenetic control of normal development. Hum Mol Genet 2003;12(Spec No 1): R61–R68.

20 Morgan HD, Santos F, Green K, et al: Epigenetic reprogramming in mammals. Hum Mol Genet 2005;14(Spec No 1):R47–R58.

21 Waterland RA, Jirtle RL: Early nutrition, epigenetic changes at transposons and imprinted genes, and enhanced susceptibility to adult chronic diseases. Nutrition 2004;20:63–68.

22 Oates NA, van Vliet J, Duffy DL, et al: Increased DNA methylation at the AXIN1 gene in a monozygotic twin from a pair discordant for a caudal duplication anomaly. Am J Hum Genet 2006;79:155–162.

23 Weaver IC, Cervoni N, Champagne FA, et al: Epigenetic programming by maternal behavior. Nat Neurosci 2004;7:847–854.

24 Issa JP, Ottaviano YL, Celano P, et al: Methylation of the oestrogen receptor CpG island links ageing and neoplasia in human colon. Nat Genet 1994;7:536–540.

25 Waterland RA, Lin JR, Smith CA, Jirtle RL: Post-weaning diet affects genomic imprinting at the insulin-like growth factor 2 (Igf2) locus. Hum Mol Genet 2006;15:705–716.

26 Waterland RA, Michels KB: Epigenetic epidemiology of the developmental origins hypothesis. Annu Rev Nutr 2007;27:363–388.

27 Waterland RA, Jirtle RL: Transposable elements: targets for early nutritional effects on epigenetic gene regulation. Mol Cell Biol 2003;23:5293–5300.

28 Khosla S, Dean W, Reik W, Feil R: Culture of preimplantation embryos and its long-term effects on gene expression and phenotype. Hum Reprod Update 2001;7:419–427.

29 Li T, Vu TH, Ulaner GA, et al: IVF results in de novo DNA methylation and histone methylation at an Igf2-H19 imprinting epigenetic switch. Mol Hum Reprod 2005;11:631–640.

30 DeBaun MR, Niemitz EL, Feinberg AP: Association of in vitro fertilization with Beckwith-Wiedemann syndrome and epigenetic alterations of LIT1 and H19. Am J Hum Genet 2003;72: 156–160.

31 Choi SW, Stickel F, Baik HW, et al: Chronic alcohol consumption induces genomic but not p53-specific DNA hypomethylation in rat colon. J Nutr 1999;129:1945–1950.

32 Heijmans BT, Kremer D, Tobi EW, et al: Heritable rather than age-related environmental and stochastic factors dominate variation in DNA methylation of the human IGF2/H19 locus. Hum Mol Genet 2007;16:547–554.

33 Castro R, Rivera I, Ravasco P, et al: 5,10-Methylenetetrahydrofolate reductase (MTHFR) 677C→T and 1298A→C mutations are associated with DNA hypomethylation. J Med Genet 2004;41:454–458.

34 Reik W, Dean W, Walter J: Epigenetic reprogramming in mammalian development. Science 2001;293:1089–1093.

35 Chong S, Whitelaw E: Epigenetic germline inheritance. Curr Opin Genet Dev 2004;14: 692–696.

36 Chan TL, Yuen ST, Kong CK, et al: Heritable germline epimutation of MSH2 in a family with hereditary nonpolyposis colorectal cancer. Nat Genet 2006;38:1178–1183.

37 Hitchins MP, Wong JJ, Suthers G, et al: Inheritance of a cancer-associated MLH1 germ-line epimutation. N Engl J Med 2007;356:697–705.

38 Chong S, Youngson NA, Whitelaw E: Heritable germline epimutation is not the same as transgenerational epigenetic inheritance. Nat Genet 2007;39:574–575; author reply 575–576.

39 Egger G, Liang G, Aparicio A, Jones PA: Epigenetics in human disease and prospects for epigenetic therapy. Nature 2004;429:457–463.

Discussion

Dr. Lagercrantz: Can you say anything more about critical windows? Are they due to epigenetic mechanisms or are there special critical windows for epigenetic mechanisms? Is demethylation also important for epigenetic mechanisms?

Dr. Waterland: In terms of the critical windows, certainly various critical windows may be associated with specific developmental periods during which epigenetic mechanisms are being established. But I would like to stress that epigenetic mechanisms are not the only mechanisms that can lead to critical windows of development. For example, yesterday we discussed the hypothalamic development studies of Bouret et al. [1]. I think that work provides a very nice example where, in the mouse at least, there is a postnatal period during which hypothalamic innervation must occur. If it doesn't occur properly during this specific period, the animal is left with a permanent change in its ability to maintain energy homeostasis. So, although people increasingly seem to equate developmental plasticity with epigenetics, that is not appropriate; epigenetic mechanisms are just one potential class of mechanisms that can lead to this type of developmental plasticity. Regarding demethylation, that is one of the things we looked at in our microarray studies and showed that in the postnatal liver there were not only increases in methylation but also genes undergoing demethylation. When we looked at the temporal relationships between methylation and expression, in every case the transcriptional changes preceded methylation changes. So in the case of hypomethylation it appeared that transcription could override methylation and lead to a gene activation, and this activation subsequently led to hypomethylation. I am certainly not saying DNA methylation is not important, but rather that it probably serves to maintain transcriptionally active or inactive states.

Dr. Gluckman: About tissue specificity, you mentioned that it is a very important part of the story. For example, I showed yesterday and in our paradigm, fat and muscle can be seen to move in totally different directions under leptin induction, with PPARα going up with leptin in one and demethylated in the other. So I think that the confusion in experiments is going to be very much driven by the problems of what tissue under what circumstance to look at. Even within tissues I suspect that one needs to look at individual cell types, which is going to make matters even more difficult, which is going to come down to the issues of how we look at individual cells and the methylation patterns in individual cells and whether we can actually use amplification techniques accurately. How do you feel about the use of amplification technology for single cell methylation analysis?

Dr. Waterland: As far as I know that is currently not possible because once the DNA is amplified, all the methylation information is lost. So either some type of methylation-sensitive enzyme digest or bisulfate modification must be done before amplification. As far as starting with DNA from one cell as a template, I think theoretically that may be possible but the tools are certainly not yet available.

Dr. Gluckman: If we just use the example of Weaver et al. [2], just to make the point, how do you think that so much specificity is given on these mechanisms? Weaver's model, your model, our model, all are very gross stimuli whether leptin or your cocktail of methylation donors are given, or whether grooming experiments are done, and yet it all comes down to very few CpG islands, and indeed within one gene in Weaver's case where the 5′ is affected and the 3′ isn't. There is a lot of complexity and we all just say it must be small RNAs or something. Do you have a view on how that specificity of CpG island control is so precisely regulated?

Dr. Waterland: We really don't know how these various environmental stimuli are altering methylation. Even in our mouse studies, in which we are feeding a diet that provides more methyl donors and should lead to hypermethylation by 'mass action', is perhaps not so simple. It may be that the environmental stimuli are inducing transcriptional changes which are then causing secondary changes in methylation. That is very consistent with the results of the study by Weaver et al. [2] in which the one CG site that is affected happens to be within a key transcription factor-binding site.

Dr. Gluckman: In the work we have been doing with Mark Hanson, we found one of the genes that most consistently regulated itself by methylation is *Dnmt1*, which is one of the key enzymes involved in actual methylation. So it does raise the issue of a hierarchy of control where methylation itself has been regulated; there are epigenetic changes in the enzymes actually regulating methylation. While we understand a lot about methylation, we don't actually understand very much about the demethylation pathways. What is the mechanism, because I don't think the demethylase has been unequivocally demonstrated?

Dr. Waterland: That is correct. Several years ago Bhattacharya et al. [3] reportedly identified the demethylase activity, but those results have not been corroborated. In our studies of postnatal hepatic development, when rapid DNA replication is occurring and methylation can be lost passively, demethylation appears to always follow transcriptional activation of a gene. Again, I don't mean to take away from the importance of DNA methylation because I think it serves a critical stabilizing role in the differentiation process.

Dr. Berry: There are a few rare patients with hereditary defects in methionine synthesis or adenosylmethionine production, and I believe there is at least one report. Have you performed a genome-wide analysis to see whether the methylation defects are consistent with your hypothesis? Some patients with a complete absence of 5,10-methylenetetrahydrofolate reductase activity really should be unable to synthesize any S-adenosylmethionine beside what the betaine pathway might afford, although that probably wouldn't be operative as well, so they really should have no methylation present. Have you had a chance to study that?

Dr. Waterland: Don't disregard the betaine-homeocysteine methyltransferase pathway; that can compensate for a methionine synthase deficiency and provide a fungible source of methyl donors.

Dr. Berry: I was actually interested in that as well. It is not clear why the betaine pathway exists in the first place. Is it more important developmentally than in postnatal life when the more traditional methionine pathway would take over?

Dr. Waterland: I don't know if it is possible to say which is more important but I think it is a good example of the redundancy that is built into many of these critical pathways. To address your original question, I don't know of any genome-wide studies looking at methylation changes in individuals with inborn errors; that would be very interesting. What is also interesting is that when people look at global methylation, just taking overall 5-methylcytosine content of the genome in situations where we would expect to see a profound hypomethylation, in several cases just the opposite has been reported. So there appears to be not only redundancy but also compensatory mechanisms that kick in and can lead to counter-intuitive effects.

Dr. Berry: With regard to prenatal methylation, is this a binary process or more of a continuous one? In other words if a methyltransferase is destined to methylate a particular area of DNA, does it or doesn't it happen, or does it happen sometimes in a partial way? For instance, if you need more than one cytosine moiety in an area that can bind to a transcription factor, do they all get methylated to do the job or does it happen where maybe only one or two of a group of four that will necessarily get methylated?

Dr. Waterland: It depends on the specific genomic region you are talking about. For the last decade or so a great deal of attention has been focused on CpG islands, which are CG-rich areas that are often found in the promoter regions of genes. In most cases at CpG islands, you get the kind of all or nothing methylation pattern you are talking about, either you get hypermethylation and silencing or you don't. But increasingly we are finding that also methylation at CpG sites not within CpG islands can also be critical, even at single sites such as found by Weaver et al. [2]. There are other examples where methylation at a single CG site, for example within an intron of a gene, is correlated with expression of that gene.

Dr. Björkstén: I have a philosophical question. We always learned that Darwin was 100% right and Lamarck was 100% wrong. As I understand epigenetics this is not quite the case and this is really a paradigm shift. Lysenko's research in the Soviet Union used to be ridiculed. Today it seems to make slightly more sense based on what we have learned on epigenetics.

Dr. Waterland: I will take your question as an opportunity to comment on Lamarckianism. For anybody who is not familiar with that, the idea is that environmentally induced adaptations can be inherited from one generation to the next. Of course, epigenetic inheritance provides a potential mechanism by which that could occur. We have shown in our studies that the environment in one generation can alter epigenotype; if that information can be conveyed to subsequent generations then you have a mechanism for this adaptive evolution that Lamarck proposed. We actually tested for that type of transgenerational epigenetic inheritance recently [4]. In the A^{vy} model we expected that the effects of diet on epigenetic regulation of A^{vy} would be inherited from one generation to the next and would provide a proof of principle for inheritance of acquired traits. But actually we found that the diet-induced changes at A^{vy} were not inherited. So in the A^{vy} mouse at least, it appears that the germline is protected from environmentally induced changes being transmitted from one generation to the next. But I do agree that this whole area opens up a potential paradigm shift in biology and it might turn out that Lamarck was just a little bit right after all.

Dr. Gluckman: Lamarck is not what we are talking about here. Lamarck was talking about the evolution of acquired characteristics. What Dr. Waterland is showing is inheritance to the environmental memory; the echo of the environment of one generation being transmitted to another. I think it was very unfortunate that Eva Jablonka, who is really the mother of this field in many ways, called her book Neo-Lamarckism and I think it has caused a delay in the understanding of the biology that is involved here. In terms of Lysenko, there is actually a recent paper showing that vernalization does lead to epigenetic changes in some of the genes in maize or corn. Of course that is not really what Lysenko was really doing; he was doing other things which were much more horrible.

Dr. Lau: Some people define the epigenetic code to include more than just DNA methylation, including the histone methylation pattern, etc. How tightly are those two processes co-regulated and, if so, are we missing something if we only look at the DNA methylation pattern?

Dr. Waterland: Epigenetics is not just about DNA methylation. Additional mechanisms including numerous modifications to the histone proteins and various autoregulatory DNA-binding proteins participate in maintaining the overall epigenetic state of a genomic region. Many people would add micro-RNAs to this list of mechanisms because in plants there are a lot of good data indicating a role for micro-RNAs, but that remains unclear in mammals. I certainly don't mean to imply that DNA methylation is the only thing that is important, but what is really nice about DNA methylation is that it is relatively simple to measure; on each allele, a specific CG site is either methylated or it is not. For histone modifications, on the other hand, while it is proposed that there is a histone code, the list of participating modifications just becomes longer and longer every year and the correspondence between a given modification and transcriptional activity becomes less and less clear. Another great advantage of studying DNA methylation is that of all the epigenetic mechanisms it is the most stable, so it has the potential to act as a persistent mechanism that might be able to transduce a memory all the way from infancy or embryonic development into adulthood, unlike histone modifications which are relatively dynamic.

Dr. Adlerberth: Could it be possible that contact with microbes or infectious diseases may have some influence on methylation patterns?

Dr. Waterland: Yes certainly, from almost any perspective imaginable there are interesting questions in developmental biology that now can be viewed from this molecular epigenetic perspective. In fact I have a GI fellow, Richard Kellermayer, who is very interested in exploring the role of epigenetic mechanisms in gut development. He is currently working on characterizing the ontogeny of these processes and examining what types of environmental stimuli during critical periods of development might affect epigenetic outcomes relevant to GI pathology. Just perhaps a closing comment, it is interesting that even though Lamarck is most known for the inheritance of acquired traits, which is his fourth evolutionary law, his first evolutionary law may actually be most relevant today. It says that, 'Life by its own forces tends continually to increase the volume of every body that proposes it, as well as to increase the size of all parts of the body up to a limit which it imposes upon itself'. In the context of the worldwide obesity epidemic, I would say that Lamarck's first law is strikingly prescient.

Dr. Walker: Just to come back to your comment, microbes can ferment undigested oligosaccharides causing short-chain fatty acids to be produced. One fatty acid, butyrate, is thought to cause histone deacetylation which may be a transient phenomenon. This may not be similar to epigenetic changes but I think there may be some associations.

Dr. Waterland: Certainly the histone deacetylase inhibition caused by butyric acid in the gut could lead to changes in transcription and then lead to a more stabilized epigenetic state at a given locus. So yes, the intersection of all these different mechanisms is going to need to be considered.

Dr. Hernell: You talked about those windows and that there is a critical postnatal period, but how long could that period actually be? In the twin studies you also showed that differences can be found later. We know that mutations increase in elderly people. Would it be possible that there is an increase in epigenetic effects in elderly people?

Dr. Waterland: Yes, certainly the aging process is another source of epigenetic variation and the most classic study of that is from Issa et al. [5] back in the 1990s. They showed that the estrogen receptor gene promoter in the colon shows a very nice progression of hypermethylation with age. Hypermethylation of this gene appears to play a role in colon tumorigenesis. So yes, you are correct, aging is certainly another very important factor relating to epigenetic variation and disease.

Dr. Corsello: What is your opinion on the risk of epigenetic variation and abnormalities during assisted reproductive technologies (ARTs), and do you think it should be predicted?

Dr. Waterland: Yes, that is a very important question right now. Increasingly, epidemiological studies are showing that there is a higher incidence of several epigenetically based developmental diseases such as Beckwith-Wiedemann syndrome in individuals who have been conceived by ARTs [6]. These types of outcomes are consistent with studies that have shown that culturing the early embryo in vitro leads to persistent epigenetic changes. So essentially we have underway a huge human experiment on the long-tern effects of ARTs and, alarmingly, these technologies are becoming increasingly popular. While many people say that everything is fine, that obviously there is no big problem, one has to consider that the oldest individual who was conceived by ARTs is only about 30 years old. It is quite possible that these relatively rare early developmental syndromes are only the tip of an iceberg. When these individuals are in their 50s and 60s, we don't know what might happen as far as susceptibility to cancer and other diseases related to epigenetic dysregulation is concerned.

References

1   Bouret SG, Draper SJ, Simerly RB: Trophic action of leptin on hypothalamic neurons that regulate feeding. Science 2004;304:108–110.
2   Weaver IC, Cervoni N, Champagne FA, et al: Epigenetic programming by maternal behavior. Nat Neurosci 2004;7:847–854.
3   Bhattacharya SK, Ramchandani S, Cervoni N, Szyf M: A mammalian protein with specific demethylase activity for mCpG DNA. Nature 1999;397:579–583.
4   Waterland RA, Travisano M, Tahiliani KG: Diet-induced hypermethylation at agouti viable yellow is not inherited transgenerationally through the female. FASEB J 2007;21:3380–3385.
5   Issa JP, Ottaviano YL, Celano P, et al: Methylation of the oestrogen receptor CpG island links ageing and neoplasia in human colon. Nat Genet 1994;7:536–540.
6   Niemitz EL, Feinberg AP: Epigenetics and assisted reproductive technology: a call for investigation. Am J Hum Genet 2004;74:599–609.

Bier DM, German JB, Lönnerdal B (eds): Personalized Nutrition for the Diverse Needs of Infants and Children.
Nestlé Nutr Workshop Ser Pediatr Program, vol 62, pp 157–172,
Nestec Ltd., Vevey/S. Karger AG, Basel, © 2008.

Interaction of Early Infant Feeding, Heredity and Other Environmental Factors as Determinants in the Development of Allergy and Sensitization

Erkki Savilahti

Hospital for Children and Adolescents, University of Helsinki, Helsinki, Finland

Abstract

The role of early infant nutrition in the development of allergic symptoms and allergic sensitization has been disputed for 70 years. Interaction between genetic factors and infant feeding has been limited to studies on parental heredity of allergy and length of breastfeeding, as well as the qualities of breast milk. In the 10 original studies comparing the development of allergic symptoms among children in whom breast-feeding duration was used as a risk factor separately among those with either positive or negative parental heredity for atopy, no definite answer could be found. The effect of early feeding was even changed in both heredity negative and positive groups when looking at symptoms at ages 2 and 5 years. Of 9 possible combinations, 6 were present in the studies, and none in more than 2 studies. For sensitization, long breastfeeding was a risk in 3 of 5 reports if the family history of allergy was positive, and in 2 if negative. Low levels of soluble CD14 and cow's milk-specific IgA antibodies in breast milk may increase an infant's risk of developing allergy.

Introduction

The role of early infant nutrition in the development of allergic symptoms and allergic sensitization has been disputed for 70 years, as cited in a review by Zeiger and Friedman [1] on the issue. Complex properties of breast milk (BM) have developed over thousands of generations to protect the newborn infant from a hostile environment. Major threats to the infant are infections, the weakest point of resistance being the gastrointestinal tract. The need for

157

effective absorption of nutrients makes mechanical defense impossible and only a single epithelial layer separates the contents of the gastrointestinal tract from a well-developed vascular bed in the intestine. The properties of BM have developed in order to offer the newborn infant protection from pathogenic microorganisms in several ways [2]. BM contains factors which in nonspecific ways act as antimicrobial agents, and it contains IgA antibodies to microorganisms the mother has contact with, which effectively reduces intestinal infections even in developed countries [3]. BM also contains IgA antibodies to food proteins and at the same time small amounts of food antigens, but how these relate to the development of immune responses to food antigens is poorly understood. BM contains large amounts of non-digestible oligosaccharides, which are important in selecting the type of commensal microflora in the gut. Intestinal commensal microflora prevents proliferation of pathogenic bacteria and is the most important stimulus for innate immunity, the latter directing the development of specific immune responses. Regulatory and immunomodulatory substances in BM directly affect the development of gut-associated lymphoid tissue, as well as morphologic development of the intestine. Immunomodulation aims to advance non-inflammatory defense as local inflammation in the intestine would weaken absorptive function.

Early Infant Nutrition and Heredity for Allergy

How a mother through this delicate system, in addition to providing complete nutrition, contributes to an infant's immunomodulation and the maturation of its regulatory system and how this relates to the infant's hereditary predisposition for an allergic immune response are mostly unexplored. Interactions between genes and environmental conditions for the development of allergies have been explored since the 1990s and seem to be complicated [4]. The same genotype may lead to either an increased or decreased prevalence of asthma depending on environmental conditions, such as exposure to a high endotoxin concentration during infancy. The interaction between genetic factors and infant feeding has been limited to studies on parental heredity for allergy and the length of breastfeeding (BF), as well as the qualities of BM.

In a nutrition study we noted that allergic symptoms, mostly atopic dermatitis, occurred during the first year of life more frequently among infants who had received exclusive BF for longer than 9 months. According to a questionnaire about symptoms to age 2, a similar number of new symptomatic cases developed in the group that was breastfed for <3.5 months and those breastfed for >9 months. During the first 2 years, among those with a positive family history of allergy (FHA), the length of exclusive BF did not influence the prevalence of allergic symptoms (table 1); while among those without FHA, those with short exclusive BF (<3.5 months) tended to have

Table 1. Allergic symptoms in a population-based cohort at ages 2, 5 and 20 years

Exclusive BF months	Allergic symptoms at age 2 years [3]	
	FHA pos. (n = 70)	FHA neg. (n = 108)
<3.5	3/12 (25%)	1/19* (5%)
3.5–6	3/15 (20%)	4/30 (13%)
>6	13/43 (30%)	12/59 (20%)
>9	4/13 (31%)	5/18* (28%)

Exclusive BF months	Allergic symptoms at age 5 years [5]		Allergic symptoms at age 20 years	
	FHA pos (n = 72)	FHA neg. (n = 88)	FHA pos (n = 67)	FHA neg. (n = 97)
<2	5/14 (36%)	1/14 (7%)	6/12 (50%)	8/15 (53%)
2–6	3/15 (20%)	3/18 (17%)	9/17 (53%)	12/22 (55%)
6–9	8/27 (30%)	6/38 (16%)	18/25 (72%)	17/41 (41%)
>9	9/16 (56%)	5/18 (28%)	8/13 (62%)	7/19 (37%)

BF = Breastfeeding; FHA = family history of allergy.
*p = 0.06 by χ^2 test.

Table 2. Summary of the effect of long vs. short breastfeeding on allergic symptoms in children with or without a family history of allergy (FHA)

FHA positive	FHA negative	Study
↔	↑	Savilahti et al. [3]
↑	↔	Pesonen et al. [5]
↓	↑	Siltanen et al. [6]
↑[a]	↔	Wright et al. [7]
↑	↑	Sears et al. [9]
↓	↓	Oddy et al. [15]
↔	↓	Kull et al. [11]
↔	↑	Miyake et al. [12]
↓	↑	Benn et al. [13]
↔	↓	Obihara et al. [14]

↓ = Significant decrease in allergic symptoms in children who were breastfed long; ↑ = significant increase, ↔ = no significant change in allergic symptoms.
[a]Maternal asthma, paternal asthma did not have an effect.

allergic symptoms less often than those with long exclusive BF (>9 months) [3]. The same group was again studied at ages 5, 11 and 20 years [5]. At age 5 the prevalence of allergic symptoms was highest (41%) among the children who had received exclusive BF over 9 months. The risk for allergic symptoms among those with a positive FHA and exclusive BF for >9 months was 6.1 (95% CI 1.5–24.8; p = 0.01), compared to those with shorter BF (table 2). Among those with a negative FHA the same risk was nonsignificant (1.4; 95% CI 0.3–7.3). At age 20 years, the length of BF had no effect on the prevalence of allergic symptoms either in the whole group or in groups divided according to FHA [5]. Skin prick test (SPT) with 11 most common food and inhalant allergens was done at ages 5, 11 and 20 years. BF length did not have any effect on the prevalence of sensitization to the allergens at any age. In this population-based group, the length of exclusive BF showed different association with allergic symptoms during infancy and childhood. During infancy (to age 2 years) long exclusive BF was associated with an increased incidence of allergic symptoms among those with a negative FHA; it did not affect the incidence among those with a positive FHA [3], while at age 5 years long exclusive BF increased the risk atopic eczema among those with a positive FHA and the effect was nonsignificant among those without FHA. Milk feeding during infancy was not associated with allergic symptoms at age 20 years.

More recently, we looked at the effect of early feeding based on large population of 4,674 children born in 1994–1995, whose early feeding we recorded carefully from birth. We selected 4 groups, 2 with the longest exclusive BF in the cohort with and without a FHA; everyone in these 2 groups had been exclusively breastfed for at least 4 (range 4–6.5) months. The 2 other groups had been given a cow's milk (CM)-based adapted formula already during first 2 weeks of life; again one group with a positive and the other with a negative FHA [6]. These 285 children visited the outpatient clinic at age 4 years and were studied for allergic symptoms and sensitization both by SPT and specific IgE levels. Logistic regression analysis showed a significant interaction between FHA and length of BF to the effect on atopic eczema (p = 0.022) and symptomatic allergy (asthma, allergic rhinitis and atopic eczema; p = 0.006). When children were stratified by FHA, those with a positive FHA and long BF had a significantly lower risk of allergic rhinitis (OR = 0.41; 95% CI 0.18–0.95) for positive SPT to dog and cat and for a high level of cat-specific IgE than those with short BF. In contrast, among those with a negative FHA, long exclusive BF significantly increased the risk of atopic eczema (OR = 2.37; 95% CI 1.03–5.5), for any symptoms of allergy (OR = 2.6; 95% CI 1.2–5.7) and for high (>130 kU/l) total serum IgE. When children were stratified by early feeding pattern, the effect of FHA was a highly significant risk of several allergic symptoms among those with short exclusive BF. For any allergic symptom the OR for FHA-positive children was 6.4 (95% CI 2.9–14) and for any positive SPT 8.3 (95% CI 2.3–30). Among those with long BF, the effect of FHA was weaker and significant only for any positive SPT. We concluded that the interaction between BF and FHA was significant and resulted in a more distinct effect of FHA on children with short BF, whereas long exclusive BF seemed partly to protect children from the allergy-promoting effect of heredity [6].

Wright et al. [7] followed 1,246 children with questionnaires to the age of 13 years. They found that exclusive BF for >4 months was associated with a higher incidence of asthma to age 13 years among those whose mothers had asthma. Among those with short BF asthmatic symptoms were reported by 23.5%, and among those with long BF by 45.9%. Exclusive BF for >4 months in children whose mothers had asthma resulted in a significantly increased odds ratio for asthma (OR 8.7; 95% CI 3.4–22). Maternal asthma in the absence of exclusive BF was associated with a borderline increase in risk (OR 2.1; 95% CI 0.9–5.1). Among those with paternal asthma, the length of BF did not have an effect on the incidence of asthma. Children were classified to atopics and non-atopics on the basis of SPT at age 6 years, the effect of long BF on the incidence of asthma was seen among atopic children.

In the same group, Wright et al. [8] found that total serum IgE levels at ages 6 and 11 years depended on the IgE levels of the mothers and the length of BF. Children of mothers with high IgE levels, those in the highest IgE tertile, who had been exclusively breastfed for 4 months or longer had significantly higher IgE levels at age 6 years than those who had never been breastfed; the difference persisted at age 11 years, but was not significant. In contrast, BF of any duration among those children with mothers in the 2 lower IgE tertiles resulted in lower total IgE levels at ages 6 and 11 years. No data are given on the association of IgE levels and the clinical status of children in the study.

Sears et al. [9] compared 504 children with a total BF of >4 weeks with 533 children with BF of <4 weeks, born in 1972–1973 in New Zealand. Children were assessed at ages 9, 11, 13, 15 and 21 years and sensitization with several allergens was studied by SPT at 13 and 21 years. At age 13 years sensitization to cat, house dust mite, grass and *Alternaria* were significantly more frequent among those with BF than those without BF; at age 21 years the finding was the same. When they looked separately children with and without FHA; BF increased the odds ratios for sensitization to the same degree. Asthma was significantly more frequent at all ages and at the time of the study (age 26 years) among those with longer BF than among those with short BF. The result was the same when only those with airway hyper-responsiveness were compared: risk of having asthma with airway hyper-responsiveness was greater at ages 9, 11, 13, 15, and 21 years among those with BF for >4 weeks than among those with short BF. The effect of BF on asthma was not affected by FHA at 9 years or after. Those with a positive FHA were more often sensitized at 13 and 21 years and more often had asthma at 9 years. BF significantly increased the risk for both sensitization and asthma among the FHA positive and negative groups of the cohort [9].

In a cohort of 1,980 children from western Australia, the risk of childhood asthma increased if exclusive BF was stopped before 4 months (OR 1.28; 95% CI 1.01–1.82). Maternal asthma status did not modify the effect. No evidence of a formal interaction in the logistic regression was found between BF and maternal asthma status for the child's asthma at age 6 years [10].

Kull et al. [11] followed a cohort of 4,089 newborns to age 4 years for the role of BF on the development of asthma and other allergic diseases. They found that BF, both exclusive and partial, was protective against the development of asthma. The prevalence of asthma at the age of 4 years was 9.1% among children who had been exclusively breastfed for <4 months, and 6.4% among those breastfed for >4 months (OR 0.72; 95% CI 0.53–0.97). The effect tended to be stronger in children without FHA; among those without FHA exclusive BF for 4 months or more was associated with an OR of 0.58 (95% CI 0.38–0.88) for asthma relative to those with exclusive BF for <2 months. Among those with FHA, the same OR was 0.73 (95% CI 0.43–1.2). Kull et al. [11] also studied sensitization to air-borne allergens by measuring specific IgE antibodies with a multi-allergen test; sensitization was present in 15%. BF did not have any effect on the rate of sensitization; OR for sensitization of children with long exclusive BF was 0.93 (95% CI 0.7–1.22).

Based on questionnaire, Miyake et al. [12] found that atopic eczema at age 12–15 years was associated with feeding in infancy. The prevalence of wheeze during past 12 months was 6.7%, that of rhinoconjunctivitis 23.9%, and atopic eczema 14.5%. BF in comparison to artificial feeding increased the incidence of eczema significantly (OR 1.56; 95% CI 1.13–2.22). When children were divided according to FHA, only among those with a negative FHA did BF during first 3 months significantly increase the risk when compared to those fed artificially (OR 1.9; 95% CI 1.1–3.6). Among those with positive FHA the OR was 1.4 (95% CI 0.97–2.2).

According to telephone interviews, 1,770 of 15,430 full-term Danish infants (11.5%) had atopic dermatitis at age 18 months [13]. Exclusive BF for at least 4 months did not have an overall effect on the risk of atopic dermatitis occurring between ages 4 and 18 months, but the effect depended on the FHA. If neither parent had allergy, exclusive BF at 4 months of age increased the risk for atopic dermatitis (RR 1.3; 95% CI 1.1–1.6) appearing between ages 4 and 18 months; in contrast if the FHA was strong, both parents and a sibling had allergy, BF was protective (RR 0.7; 95% CI 0.5–1.0).

Among poor urban children in South Africa, Obihara et al. [14] found that long exclusive BF had a protective effect on the development of allergic diseases at age 6–14 years. Among 884 children, altogether 213 had symptoms of allergic diseases. BF protected from allergic symptoms if neither mother nor father had had allergic symptoms, An inverse linear association existed between the prevalence of allergic symptoms and the duration of BF in these groups and the association was significant for hay fever; for asthma or eczema the association was not significant. No association between allergic symptoms and length BF was found among those children with positive FHA [14].

Wegienka et al. [16] examined the prevalence and risk factors for sensitization to inhalant allergens at 6–7 years among 484 children. Children who were breastfed only, regardless of the length of BF, had higher risk (RR 1.5; 95% CI 1.1–2.1) of allergic sensitization than those fed formula only. The risk was greater for children with a mother reporting a history of allergy than for those with a mother without an allergic history, though the confidence intervals overlapped. The effect of infant feeding was effected also by the presence or absence of pets: among those with multiple pets in the household, an elevated risk was not found for any level of BF. Also the birth order modified the risk. Table 3 gives a summary of studies on the association of infant feeding and sensitization in children with and without FHA.

Interaction between Early Infant Nutrition and Other Environmental Factors

Among 7,766 children the prevalence of physician diagnosed asthma between ages 2 months and 6 years was 5.9% [17]. Children breastfed for >4 months regardless of exclusivity, were less likely to be diagnosed with asthma than those fed the shorter duration (hazard ratio 0.61; 95% CI 0.4–0.9). If the household had one or more smoker, the protective effect was striking: the hazard ratio among those breastfed exclusively compared to those never

Table 3. Summary of the effect of long vs. short breastfeeding on sensitization in children with or without a family history of allergy (FHA)

FHA positive	FHA negative	Study
↔	↔	Pesonen et al. [5]
↓	↑	Siltanen et al. [6]
↑a	↓	Wright et al. [8]
↑	↑	Sears et al. [9]
↑	↔	Wegienka et al. [16]

↓ = Significant decrease in sensitization in children who were breastfed long; ↑ = significant increase; ↔ = no significant change in sensitization.
aOn total IgE level.

breastfed was 0.27 (95% CI 0.1–0.99). The authors speculate that BF may reduce the tobacco smoke-related asthma by interfering with the gene–environmental interaction [17].

Interaction between the effect of BF and the level of dichorodiphenyl dicholoroethylene (DDE) was described in 338 children studied at age 7–8 years [18]. BF longer than 12 weeks was protective against asthma; OR 0.3 (95% CI 0.11–0.9) for ever having had asthma. The protective effect became stronger in children with a DDE blood level below the median value, and among those with higher values the protective effect was lost.

Immunologic Factors in Breast Milk and Development of Allergies

Several studies [5, 8, 10] have shown that maternal heredity is a stronger determinant for the development of allergy than paternal heredity. This has given rise to the assumption that BM properties account for this difference. Further, higher concentrations of IL-4, IL-8 and RANTES were found in milks from allergic than non-allergic mothers [19, 20]. The findings of the associations between immunologic factors in BM and the development of allergic symptoms in infants and children are presented in table 4. Findings on both total and antigen-specific IgA antibodies on the development of CM allergy are contradictory. Our recent study shows associations between low IgA CM-specific antibodies and the development of allergies by age 4 years [21].

TGFβs, both 1 and 2, are plentiful in BM. Associations between their levels and the development of allergic symptoms is again contradictory (table 4). TGFβ1 was lower in samples of mothers of infants with IgE-mediated CM allergy than in those from mother of infants with non-IgE-mediated CM

Table 4. Immunologic properties of breast milk and the development of allergies

Breast milk component	Observed effect	No effect
Total IgA	Low Development of cow's milk allergy [26, 27]	Appearance of cow's milk allergy [22]
Specific IgA antibodies	Low Symptoms suggestive of cow's milk allergy [28] Development of cow's milk allergy [27] Sensitization and allergic symptoms at age 4 [21]	Appearance of cow's milk allergy [22]
TGFβ1	Low Development of IgE-mediated cow's milk allergy [22] More frequent wheezing during 1 year [23]	Allergic symptoms and sensitization at age 2 [20] Allergic symptoms or sensitization at age 4 [21]
TGFβ2		Allergic symptoms and sensitization at age 2 [20] Allergic symptoms and sensitization at age 4 [21]
Soluble CD14	Low Eczema by age 6 months [24] Asthma by age 2 among long BF and mothers without atopy [25] Verified atopy at age 4 [21]	

allergy; the levels of controls were between the patient groups and did not differ significantly from either group [22]. Oddy et al. [23] found an inverse relationship between the dose of TGFβ1 infants received in the BM and the percentage of infants with wheezing during first years of life. Böttcher et al. [20] looked for a relation between allergic symptoms and sensitization at age 2 years and the BM content of IgA antibodies, several cytokines, including TGFβ1 and TGFβ2, as well as some chemokines, but found no significant associations. We also did not find any difference between the levels of TGFβ1 or TGFβ2 in colostrum samples of mothers of infants who at age 4 years either had allergic symptoms, were sensitized to common allergens or both, compared to those of mothers of non-allergic children [21]. Soluble CD14, a co-receptor with a Toll-like receptor-4, is also plentiful in BM and colostrum. Its low concentration is associated with the development of eczema by age 6 months [24]. Rothenbacher et al. [25] found an interaction between the length

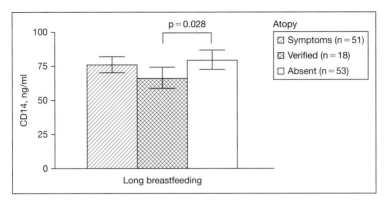

Fig. 1. Geometric mean and 95% confidence interval of the concentration of soluble CD14 (ng/ml) in the colostrum of mothers of children with symptoms of atopy (n = 51), verified atopy (n = 18) and no symptoms (n = 53) at age 4 years.

of BF, a maternal history of atopic disease, and concentrations of soluble CD14 in BM at 6 weeks postpartum and the cumulative incidence of asthma at age 2 years. Among mothers without atopic diseases, a significant negative trend (p = 0.02) existed between the length of BF and the cumulative incidence of asthma by age 2 years. In this group those with mothers with soluble CD14 concentrations below the median tended to have a higher incidence of asthma (21.6%) than those with a higher content (14%; p = 0.07). Rothenbacher et al. [25] concluded that the protective effect of BF seems to be synergistic with soluble CD14 concentrations in BM. We also found that children without atopy at age 4 years who had long BF received BM with a significantly higher soluble CD14 concentration than children with allergic symptoms and sensitization (fig. 1) [21].

Conclusions

Upon examination, the results of the original studies cited do not allow any straight forward conclusions. My idea was that within a single study definitions for BF, for heredity as well as allergic symptoms and sensitization are the same, and the interaction between the factors should not depend on the variability of definitions, ways of diagnosing the diseases and sensitization. If any interaction exists, such studies might be the answer. The cited studies show all types of combinations on the interaction: long vs. short BF being either beneficial, having no effect or being detrimental for the development of allergies or sensitization when combined with the knowledge of parental heredity for allergy. None of the possible 9 combinations is found in more than 2 studies. Complexities of genetic and environmental interactions, together with epigenetic influences, make one think that it is not possible that such a simplified association would exist and as such the above analysis is valid. Further, the content of immunologically active substances in BM varies widely. They again have an independent influence on the development of a child's allergies. Analysis concerning infant nutrition as an environmental factor interacting with the genes needs to be much more focused than the studies published so far. Both the nutrition parameters and the disease endpoints need to be carefully defined, and great care should be taken to have in all other aspects a similar environment for the study population to allow analysis of an interaction with genetic factors.

References

1 Zeiger RS, Friedman NJ: The relationship of breastfeeding to the development of atopic disorders; in Lucas A, Sampson, HA (eds): Primary Prevention by Nutrition Intervention in Infancy and Childhood. Basel, Karger, 2006, pp 93–105.
2 Labbok MH, Clark D, Goldman AS: Breastfeeding: maintaining an irreplaceable immunological resource. Nat Rev Immunol 2004;4:565–572.
3 Savilahti E, Tainio VM, Salmenperä L, et al: Prolonged exclusive breast feeding and heredity as determinants in infantile atopy. Arch Dis Child 1987;62:269–273.
4 Martinez FD: Genes, environments, development and asthma: a reappraisal. Eur Respir J 2007;29:179–184.
5 Pesonen M, Kallio MJ, Ranki A, Siimes MA: Prolonged exclusive breastfeeding is associated with increased atopic dermatitis: a prospective follow-up study of unselected healthy newborns from birth to age 20 years. Clin Exp Allergy 2006;36:1011–1018.
6 Siltanen M, Kajosaari M, Poussa T, et al: A dual long-term effect of breastfeeding on atopy in relation to heredity in children at 4 years of age. Allergy 2003;58:524–530.
7 Wright AL, Holberg CJ, Taussig LM, Martinez FD: Factors influencing the relation of infant feeding to asthma and recurrent wheeze in childhood. Thorax 2001;56:192–197.
8 Wright AL, Sherrill D, Holberg CJ, et al: Breast-feeding, maternal IgE, and total serum IgE in childhood. J Allergy Clin Immunol 1999;104:589–594.
9 Sears MR, Greene JM, Willan AR, et al: Long-term relation between breastfeeding and development of atopy and asthma in children and young adults: a longitudinal study. Lancet 2002;360:901–907.
10 Oddy WH, Peat JK, de Klerk NH: Maternal asthma, infant feeding, and the risk of asthma in childhood. J Allergy Clin Immunol 2002;110:65–67.
11 Kull I, Almqvist C, Lilja G, et al: Breast-feeding reduces the risk of asthma during the first 4 years of life. J Allergy Clin Immunol 2004;114:755–760.
12 Miyake Y, Yura A, Iki M: Breastfeeding and the prevalence of symptoms of allergic disorders in Japanese adolescents. Clin Exp Allergy 2003;33:312–316.
13 Benn CS, Wohlfahrt J, Aaby P, et al: Breastfeeding and risk of atopic dermatitis, by parental history of allergy, during the first 18 months of life. Am J Epidemiol 2004;160:217–223.
14 Obihara CC, Marais BJ, Gie RP, et al: The association of prolonged breastfeeding and allergic disease in poor urban children. Eur Respir J 2005;25:970–977.
15 Oddy WH, de Klerk NH, Sly PD, Holt PG: The effects of respiratory infections, atopy, and breastfeeding on childhood asthma. Eur Respir J 2002;19:899–905.
16 Wegienka G, Ownby DR, Havstad S, et al: Breastfeeding history and childhood allergic status in a prospective birth cohort. Ann Allergy Asthma Immunol 2006;97:78–83.
17 Chulada PC, Arbes SJ Jr, Dunson D, Zeldin DC: Breast-feeding and the prevalence of asthma and wheeze in children: analyses from the Third National Health and Nutrition Examination Survey, 1988–1994. J Allergy Clin Immunol 2003;111:328–336.

18 Karmaus W, Davis S, Chen Q, et al: Atopic manifestations, breast-feeding protection and the adverse effect of DDE. Paediatr Perinat Epidemiol 2003;17:212–220.
19 Böttcher MF, Jenmalm MC, Garofalo RP, Björkstén B: Cytokines in breast milk from allergic and nonallergic mothers. Pediatr Res 2000;47:157–162.
20 Böttcher MF, Jenmalm MC, Björkstén B: Cytokine, chemokine and secretory IgA levels in human milk in relation to atopic disease and IgA production in infants. Pediatr Allergy Immunol 2003;14:35–41.
21 Savilahti E, Siltanen M, Kajosaari M, et al: IgA antibodies, TGF-beta1 and -beta2, and soluble CD14 in the colostrum and development of atopy by age 4. Pediatr Res 2005;58:1300–1305.
22 Saarinen KM, Vaarala O, Klemetti P, Savilahti E: Transforming growth factor-β1 in mothers' colostrum and immune responses to cows' milk proteins in infants with cows' milk allergy. J Allergy Clin Immunol 1999;104:1093–1098.
23 Oddy WH, Halonen M, Martinez FD, et al: TGF-beta in human milk is associated with wheeze in infancy. J Allergy Clin Immunol 2003;112:723–728.
24 Jones CA, Holloway JA, Popplewell EJ, et al: Reduced soluble CD14 levels in amniotic fluid and breast milk are associated with the subsequent development of atopy, eczema, or both. J Allergy Clin Immunol 2002;109:858–866.
25 Rothenbacher D, Weyermann M, Beermann C, Brenner H: Breastfeeding, soluble CD14 concentration in breast milk and risk of atopic dermatitis and asthma in early childhood: birth cohort study. Clin Exp Allergy 2005;35:1014–1021.
26 Savilahti E, Tainio VM, Salmenperä L, et al: Low colostral IgA associated with cow's milk allergy. Acta Paediatr Scand 1991;80:1207–1213.
27 Järvinen KM, Laine ST, Järvenpää AL, Suomalainen HK: Does low IgA in human milk predispose the infant to development of cow's milk allergy? Pediatr Res 2000;48:457–462.
28 Machtinger S, Moss R: Cow's milk allergy in breast-fed infants: the role of allergen and maternal secretory IgA antibody. J Allergy Clin Immunol 1986;77:341–347.

Discussion

Dr. Nassar: We did similar work in Egypt and found that maternal diet is the most determinant factor in early infant sensitization since the mothers who received cow's milk were the ones who had sensitized children regardless of the family history of allergy [1]. In your study and in the other studies you mentioned, was maternal nutrition taken into consideration as a risk factor for early sensitization?

Dr. Savilahti: There are several Swedish studies looking at this question of eliminating certain factors from the mother's diet. I think that Dr. Björkstén may be better able to comment on these studies which did not find any effect when eliminating at least certain factors from the mother's diet. I don't have any personal experience on this matter but the general opinion is that it doesn't have an effect on the development of allergy.

Dr. Björkstén: Could I comment on that since we studied this in Sweden. Elimination of all fish, egg and milk products from the maternal diet during the last trimester of pregnancy had no protective effect. In contrast, there were 5 of about 200 children who still retained their clinically relevant cow's milk allergy at the age of 5 years. As fetuses all these 5 children had been subject to the maternal avoidance diet and not been exposed to milk. In another study we actually looked at the same elimination diet but starting after birth and continuing through the first 3 months of lactation. Babies in the avoidance diet group were not sensitized at 3 months, but when milk was then introduced the first positive skin prick test appeared within 2 weeks and there was no maternal effect on the clinical outcome with time. So we concluded that it is clearly not worthwhile to manipulate the diet either during pregnancy or lactation.

Dr. Prescott: I agree that there is certainly no doubt about the benefits of breast-feeding but it seems, as Dr. Björkstén pointed out, that there is increasing controversy over whether this should be exclusive and when solids should be introduced. Certainly based on animal studies there is a growing school of thought that in fact earlier and regular exposure to allergens may actually be protective as this may promote tolerance and prevent sensitization. The fact that we have been recommending avoidance and delayed feeding for many years may actually be doing our patients a disservice. Would you care to comment on that?

Dr. Savilahti: I quite agree that it might be the right direction. Breastfeeding is good and the best nutrition for the newborn but I don't think that allergy as such should be used as an argument to promote breastfeeding because, as you said, we don't actually know how it should be done, whether certain nutrients should be introduced earlier and at what age. There is a lot of work to be done before we will know this.

Dr. Walker: My question is similar to what Dr. Prescott asked. Have you compared infants exposed to formula versus breast milk as opposed to hydrolysate? How would it stand up if you compared hydrolyzed formula in allergy-prone infants initially versus breastfeeding?

Dr. Savilahti: Yes, many intervention studies have been done and work on much the same level, as has been summarized for instance in the review by Zeiger et al. [2]. It is an effective intervention but I don't think it could be used on a population basis, only in selective cases. But again, we don't really know what happens in the long run in those children who have been on the hydrolyzed formula because, as Dr. Prescott pointed out, we also need stimulation of the immune system by foreign antigens, which might be important for the development and balance of the immune system. There are so many unknown questions, and there may be some danger if we eliminate everything for a very long time from the intestine, we don't really know what happens, and that is the difficulty.

Dr. Koletzko: A comment in response to the point that Dr. Prescott raised: I could not agree more with your conclusion. The Committee of Nutrition of ESPGAN has recently reviewed the evidence on complementary feeding, time of introduction and choice of products, and has written a comment which is to be published in the *Journal of Pediatric Gastroenterology and Nutrition.* It is looking not only at allergy but also many other aspects, also considering the data available on allergy. The conclusion was that the interaction of complementary feeding in the European setting, where there is little risk of infections from early introduction, should occur between 17 and 26 weeks and not only from the first day of the 7th month onward. With respect to your review of these numerous data in which you point out that apparently there is an effect of family history and genetics, even though it is difficult to interpret exactly, the question is what information is available on infection as a confounder? Obviously we are all impressed by the hygiene hypothesis identifying early infections and the exposure to infectious agents as a strong predictor of later allergy risk. There are numerous data showing that breastfeeding reduces the risk particularly of gastrointestinal infections. The recent reviews of WHO, the Dutch State Institute of Population Health and the US Agency of Healthcare and Quality have shown a very strong reduction in diarrhea with breastfeeding, but it is not the same in all populations. Is there any information to identify to which extent that might be a relevant interaction for allergy?

Dr. Savilahti: There are very extensive data available on that question. I am not an expert, but certainly infections cannot be taken as one entity. There are several specific infections which increase the rate of allergies, some are viral infections, and then there are some viral infections which are associated with a decreased prevalence of allergies. This is a very complicated question and I am not really an expert, but certainly it is an important cofactor, probably more important than feeding itself.

169

Dr. Koletzko: Couldn't one assume that this interaction would be different in various populations? For instance in a country like Finland where the risk of early infection is rather low, one might assume that the interaction between breastfeeding, infection and allergy is different than in a country where infection reduction by breastfeeding is very strong?

Dr. Savilahti: Yes, you are quite right; it is really what I was trying to look at in these papers, but it is usually not taken as a confounding factor in the studies. This neglect is one reason why these studies are so conflicting; so much data and knowledge are missing on the other environmental factors which might be important in this development. I am saying that diet per se is not important, but it might be associated with some factors that haven't been described in these studies.

Dr. Björkstén: We heard yesterday that the gut flora is not that different between breastfed babies and babies fed a modern formula. As some of you might remember, in the 1950s and 1960s when the first-born infants received formula, their stools looked and smelled like adult feces. This may explain why we do not see any differences in allergy development between breastfed babies and infants fed a modern formula. You have a point regarding the gut microbiota in that way. On the other hand, I question that respiratory infections could play any significant role in this context because they do cause wheezing and they do not affect allergy atopy or sensitization. I suggest that one should look along your lines, but rather at the gut microbiota.

Dr. Strandvik: It is perhaps a little dangerous for me to disagree with two authorities like Dr. Savilahti and Dr. Björkstén, but I am very surprised that they say that the diet has no influence. I am sure it has, but we have not yet studied all the components which could be of importance. Is there a difference in parity; is allergy more common in siblings or in the first child? Has anyone looked at that?

Dr. Savilahti: To answer your first question it was actually the basis for the hygiene hypothesis by Strachan [3] in 1989. In one of the first studies, he found that allergies were more common in older siblings, in the first child. Dr. Björkstén has published data on that.

Dr. Strandvik: One very important thing is that we haven't looked at the ratio of the essential fatty acids in breast milk and it varies a lot, and with time. In long-term breastfeeding, the ratio between n-6 and n-3 changes remarkably in the infants [4]. We have also done studies in rats [5, 6] showing that both the amount of essential fatty acids in the rat mothers' diet and the ratio between n-6 and n-3 have a profound influence on the development of oral tolerance and also the development of IgE antibodies in the pups. So I would say that when we study the diet and say how much fish we eat, we don't take into consideration how much vegetable oil is ingested at the same time, because this ratio is probably more important for the immunological system, i.e. whether it will have Th1 or Th2 dominance. Please don't say that this has no influence. We need to study the relation between the fatty acid content of the mothers' breast milk and the development of allergy before we can say this.

Dr. Björkstén: We have shown that a low n-3 to n-6 ratio in colostrum and early milk is associated with an increased risk of allergy in children. The same person who did these studies in my laboratory is now doing a placebo-controlled intervention study with PUFA. The data are not available yet but the 6-month data are extremely encouraging.

Dr. Venter: Some of the children in your study were exclusively breastfed for longer than 9 months. How did you define exclusive breastfeeding?

Dr. Savilahti: They were allowed to have water and vitamin D supplementation. There were also some infants who had extended exclusive breastfeeding up to 12 months of age.

Dr. Venter: Does that actually mean that there were some infants who had no solids introduced into their diets up to the age of 12 months, or was that breastfeeding plus solid food?

Dr. Savilahti: No, only breastfeeding.

Dr. Lönnerdal: I am not an expert on allergy but I would like to share an observation with you because I think that breastfed groups may not be as homogenous as many believe. We did a study a few years ago which unfortunately has not yet been published. For those of you in the allergy field I am sure you remember the publications on cow's milk proteins appearing in breast milk. We followed up on those observations and developed sensitive assays for bovine β-lactoglobulin and bovine α-casein. We followed 30 women and looked at the penetrance of the cow's milk antigens into the breast milk. There were 'penetrators' or 'non-penetrators', and there was no correlation between the two proteins. Of these 30 women, 15 had the cow's milk antigens in their breast milk, and 15 had not. When we put the women with antigens in their milk on a cow's milk elimination diet, the concentrations of antigens went down but the rate of that varied a lot individually. As a biochemist and biologist, I have a hard time understanding how these antigens penetrate into the breast milk but there was no doubt that cow's milk proteins were in the breast milk of some women but not all and, depending on the exclusively breastfed population, some breastfed infants may be exposed to cow's milk proteins which may be a confounder in the interpretation of the results.

Dr. Savilahti: Certainly it is a well-known phenomenon that breast milk contains these antigens and it is probably also very important for the development of the response to food antigens that they are there because they are complexed IgA antibodies. It may be that nature has thought that they should be in connection with the mother's breast milk antibodies. This is a phenomenon which we probably see for all antigens. More recently there has been much data importantly showing that these food antigens might penetrate the skin or may be inhaled. There are many ways in which infants can probably come in contact with these foreign antigens; not only the food eaten. But I think that in breast milk they are meant to be there for the development of the immune response of the infants.

Dr. Björkstén: Breast milk was designed by evolution for very particular reasons. Allergy and diabetes were not among those. Mothers are extremely prone to guilt feelings. If the child develops an allergy, the mother will blame herself for not having breastfed or for not doing it long enough. We have an obligation to be very careful with advice that would add to those guilt feelings. The fact is that breastfeeding does not prevent allergy, although it modestly reduces infant wheezing.

Dr. Salminen: I couldn't agree more with your statement on the fat side because it is also very important to look at the microbiota in early colonization. The mother's breast milk fatty acid composition has a profound effect on what kind of microbes actually enter and adhere to the newborn intestine and you see very quickly that the diet is reflected in the breast milk fatty acid composition. I think it is one of the important factors that has been neglected.

Dr. Adlerberth: I would like to come back to the role of the intestinal flora and I want to point out that, although the differences in the intestinal microbiota between breastfed and bottle-fed infants are not so big today, there is a tremendous difference with regard to how these bacteria are encountered by breastfed and bottle-fed infants. If an infant is breastfed, it will have enormous amounts of secretory IgA present in the gut which will prevent bacteria from translocating over the epithelium and coming in contact with the immune system. That is a main function of breast milk, to protect the infant from microbes, and breastfeeding efficiently protects from septicemia and other infections. However, according to the hygiene hypothesis, microbial stimulation might protect from allergy, and then breastfeeding could actually be a risk factor for allergy as it prevents translocation of intestinal bacteria. At the same time breast milk contain numerous factors which could possibly influence maturation of the immune system and in that way breastfeeding could be protective.

Savilahti

Dr. Savilahti: I quite agree that it is really important for the defense against these pathogens in the intestine, that is the main function of these protective factors, it is not against allergy.

Dr. Björkstén: As one of the few allergy-trained people here, there are two things that our fellow allergists may be saying. One is that sensitization is a risk factor because when there is an immune response then tolerance is induced. A positive prick test in early infancy is only showing an immune response, and from that point, avoidance is not always necessary.

References

1   Nassar M: Different infant feeding patterns in the first 6 months of life and predictability of early atopy. Egypt J Pediatr 2006;23:403–418.
2   Zeiger RS, Heller S, Mellon M, et al: Effectiveness of dietary manipulation in the prevention of food allergy in infants. J Allergy Clin Immunol 1986;78:224–238.
3   Strachan DP: Hay fever, hygiene, and household size. BMJ 1989;299:1259–1260.
4   Peng YM, Zhang TY, Wang Q, et al: Fatty acid composition in breast milk and serum phospholipids of healthy term Chinese infants during first 6 weeks of life. Acta Paediatr 2007;96: 1640–1645.
5   Korotkova M, Telemo E, Yamashiro Y, et al: The ratio of n-6 to n-3 fatty acids in maternal diet influences the induction of neonatal immunological tolerance to ovalbumin. Clin Exp Immunol 2004;137:237–244.
6   Korotkova M, Telemo E, Hanson LA, Strandvik B: Modulation of neonatal immunological tolerance to ovalbumin by maternal essential fatty acid intake. Pediatr Allergy Immunol 2004;15: 112–122.

Bier DM, German JB, Lönnerdal B (eds): Personalized Nutrition for the Diverse Needs of Infants and Children.
Nestlé Nutr Workshop Ser Pediatr Program, vol 62, pp 173–188,
Nestec Ltd., Vevey/S. Karger AG, Basel, © 2008.

Personalized Care of Pediatric Cancer Patients

Karen Rabin, Tsz-Kwong Man, Ching C. Lau

Texas Children's Cancer Center, Baylor College of Medicine, Houston, TX, USA

Abstract

One of the great success stories of clinical oncology is the improvement in the cure rates of pediatric acute lymphoblastic leukemia (ALL) from around 10% in the 1960s to nearly 90% today. The primary factor responsible for this remarkable improvement is the personalization of treatment, with stratification of patients based on both disease and host characteristics in order to optimize therapy. While age, WBC, and immunophenotype provide a rudimentary system for classification of ALL, molecular factors are playing an increasingly important role in further individualization of ALL therapy. Such risk-based stratification strategies are also increasingly being used in the treatment of children with solid tumors. In addition, genomic technologies are now being used to identify new molecular markers or signatures for both diagnostic and prognostic purposes. Recently we reported the analysis of pediatric osteosarcoma by expression profiling in an attempt to identify a molecular signature that could predict the chemoresistance of a tumor before treatment is initiated. We identified a 45-gene signature that discriminates between good and poor responders to chemotherapy in osteosarcoma. Using this classifier, we can predict with 100% accuracy the chemoresponse of osteosarcoma patients prior to the initiation of treatment. These encouraging results suggest that the genomic approach will revolutionize the diagnosis and prognosis of pediatric cancer patients and improve their outcome through predictive, personalized care.

Introduction

It has always been the goal in oncology to customize therapy for cancer patients in order to optimize long-term survival while minimizing the side effects of therapy. This is particularly important in the treatment of children with cancer because the potential side effects of therapy on the rest of the patient's rapidly growing body could be unacceptable or irreversible. Such personalization of treatment is usually based on the assessment of the aggressiveness of the cancer as well as the potential response of the cancer and the rest of the body to treatment. The former assessment is traditionally based on the extent of the spread of the disease at diagnosis as well as histologic subtypes within the same diagnostic group that are associated with poor outcome. The latter assessment is based on our previous observations of the response of a particular cancer type to standard therapy and the severity of toxicity patients had experienced. However, it has been difficult to predict the response to treatment or the side effects in a particular patient before therapy is initiated. Here, we will use pediatric acute lymphoblastic leukemia (ALL) and osteosarcoma to highlight the impact of personalized treatment in the clinical outcome of patients, and to illustrate how we have begun to augment the risk assessment of cancer patients by including novel molecular signatures identified by genomic technologies.

Acute Lymphoblastic Leukemia

ALL is the most common childhood cancer, with a peak incidence between 2 and 5 years of 4–5 per 100,000. Treatment of pediatric ALL is one of the great success stories of clinical oncology over the past several decades. ALL was a generally fatal diagnosis in the 1960s, with cure rates around 10%. In the decades that followed, the cure rate has steadily risen and today is approaching 90% [1]. One of the primary factors responsible for this remarkable improvement is the personalization of treatment, with stratification of patients based on both host and disease characteristics in order to optimize therapy (table 1).

Initial Classification

The cornerstone of ALL therapy is stratification of patients into different risk groups based on a combination of clinical, laboratory, and molecular features, so that the type and intensity of therapy may be tailored appropriately. The initial classification as high versus standard risk is made on the basis of age and initial white blood count (WBC), two powerful and independent prognostic factors. High risk is defined by age <1 or >10 years, and/or initial WBC $>50,000/\mu l$ [2]. Immunophenotype also plays an important role in determining the choice of therapeutic regimen: T-cell ALL regimens differ somewhat from B-precursor ALL regimens based on the differential chemosensitivity of T-lineage lymphoblasts. Mature B-cell (Burkitt's) leukemia therapy is unique in its short duration and high intensity, tailored to the unique, aggressive biologic features of this subtype.

While age, WBC, and immunophenotype provide a rudimentary system for categorization of ALL, numerous other factors are playing an increasingly important role in further individualization of ALL therapy.

Table 1. Factors with potential influence on ALL therapy

Disease factors
  At diagnosis
    Initial white blood count (WBC)
    Immunophenotype
    Molecular genetics
    Gene expression profiling
  Response to therapy
    Marrow morphology
    Marrow minimal residual disease (MRD)
    Gene expression profiling
Host factors
    Age
    Gender
    Race
    Down syndrome
    Gene polymorphisms

Disease Factors

Molecular Genetics

An understanding of molecular genetics has played a key role in optimizing therapy in pediatric ALL, defining low-risk subgroups which can be spared unnecessary toxicity, and high-risk subgroups which require more intensive therapy to increase the likelihood of cure. Approximately 75% of pediatric ALL cases bear a recurrent chromosomal abnormality with known prognostic relevance [3].

Abnormalities of Chromosome Number (Ploidy)

Hyperdiploid cases, with more than 46 chromosomes, constitute about 35% of pediatric ALL. Hyperdiploidy has an independent positive prognostic value, which was recently recognized as being attributable to specific trisomies, with the most favorable being chromosomes 4, 10, and 17, and not simply total chromosome number [4]. Hypodiploid cases, with fewer than 45 chromosomes, have significantly worse outcome than diploid or hyperdiploid ALL, with the worst outcome in near-haploid cases (24–28 chromosomes).

Abnormalities of Chromosome Structure in ALL

Chromosomal translocations are a cardinal feature of ALL. Most often the translocation brings a proto-oncogene into proximity with a T-cell receptor or immunoglobulin locus, causing overexpression of the intact gene; or genes at the translocation breakpoints, often transcription factors, may fuse to form a

175

Table 2. Common chromosomal abnormalities in pediatric ALL

Chromosomal abnormality	Genes involved	Frequency (%)	Prognostic impact
t(12;21)(p13;q22)	TEL-AML1	25	Favorable
9p21 deletion	p15, p16	10	Uncertain
t(4;11)(q21;q23)	MLL-AF4	8	Poor
t(1;19)(q23;p13)	E2A-PBX1	6	Formerly poor; negated by intensive therapy
t(9;22)(q34;q11)	BCR-ABL	3	Poor
t(8;14)(q24;q32)	MYC, IgH	2	Poor; partly negated by Burkitt's-directed therapy

new, chimeric protein with oncogenic effects [5]. The most common prognostically significant chromosomal translocations associated with pediatric ALL are listed in table 2.

The TEL-AML1 fusion protein formed by the t(12;21)(p13;q22) translocation occurs in approximately 25% of childhood ALL, making it the most frequent abnormality in childhood ALL. TEL-AML1 is generally associated with a more favorable prognosis, although late relapses are relatively frequent. However, relapsed TEL-AML1+ ALL generally demonstrates an excellent chemosensitivity and salvage rate.

The E2A-PBX1 fusion protein, associated with the t(1;19)(q23;p13) translocation, is the second most common translocation in pediatric ALL, occurring in approximately 6% of pediatric pre-B ALL. The E2A-PBX1 fusion protein tends to be associated with other known high-risk factors. In early studies it was found to have an independent adverse prognostic impact, but on modern intensive treatment regimens, survival is equivalent.

The t(9;22) translocation, known as the Philadelphia chromosome (Ph), is an essential criterion in the diagnosis of chronic myeloid leukemia (CML) and the most frequent abnormality in adult ALL, but occurs in only about 3% of pediatric ALL. Ph is an adverse prognostic marker, with significantly lower induction rates, more frequent and earlier relapse, and poorer overall survival. Allogeneic stem cell transplant has generally been regarded as the only curative therapy, and is generally recommended in first complete remission. Treatment of CML and Ph+ ALL was revolutionized by the advent of imatinib mesylate, also known as Gleevec, in 2001 [6]. Imatinib, a selective tyrosine kinase inhibitor, was the first molecularly targeted therapy to attain large-scale clinical success, fulfilling the goals of antitumor selectivity and low systemic toxicity. Despite its success, it has not been effective as a single agent due to the rapid development of resistance, and allogeneic stem cell transplant in first complete remission remains the optimal curative therapy.

MLL gene rearrangements occur in 8% of pediatric ALL and 60–70% of infant ALL. Over 40 MLL fusion partners have been identified, but the MLL-AF4 fusion formed by t(4;11) is the most common in ALL. MLL rearrangement in infant ALL is a poor prognostic factor, associated with frequent early relapse. Gene expression studies have revealed that the receptor tyrosine kinase FLT3 is highly expressed in MLL-rearranged ALL, and targeted FLT3 inhibitor therapy for MLL-rearranged ALL is an area of active investigation [7, 8].

The t(8;14)(q24;q32) translocation places the c-MYC oncogene under control of the immunoglobulin heavy chain promoter, resulting in constitutive c-MYC overexpression. MYC dysregulation is an essential feature of mature B cell, also known as Burkitt's lymphoma and leukemia. Outcomes have markedly improved since the recognition that this molecular abnormality defines a group of diseases that require specific, short and highly intensive chemotherapy [9, 10].

Microarray-based analysis of gene expression patterns is emerging as an additional powerful tool for defining ALL subgroups. Expression arrays have identified highly overexpressed genes which are candidate targets for development of new therapies, such as FLT3 in MLL [7]. Microarray analysis has also characterized gene expression changes in response to particular chemotherapeutic agents [11, 12] and identified expression patterns associated with chemotherapy sensitivity versus resistance [13].

Response to Therapy

Early response to therapy is a powerful, independent predictor of prognosis, and is used on many current protocols as a determinant of subsequent therapy. Response to therapy is assessed both by marrow morphology, typically after 1–2 weeks of induction therapy, and by minimal residual disease (MRD) assessment, typically at the conclusion of the month-long induction regimen. MRD, based on flow cytometry or PCR-based assays, is far more sensitive than morphology and has been shown to identify patients at risk of ultimate morphologic relapse [14]. Conversely, rapid achievement of MRD negativity before the end of induction identifies a favorable prognosis group with a high probability of cure, who might be spared the adverse effects of high-intensity regimens.

Host Factors

Gender is a basic host factor long recognized as affecting prognosis, with males having a survival disadvantage, at least in part due to the testicles being a sanctuary site to chemotherapy and therefore a frequent site of relapse. In the current US Children's Oncology Group protocol, males are treated for a full year longer than females to compensate for the gender discrepancy in prognosis.

Race also has an impact on prognosis, with African-Americans and, to a lesser extent, Hispanics doing somewhat more poorly than Caucasians [15]. This appears to be due in part to more frequent high-risk molecular and clinical features, and less frequent low-risk features among these ethnicities. However, even within each risk category, African-Americans and Hispanics seem to do somewhat more poorly.

Pharmacogenetic factors are increasingly recognized as important determinants of prognosis in oncology. A prime example is the effect of host polymorphisms in thiopurine methyltransferase (TPMT), a key enzyme involved in inactivation of mercaptopurine, a mainstay of ALL maintenance chemotherapy [16]. Several gene polymorphisms cause decreased TPMT activity and hence increased exposure to active drug, which leads to both a greater antileukemic effect and greater systemic toxicity, including myelosuppression and increased long-term risk of second malignancy. It is now standard practice to perform TPMT genotyping either in all patients prior to therapy, or in those patients exhibiting severe myelosuppression, to identify those who require mercaptopurine dose modification.

Patients with Down syndrome constitute another group in which pharmacogenetic factors play an important role in modulating therapy. Methotrexate has long been noted to cause increased toxicity in Down syndrome patients, apparently due to an extra copy of the reduced folate carrier gene on chromosome 21, which is responsible for intracellular transport of methotrexate, leading to higher intracellular methotrexate levels at a given dose level compared to non-Down syndrome patients, and hence increased somatic toxicity. To minimize toxicity, a substantial reduction in methotrexate dosing in Down syndrome patients has been adopted in many current protocols.

Glutathione S-transferases, which inactivate many ALL chemotherapeutic agents, harbor frequent polymorphisms which have also not surprisingly been associated with increases both in chemotherapeutic efficacy and in toxicities such as second malignancies [17]. Polymorphisms in thymidylate synthase, a target of methotrexate, have been associated with an increased risk of relapse. The effects of these gene polymorphisms vary somewhat across studies, suggesting that effects are likely influenced by treatment and other factors.

Osteosarcoma

We have much experience customizing therapy for leukemia patients based on risk assessment as described above. However, such therapeutic strategies have not been as well developed in the treatment of solid tumors until very recently because of the lack of validated prognostic makers. In the past few years, we and others have tested the feasibility of using comprehensive molecular profiling technologies to identify biomarkers for both diagnostic and prognostic purposes. Using osteosarcoma as an example, we will

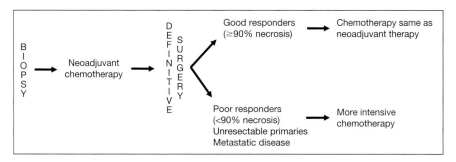

Fig. 1. Treatment scheme for osteosarcoma. All patients with localized disease and good response to preoperative chemotherapy will receive the same chemotherapeutic agents in postoperative chemotherapy. Poor risk patients including the poor responders and those who have unresectable primary tumors or metastatic disease will receive more intensive chemotherapy as postoperative therapy.

illustrate how these biomarkers have been identified and validated. One such application is the use of a multi-gene signature to predict the response to chemotherapy at the time of diagnosis prior to the initiation of therapy.

Osteosarcoma is the most common malignant bone tumor in children and accounts for approximately 60% of malignant bone tumors diagnosed in the first 2 decades of life [18]. After the diagnosis is made by an initial biopsy (IB), standard treatment involves the use of multi-agent chemotherapy, definitive surgery (DS) of the primary tumor, and postoperative chemotherapy (fig. 1). At the time of DS, the resected tumor specimen is assessed for the degree of necrosis which is used to guide the choice of postoperative chemotherapy. The degree of necrosis at the time of DS is a reliable and only significant prognostic factor in patients with non-metastatic disease. Patients whose tumors display ≥90% necrosis (good or favorable response) have an excellent prognosis and continue to receive chemotherapy similar to the preoperative regimen. Patients whose tumors display <90% necrosis (poor or unfavorable response) have a much higher risk of relapse and poor outcome even after complete resection of the primary tumor [19]. To improve the outcome of the poor responders, attempts are usually made to use postoperative chemotherapy regimens that are different from the preoperative regimen by the addition or replacement of a chemotherapeutic agent. In the past such attempts have been unsuccessful [18, 20], partly because the degree of necrosis is known only after 8–10 weeks of preoperative therapy. It is possible that resistant tumor cells have additional time to either metastasize to the lungs or to evolve further during the period when ineffective pre-operative chemotherapy is given. Therefore, at the time of initial diagnosis, there is a need to identify the patients who are likely to have a poor response to standard preoperative therapy and therefore a poor outcome eventually. Therapies tailored to improve the outcome of those patients identified at the time of diagnosis to have a poor outcome can then be instituted at the outset when the chance for success is potentially higher. Although a number of other prognostic factors have been proposed for predicting the long-term outcome of osteosarcoma patients, most are still controversial or have not been tested in large prospective studies [21–28].

Expression Profiling of Osteosarcoma

Recently we reported the analysis of 34 pediatric osteosarcoma samples by expression profiling [29]. With the goal of identifying molecular signatures that can predict the chemoresistance of osteosarcoma, we first attempted to determine the expression profiles of resistant versus sensitive osteosarcoma cells. We hypothesized that the DS samples from the poor responders (PR) should be enriched for resistant tumor cells. Using expression profiles from DS samples would therefore enhance the sensitivity and power to detect the difference between chemosensitive and resistant cell populations as compared to using IB samples in which resistant cells may only be present as a small fraction. Therefore, we predicted that using DS samples would increase the chance of identifying a molecular signature of chemoresistance and, if this signature is valid, it could be used to identify the good responders (GR) and PR in the IB samples. To test this hypothesis, we examined if we could classify GR and PR using DS specimens only. We divided the DS samples from 20 patients into 2 groups, GR (n = 7) and PR (n = 13). We first identified a set of 45 predictor genes that could discriminate the two classes (GR and PR) in the DS samples using a 2-sample t test with a significant cutoff (p = 0.005). Figure 2 shows the relative expressions of these 45 predictor genes in GR and PR. Most of these genes (91%) were overexpressed in PR specimens.

Various supervised classification algorithms, Compound Covariate Predictor, K-Nearest Neighbor, Nearest Centroid, Support Vector Machine (SVM), and Linear Discriminant Analysis,, were then applied to the training set to test if they could classify GR and PR using a p value of 0.005. The Leave-One-Out Cross-Validation (LOOCV) method was used to test the robustness of each classifier in the training set (table 3). The correct classification rates of LOOCV using these algorithms were 65–70%. Among the 6 algorithms, SVM had one of the best performances (70% correct classification). Three GR and three PR were misclassified using SVM. Two of the GR (No. 300 and 394) that were misclassified as PR by the SVM classifier developed recurrent disease 11 and 9 months, respectively, after completion of therapy. This suggests that there may be some residual resistant cells in the DS specimens of these two cases that were recognized by the algorithm based on the predictor gene set. One of the PR (No. 680) that was misclassified as a GR by the SVM classifier remains free of disease after 30 months of follow-up.

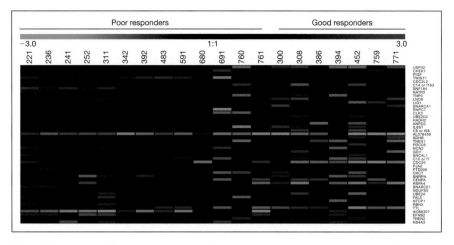

Fig. 2. The 45 predictor genes in the chemoresistance signature were selected based on a 2-sample t test to distinguish between good and poor responders in 20 definitive surgery samples at a p value of 0.005. Forty-one genes were overexpressed in poor responders, while only 4 genes were overexpressed in good responders. The color scale represents log 2 expression ratios of the genes.

The other misclassified PR (No. 761) had 86% necrosis, which is very close to our cutoff for good response.

Use of Multi-Gene Classifier to Predict Response to Preoperative Chemotherapy in IB

To test the SVM classifier, we divided our 14 IB samples into two groups. The first group consisted of six samples, which had corresponding DS samples included in the training set (paired samples). Using these six cases, we attempted to verify that our classifier built from DS samples could predict the chemoresistance of the corresponding IB samples based on the hypothesis that the molecular signature of chemoresistance as recognized in DS samples was already present in the IB at the time of diagnosis. The second group consisted of eight IB samples that did not have matched DS samples included in the training set, thus representing a totally independent set of samples that had not been used to build the classifier.

The SVM classifier misclassified one sample (of 6) in the first group of paired samples, with a correct classification rate of 83% (95% CI 36, 100; table 4). The only misclassified sample was from a patient (No. 410) who was classified as a GR based on histologic response but was predicted to be a PR by the multi-gene classifier. Interestingly, this patient initially presented with localized disease but eventually developed recurrent disease in the lungs 25 months after completion of therapy, suggesting that there were resistant cells

Table 3. Leave one out cross-validation of 20 definitive surgery osteosarcoma samples

Tumor ID	Histologic response	Concordance of classification with histological response					
		CCP	LDA	1-NN	3-NN	NC	SVM
300	GR	No	No	No	No	No	No
308	GR	Yes	Yes	Yes	Yes	Yes	Yes
386	GR	No	No	No	No	No	No
394	GR	No	No	No	No	No	No
452	GR	Yes	Yes	Yes	Yes	Yes	Yes
759	GR	Yes	Yes	Yes	Yes	Yes	Yes
771	GR	Yes	Yes	Yes	Yes	Yes	Yes
221	PR	Yes	Yes	Yes	Yes	Yes	Yes
236	PR	Yes	Yes	Yes	Yes	Yes	Yes
241	PR	Yes	Yes	Yes	Yes	Yes	Yes
252	PR	Yes	Yes	Yes	Yes	Yes	Yes
311	PR	Yes	Yes	Yes	Yes	Yes	Yes
342	PR	Yes	Yes	Yes	Yes	Yes	Yes
392	PR	Yes	Yes	Yes	Yes	Yes	Yes
483	PR	Yes	Yes	Yes	Yes	Yes	Yes
591	PR	Yes	Yes	Yes	Yes	Yes	Yes
680	PR	No	No	No	No	No	No
691	PR	No	No	No	No	No	No
760	PR	No	Yes	Yes	Yes	No	Yes
761	PR	No	No	No	No	No	No
% Correctly classified		65	70	70	70	65	70

CCP = Compound Covariate Predictor; LDA = Linear Discriminant analysis; NN = Nearest Neighbor; NC = Nearest Centroid; SVM = Support Vector Machine; GR = good responders; PR = poor responders; Yes = classification by the algorithm was correct; No = classification was wrong.

present in the IB that were recognized by the multi-gene classifier, and presumably these resistant cells metastasized to the lungs prior to DS and subsequently gave rise to the recurrent tumor. Ironically the multi-gene predictor classified this patient's DS sample (No. 452) as a GR, implying that either the DS sample used in our analysis was not representative of the primary tumor in that it did not contain the resistant cells, or that the resistant cells had already metastasized before DS and therefore were no longer detectable in the primary tumor.

In the second group of independent IB samples, the classifier correctly predicted 8 of 8 of the samples (100% correct, 95% CI 63, 100). These 8 samples included 5 PR and 3 GR. These results further indicate that the gene expression signature of the resistant cells in the DS samples was already

Table 4. Classification of initial biopsy samples using a support vector machine classifier

Tumor ID	Histologic response	Concordance with histologic response	
		paired	independent
410	GR	No	
197	PR	Yes	
207	PR	Yes	
278	GR	Yes	
289	PR	Yes	
345	GR	Yes	
204	PR		Yes
274	PR		Yes
299	GR		Yes
464	PR		Yes
479	PR		Yes
481	PR		Yes
545	GR		Yes
654	GR		Yes

GR = Good responder; PR = poor responder.

present in the IB samples at the time of diagnosis. Our result is consistent with the notion proposed by Ramaswamy et al. [30] that the metastatic signature of metastatic tumors is already present in the primary tumor. The high accuracy of our multi-gene classifier to identify GR and PR from two separate groups of IB samples suggests that response to chemotherapy can potentially be predicted at the time of diagnosis. However, due to the limited number of samples used in the study, the classifier and chemoresistant signature needs to be validated in a larger multi-institutional study. If validated, this can significantly impact the design of future therapeutic studies of osteosarcoma, in which intensified therapy could be given at the time of diagnosis to those patients who are predicted to be PR to standard therapy in order to improve their outcome.

Conclusion

As illustrated by the examples of pediatric ALL and osteosarcoma, it is apparent that molecular classification will be the driving force in the further development of individualized therapy for cancer patients. We believe that molecular profiling will provide important clues regarding critical pathways that cancer cells are dependent on to maintain their malignant phenotype. Such pathways will be ideal therapeutic targets for tumor-specific therapies. An equally important aspect of this goal will involve the continuation of ongoing efforts to cautiously decrease the intensity of potentially toxic therapies in order to reduce the morbidity of treatment in tumors that have particularly favorable risk factors based on genomic profiling. In conclusion, genomic profiling analysis offers an exciting possibility for refining the diagnosis, stratification and therapy of pediatric cancers. It is reasonable to imagine that in the near future, predictive individualized care based on molecular classification and targeted therapy will become a reality for children with cancer.

Acknowledgement

This work was supported by NIH grants CA88126, CA97874, CA109467, and CA114757 as well as grants from the John S. Dunn Research Foundation and the Robert J. Kleberg, Jr. and Helen C. Kleberg Foundation, Gillson Longenbaugh Foundation and Cancer Fighters of Houston, Inc.

References

1 Pui CH, Evans WE: Treatment of acute lymphoblastic leukemia. N Engl J Med 2006;354: 166–178.
2 Smith M, Arthur D, Camitta B, et al: Uniform approach to risk classification and treatment assignment for children with acute lymphoblastic leukemia. J Clin Oncol 1996;14:18–24.
3 Armstrong SA, Look AT: Molecular genetics of acute lymphoblastic leukemia. J Clin Oncol 2005;23:6306–6315.
4 Sutcliffe MJ, Shuster JJ, Sather HN, et al: High concordance from independent studies by the Children's Cancer Group (CCG) and Pediatric Oncology Group (POG) associating favorable prognosis with combined trisomies 4, 10, and 17 in children with NCI Standard-Risk B-precursor Acute Lymphoblastic Leukemia: a Children's Oncology Group (COG) initiative. Leukemia 2005;19:734–740.
5 Rabbitts TH: Chromosomal translocations in human cancer. Nature 1994;372:143–149.
6 Druker BJ, Sawyers CL, Kantarjian H, et al: Activity of a specific inhibitor of the BCR-ABL tyrosine kinase in the blast crisis of chronic myeloid leukemia and acute lymphoblastic leukemia with the Philadelphia chromosome. N Engl J Med 2001;344:1038–1042.
7 Armstrong SA, Kung AL, Mabon ME, et al: Inhibition of FLT3 in MLL. Validation of a therapeutic target identified by gene expression based classification. Cancer Cell 2003;3:173–183.
8 Stam RW, den Boer ML, Schneider P, et al: Targeting FLT3 in primary MLL-gene-rearranged infant acute lymphoblastic leukemia. Blood 2005;106:2484–2490.
9 Cairo MS, Sposto R, Perkins SL, et al: Burkitt's and Burkitt-like lymphoma in children and adolescents: a review of the Children's Cancer Group experience. Br J Haematol 2003;120: 660–670.
10 Blum KA, Lozanski G, Byrd JC: Adult Burkitt leukemia and lymphoma. Blood 2004;104: 3009–3020.
11 Cheok MH, Yang W, Pui CH, et al: Treatment-specific changes in gene expression discriminate in vivo drug response in human leukemia cells. Nat Genet 2003;34:85–90.
12 Zaza G, Cheok M, Yang W, et al: Gene expression and thioguanine nucleotide disposition in acute lymphoblastic leukemia after in vivo mercaptopurine treatment. Blood 2005;106:1778–1785.
13 Holleman A, Cheok MH, den Boer ML, et al: Gene-expression patterns in drug-resistant acute lymphoblastic leukemia cells and response to treatment. N Engl J Med 2004;351:533–542.

14 Cave H, van der Werff ten Bosch, Suciu S, et al: Clinical significance of minimal residual disease in childhood acute lymphoblastic leukemia. European Organization for Research and Treatment of Cancer – Childhood Leukemia Cooperative Group. N Engl J Med 1998;339: 591–598.

15 Pollock BH, DeBaun MR, Camitta BM, et al: Racial differences in the survival of childhood B-precursor acute lymphoblastic leukemia: a Pediatric Oncology Group Study. J Clin Oncol 2000;18:813–823.

16 Relling MV, Dervieux T: Pharmacogenetics and cancer therapy. Nat Rev Cancer 2001;1: 99–108.

17 Cheok MH, Evans WE: Acute lymphoblastic leukaemia: a model for the pharmacogenomics of cancer therapy. Nat Rev Cancer 2006;6:117–129.

18 Link MP, Gebhardt MC, Meyers PA: Osteosarcoma; in Pizzo P, Poplack D (eds): Principles and Practice of Pediatric Oncology, ed 5. Philadelphia, Lippincott-Williams & Wilkins, 2006, pp 1074–1115.

19 Provisor AJ, Ettinger LJ, Nachman JB, et al: Treatment of nonmetastatic osteosarcoma of the extremity with preoperative and postoperative chemotherapy: a report from the Children's Cancer Group. J Clin Oncol 1997;15:76–84.

20 Meyers PA, Heller G, Healey J, et al: Chemotherapy for nonmetastatic osteogenic sarcoma: the Memorial Sloan-Kettering experience. J Clin Oncol 1992;10:5–15.

21 Baldini N, Scotlandi K, Barbanti-Brodano G, et al: Expression of P-glycoprotein in high-grade osteosarcomas in relation to clinical outcome. N Engl J Med 1995;333:1380–1385.

22 Bacci G, Longhi A, Ferrari S, et al: Prognostic significance of serum alkaline phosphatase in osteosarcoma of the extremity treated with neoadjuvant chemotherapy: recent experience at Rizzoli Institute. Oncol Rep 2002;9:171–175.

23 Gorlick R, Huvos AG, Heller G, et al: Expression of HER2/erbB-2 correlates with survival in osteosarcoma. J Clin Oncol 1999;17:2781–2788.

24 Bielack SS, Kempf-Bielack B, Delling G, et al: Prognostic factors in high-grade osteosarcoma of the extremities or trunk: an analysis of 1,702 patients treated on neoadjuvant cooperative osteosarcoma study group protocols. J Clin Oncol 2002;20:776–790.

25 Davis AM, Bell RS, Goodwin PJ: Prognostic factors in osteosarcoma: a critical review. J Clin Oncol 1994;12:423–431.

26 Feugeas O, Guriec N, Babin-Boilletot A, et al: Loss of heterozygosity of the RB gene is a poor prognostic factor in patients with osteosarcoma. J Clin Oncol 1996;14:467–472.

27 Franzius C, Bielack S, Flege S, et al: Prognostic significance of (18)F-FDG and (99m)Tc-methylene diphosphonate uptake in primary osteosarcoma. J Nucl Med 2002;43:1012–1017.

28 Ulaner GA, Huang HY, Otero J, et al: Absence of a telomere maintenance mechanism as a favorable prognostic factor in patients with osteosarcoma. Cancer Res 2003;63:1759–1763.

29 Man TK, Chintagumpala M, Visvanathan J, et al: Expression profiles of osteosarcoma that can predict response to chemotherapy. Cancer Res 2005;65:8142–8150.

30 Ramaswamy S, Ross KN, Lander ES, Golub TR: A molecular signature of metastasis in primary solid tumors. Nat Genet 2003;33:49–54.

Discussion

Dr. Haschke: This is probably a question which will be very difficult to answer. Using the genetic profiling of a tumor to look at aggressiveness and then designing tailor-made therapy, there is very little time so the profile is looked at only once because, for example in leukemia, it makes a difference whether therapy is started 5 days later or earlier. Could it be possible that the genetic profiling of the tumor could be changed if, for example, there were a few days time just to improve the nutritional status of the patient and see if the patient's immune response could be changed? Is this possible; are there animal models showing that the profiling of the tumor could be changed or modified? I know this is not possible because most tumors are not subjected to primary surgery but primarily to chemotherapy, so there is no time. But would it be possible or are there animal models showing that this profiling could change?

Dr. Lau: Actually this type of study has been done in animals and initially the profiles were quite sensitive to all kinds of perturbations, but with the more recent improvements in the platforms these profiles are rather robust now. So it can actually be done at multiple time points in animal models, and nearly exactly the same results are obtained. It is true that with leukemia we actually have the luxury of doing that. A peripheral blood sample can be taken where there are leukemic blasts and at multiple time points, and very similar results are seen. With solid tumors we don't have that luxury.

Dr. Alhaffar: You mentioned a lot about chromosomal studies and gene locations in patients who had the disease. When you are doing a random study for chromosomes, especially for Down syndrome for instance, in pregnant women, and you find these dislocations and gene positions, what do you do between prediction and prevention? Do you force yourself to follow-up treatment? What do you do, you just found the gene?

Dr. Lau: That is one of the intrinsic problems of generating so much data. In clinical medicine we always say do not order a test if you are not ready to act on the data. This is precisely the problem. Some of the translocations can actually be found in children who do not have leukemia. For example the 12;21 translocation that I mentioned briefly was subsequently discovered and the same translocation can be detected in patients if you are able to retrieve the initial blood spots at the time of birth, the Guthrie spots. This suggests that the translocation has been there all along and that something else has triggered the development of these leukemic blasts into leukemia. Unfortunately or fortunately, we did controls for those studies and found that the same translocation can also be found in some Guthrie spots of otherwise normal children. So obviously this is not the only event that is required for leukemia to develop. We are still trying to find out exactly what other events need to happen in order for full-blown disease to develop. We are still at a rather infant stage in making use of these data in a clinical setting. So yes, we may be able to predict, but the prediction is not 100%.

Dr. Björkstén: How do you handle the ethical aspects of knowing which osteosarcoma patients are going to have metastases yet not being able to do anything about it?

Dr. Lau: That is why the initial study has to be done in such a way that no information is conveyed back to the treating physician or the patient, because if we are only detecting certain events that may happen in the future but without any intervention strategies that creates an ethical challenge. We are now being challenged to find alternative therapy in association with the identification of these high-risk patients. We have created a problem for ourselves because we have the diagnostic capabilities but no therapeutic strategies available yet.

Dr. Waterland: You found a relatively small number of genes in which the expression on the array seems to predict responsiveness to osteosarcoma therapy. Have you done any type of gene ontology to look for related biochemical functions of those genes in order to predict what potential changes in therapy might improve the response?

Dr. Lau: Yes, we have started looking at that, and in fact there is a series of functional studies now validating the role of these genes in both osteosarcoma cells as well as normal osteoblast cells which we think are the progenitor cells for the tumor and some of them are very interesting. For example there is a gene called *twist1* which turns out to be involved in the normal differentiation of osteoblasts, so immediately we know that it is relevant. But equally important, it was found to be associated with chemoresistance in other types of tumors; totally independent of our own findings, they are found in neuroblastoma, in colon cancer, in prostate cancer, etc. So we can land on highly relevant genes without any prior knowledge of where these genes could be.

Dr. Saavedra: This is really more of a comment and an opportunity to contrast what you just showed compared to what we were talking about previously. You have basically shown that there is at least one very good example where a predictive mechanism can be found using microarrays and very elegant genomics for a disease which is not that common. The specificity is greater than 90% and sensitivity is close to 100%, looking at an oncologic disease. In the previous discussions we were looking at using family history to predict allergy risk, which has a sensitivity of less than 25% and the specificity is high as perhaps 70%; because the majority of children who have a family history don't have allergy and most children who have allergy don't have a family history [1]. This is a challenge for us. We are using the most primitive kinds of predictive tools to analyze studies such as allergy, where we need to make important clinical decisions to curb this epidemic. This type of problem presents a challenge to us all. We need better predicitive tools or consider interventions that can be more broadly applied.

Dr. Berry: Regarding the altered genes that are expressed, do the proteomic analyses show primarily posttranslational modifications or altered levels?

Dr. Lau: So far the correlation between the genomic profiles and the proteomic profiles are not very good. This is not too surprising because it is a well-known fact in protein biochemistry that there is a very poor correlation between the RNA level and protein level, which is precisely what you were hinting at in the posttranslational modification, and now we have to worry about micro-RNA being involved, etc. But the interesting thing is that even though the levels do not correlate that well, they are actually pointing to the same pathways. In fact we actually believe that the pathway pinpointed by this profiling is more important than the individual genes or proteins because we now have the whole pathways that we can wrestle with rather than individual genes. Even though it is not the perfect correlation that everybody would like to see, I think they are pointing to the same critical pathways.

Dr. Berry: Are you struggling with being able to find internal standards to use to normalize the data within each tumor sample?

Dr. Lau: Actually it is getting less and less problematic because of the availability of the publicly available data, and we are now actually using what is out there to normalize our data. Fortunately to the result is very stable as I suggested earlier.

Dr. German: Would it be possible to use diet to enhance the diagnostic capabilities? Obviously the sensitivity and specificity are often high, but these are presumably on the background of children on varying diets. If it could actually be standardized and get that part relatively constant, would that improve your diagnostic capability?

Dr. Lau: That is a question that we all ask and that is why metabolomic profiling is being advocated and nobody can predict where it will be going. I always worry about that myself; what is the impact of the nutritional status of these patients, prior to presentation, that might affect the profiling results. We haven't done that kind of control studies yet.

Dr. Waterland: In your introduction you mentioned the potential to do some profiling on the genomic level and I am just wondering whether you eventually see the potential to do testing at birth using comparative genomic hybridization to look for duplications, deletions, the sort of thing that might eventually predict which individuals might be at risk for these types of diseases?

Dr. Lau: That is actually in planning right now. We are trying to retrieve a lot of the Guthrie spots in the State of Texas which are stored in Austin and repeat the studies and try to test that particular hypothesis. But the other thing I need to mention other than the SNP polymorphism, we now also worry about the copy number variation polymorphism as well. Some of you may or may not realize that the normal genome does not contain two copies of every gene. Close to 7,000 regions of the normal human genome have been identified that have copy numbers other than 2, and many of them actually contain known genes. Many of these genes actually are the genes that code for proteins that interact with the environment. Again for nutrition researchers like yourself you need to include that in your equation. Copy number variation may account for some of the variation that we are seeing in these infants and children in response to different nutrition challenges.

Dr. Björkstén: The potential for personalized medicine is fascinating, but I would like to reiterate the ethical issues. It is clearly unethical to predict, unless you have treatment to offer.

Reference

1   Bergmann RL, Bergmann KE, Wahn U: Can we predict atopic disease using perinatal risk factors? Clin Exp Allergy 1998;28:905–907.

Bier DM, German JB, Lönnerdal B (eds): Personalized Nutrition for the Diverse Needs of Infants and Children.
Nestlé Nutr Workshop Ser Pediatr Program, vol 62, pp 189–203,
Nestec Ltd., Vevey/S. Karger AG, Basel, © 2008.

Personalizing Nutrient Intakes of Formula-Fed Infants: Breast Milk as a Model

Bo Lönnerdal

Department of Nutrition, University of California, Davis, CA, USA

Abstract

The growth pattern of formula-fed infants is quite different from that of breastfed infants. There may be several reasons for this difference, ranging from different endocrine responses to feeding and the presence of growth factors in breast milk to different control of food intake, but it is highly likely that differences in nutrient composition of the food (breast milk or formula) have major effects on growth. In most countries infant formula is used more or less exclusively up to 6 months of age and as part of the diet up to 12 months of age and during this period its composition remains the same. In striking contrast, the nutrient composition of breast milk changes during lactation, most dramatically during early lactation, but with pronounced differences throughout lactation for many nutrients. It is a goal that the performance of formula-fed infants should be as similar to that of breastfed infants as possible, and attempts have been made to modify the composition of infant formula to achieve this goal. However, there has been no systematic attempt to gradually change the composition of infant formula in a manner similar to the changing pattern of breast milk. This represents a technical and nutritional challenge, but is now possible.

Introduction

The concept of individualizing the nutrient intake of infants originated from feeding regimens for preterm infants. It was realized that the breast milk produced by women delivering infants prematurely was often too low in energy and protein to meet their infants' requirements. Consequently, some milk banks started analyzing breast milk samples from women of premature infants [1] with the intent of adding a human milk fortifier to make the concentrations of energy and protein commensurate with their estimated requirements at each age.

Several studies documented improved growth of infants fed such 'improved' breast milk [2]. The task of analyzing breast milk from individual women and 'personalizing' the nutrient density of the milk fed is intensive work, even if some instruments (e.g. IR analyzers) have been developed for this purpose.

The 'personalized' approach of feeding preterm infants was subsequently refined to measuring the metabolic response to feeding fortified breast milk (or preterm formula). By measuring blood urea nitrogen in the infants as an indicator of protein adequacy, the feeding regimes could be adjusted on an individual basis to keep protein intake at an adequate but not excessive level [3]. This approach has also been shown to improve the growth and development of preterm infants.

It is obvious that this kind of personalized feeding strategy is unrealistic for term infants. However, as described below, there are wide discrepancies in the nutrient intakes of formula-fed infants compared to breastfed infants and new approaches are needed to lessen these differences. This, in turn, may make the growth pattern of formula-fed infants more similar to that of breastfed infants which may have long-term consequences with regard to development and chronic diseases. Instead of analyzing clinical parameters in infants as a measure of the adequacy of their nutrient intake, it may be possible to develop formulas targeted to the individual's age and consequently to his/her nutrient requirements.

The growth pattern of formula-fed infants is quite different from that of breastfed infants [4]. There may be several reasons for this difference, ranging from different endocrine responses to feeding and the presence of growth factors in breast milk to different control of food intake, but it is highly likely that differences in nutrient composition of the food (breast milk or formula) have a major effect on growth. Infant formula is in most countries used more or less exclusively up to 6 months of age and as part of the diet up to 12 months of age and during this period its composition remains the same (although some countries also use so-called 'follow-on' formula). In striking contrast, the nutrient composition of breast milk changes during the lactation period, most dramatically during early lactation, but with pronounced differences throughout lactation for many nutrients.

It has been stated as a goal that the performance of formula-fed infants should be as similar to that of breastfed infants as possible, and attempts have been made to modify the composition of infant formula to achieve this goal. However, although the concept of 'individualizing' the nutrient intake of premature infants fed their own mothers' milk has been used, there has been no systematic attempt to gradually change the composition of infant formula in a manner similar to the changing pattern of breast milk. This represents a technical and nutritional challenge, but is now possible. Although many bioactive components are unique to breast milk, present dairy technology allows isolation of bovine milk fractions that may at least provide some of the bioactivities of breast milk components. Addition of such components at physiologically relevant concentrations at each developmental period may result in improved performance of formula-fed infants.

Protein

Colostrum and milk produced during early lactation are very high in protein concentration, up to 20–30 g/l [5, 6]. Partly this is due to the low volumes being produced, but mostly due to hormonal regulation of protein synthesis. During the first month of lactation, the milk protein concentration decreases considerably, reaching levels around 9–11 g/l. These levels are then largely maintained during the entire lactation period and even after 1–2 years of lactation, which is common in developing countries, protein concentrations are around 8–10 g/l [7]. Few factors appear to affect the protein concentration of breast milk and even malnourished women produce milk with a normal protein concentration [8], even if large differences in protein intake may have short-term effects on the milk protein concentration [9].

The protein concentration of infant formula has always been considerably higher than in breast milk, in part due to the assumed lower digestibility and different amino acid composition of the formula protein source, in part to assure meeting the requirements of infants with high protein needs. During the past decades, however, there has been an overall tendency to reduce the protein level of infant formula, from the original levels of 18–20 to 15–16 g/l, and, more recently, to 12–14 g/l. Thus, the magnitude of the difference in protein level between breast milk and formula has diminished. However, combined with the higher daily volume of formula consumed by formula-fed infants (discussed below), the higher protein concentration of infant formula results in considerably higher protein intakes of formula-fed infants as compared with breastfed infants (fig. 1).

It should be noted that, with only a few exceptions, the protein level of infant formula is the same regardless whether it is fed to newborn or a 6-month-old infant. The assumed lower digestibility of infant formula proteins should be questioned; less excessive heat processing of formula and an increasing proportion of whey protein has most likely increased the digestibility of formula proteins [12]. Further, it has become more recognized that several breast milk proteins, such as lactoferrin and secretory IgA, are incompletely digested. Thus, breast milk proteins are not completely digested, in contrast to what was previously believed. Therefore, 'digestible' protein in infant formula is still considerably higher than that of breast milk, which is reflected by the fact that blood urea nitrogen levels of formula-fed infants are significantly higher than in breastfed infants, even when the protein level is reduced to 13 g/l [13].

The protein composition of breast milk also changes considerably during lactation [6]. In colostrum and early milk there is little or no casein, whereas

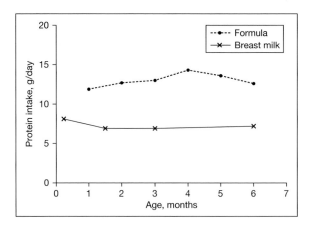

Fig. 1. Protein intakes of breastfed and formula-fed infants. Adapted from Lönnerdal et al. [10], Dewey and Lönnerdal [11] and unpublished data.

most milk-based infant formulas contain ~40% casein. Mammary gland synthesis of casein increases during early lactation so that the breast milk whey:casein ratio first reaches ~60:40 and then ~50:50 [14]. The major whey proteins in breast milk during early lactation are secretory IgA, lactoferrin and α-lactalbumin, and they are present in exceptionally high concentrations, but they remain in high concentrations throughout the lactation period. In contrast, there is very little lactoferrin and secretory IgA in infant formula, but bovine α-lactalbumin is a significant component of whey-predominant cow's milk formula. Recently, some manufacturers have started to enrich infant formulas with bovine α-lactalbumin, primarily to achieve a more balanced amino acid composition.

Human milk is known to contain a multitude of bioactive proteins [15]. Some bioactive milk proteins may be obtained from cow's milk and added to infant formula, provided that they can exert the same or partial bioactivity as their human milk counterparts. For example, it may be possible to isolate milk protein fractions with bovine secretory IgA, preferably from cows exposed to human pathogens, so that some immunoprotection may be achieved. Bovine lactoferrin is commercially available and even if it may not display all of the bioactivities of human lactoferrin, which in part are receptor-mediated, bacteriostatic/bactericidal activities may be similar. It has been shown that some bioactive proteins such as secretory IgA and lactoferrin can resist proteolytic digestion and be found in the stool of breastfed infants [16]. However, with increasing age, these proteins become digested and when added to infant formula it may only be worthwhile in products for younger infants. Further, such infants are also more likely to benefit from these bioactive components.

Carbohydrates

The major carbohydrate in breast milk is lactose which is synthesized in the mammary gland by lactose synthase, a complex between α-lactalbumin and galactosyltransferase. In colostrum and during early lactation, the lactose concentration is relatively low, but it rapidly increases to a concentration of ~5–6 g/l of mature milk, and changes little thereafter. The significant remainder of the total carbohydrate content of breast milk consists of oligosaccharides, which are largely non-digestible and therefore pass through the gastrointestinal tract of infants in intact form [17]. A major part of the oligosaccharides has been found in the stool, but there is also some intestinal absorption as about 1% is found intact in the urine, as studied with stable isotopes [18]. There are numerous types of oligosaccharides in breast milk, varying from relatively simple structures like fucosyl- and sialyllactose to very complex structures [17, 19]. Many of these vary considerably in structure among individual women as they are affected by various glycosylation pathways, such as those determining the different blood groups (Lewis, ABO). Their concentrations have been shown to vary during lactation with most of them being higher in concentration during early lactation [20]. It has been estimated that there are several hundred different oligosaccharides in breast milk, and the structures of many of them have not yet been determined. Since many of these structures are similar to oligosaccharides present on the mucosal surface of the small intestine, it has been suggested that they act as soluble 'decoys' and bind pathogens, thereby preventing their attachment and possible invasion of the host [19]. They have also been suggested to have a prebiotic function by stimulating the growth of bacteria beneficial to the host, e.g. lactobacilli and bifidobacteria, but also discouraging the growth of pathogens [19].

It is obvious that it would be very difficult to mimic the oligosaccharide composition of breast milk when manufacturing infant formula, and very few and limited attempts have been made to add single oligosaccharides found in breast milk. An alternative approach that has been used by some manufacturers is based on the presumed prebiotic activity of breast milk oligosaccharides – by adding non-digestible carbohydrates such as fructo- and galacto-oligosaccharides (FOS and GOS, respectively) to infant formula, some of the perceived benefits of breast milk oligosaccharides, e.g. prebiotic activity, may be achieved [21].

Lipids

The triglyceride content of breast milk increases rapidly during the first week of lactation [5, 22]. Colostrum is usually very low in lipids (although the contents of fat-soluble vitamins such as vitamin A and carotenoids can be high), early milk contains 1–2% lipids and when the milk has matured it is usually around 3.5–4.0% [5]. The individual fatty acids also change during lactation [5, 22], although this is affected by intake of lipids/fatty acids by the mothers and their energy balance. The major fatty acids in breast milk (C16, C18 and C18:1n-9) and the long-chain polyunsaturated fatty acids decrease during lactation, whereas the medium-chain fatty acids (C12 and C14) increase [5, 22]. Most infant formulas contain ~3.5% lipids and the fatty acid composition is usually tailored towards an 'average' breast milk composition.

Docosahexaenoic acid (DHA) and arachidonic acid (AA) have received special interest with regard to the addition of these fatty acids to infant formulas. DHA has been shown to be important for brain development (usually assessed by visual acuity) in preterm infants [23] and as breast milk from most women is substantially higher in DHA than infant formula, some manufacturers have supplemented their products for term infants with DHA. Whether DHA supplementation of infant formula is of benefit for visual acuity is still a matter of controversy, but a recent study on the increased DHA intake of infants leading to a lower BMI [24] may strengthen the argument for DHA supplementation, perhaps particularly to young term infants. The proper level of DHA to use is difficult to assess as few studies have evaluated the dose dependency of the beneficial effect of DHA and as the level of DHA in breast milk is highly variable and dependent upon maternal intake of DHA. Due to possible competition between metabolic pathways, the ratio of DHA to AA may also be an important consideration. Generally, an AA:DHA ratio of 1.5 is recommended, but there are few studies evaluating the 'optimal' ratio.

Most infant formulas use blends of vegetable oils in their lipid premix to achieve a fatty acid pattern similar to that of breast milk. Although there has been a trend towards avoiding milk fat in formulas due to its high content of saturated fatty acids, there may be a need to reconsider the possibility of using some milk fat. Conjugated linoleic acid has been shown to have some beneficial biological activities [25] and both breast milk and cow's milk contain conjugated linoleic acids, whereas most infant formulas lack these fatty acids.

Energy

The energy density of infant formula has received little interest. Virtually all infant formulas have energy contents similar to the assumed energy density of breast milk, i.e., ~670 kcal/l. However, the energy content of breast milk changes during lactation and it has also been overestimated due to erroneous assumptions, such as all carbohydrates are digestible and breast milk proteins are efficiently digested and absorbed. Further, the volume of infant formula consumed by formula-fed infants considerably exceeds the intake of milk by breastfed infants; for example, by 3 months of age most breastfed infants consume ~800 ml/day whereas formula-fed infants have an intake of ~1,000 ml/day (with

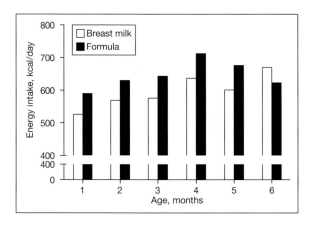

Fig. 2. Energy intakes of breastfed and formula-fed infants. Adapted from Lönnerdal et al. [10], Dewey and Lönnerdal [11] and unpublished data.

considerable individual differences). It appears that most breastfed infants are able to regulate their intake [26], whereas formula-fed infants are less capable of doing this. With an energy density of formula higher than that of breast milk, and an intake much higher than that of breastfed infants, it is obvious that the energy intake of formula-fed infants exceeds that of breastfed infants. As shown in figure 2, the calculated (Atwater factors) energy intake of formula-fed infants exceeds that of breastfed infants by ~60–80 kcal/day. It is therefore not surprising that breastfed infants gain less weight during the first 6 months and are leaner than formula-fed infants by 1 year of age [27]. The possible long-term consequences of this difference in growth pattern and weight gain are a matter of controversy. There have been a few attempts to try to limit the intake of formula-fed infants but this has proven to be difficult. Studies on lower energy content of formula are sorely lacking and may have some difficulties with regard to ethical considerations due to the current consistency in energy content of infant formulas. However, several recent studies have shown that previous calculations of energy requirements of infants were overestimates and that 'true' energy requirements are ~10–30% lower than earlier believed [28]. Thus, an evaluation of the effects of lowering the energy density of formula appears logical and desirable.

Micronutrients

Several micronutrients which are important for infant development vary considerably in the concentration in breast milk during lactation. For example, the zinc concentration of colostrum is ~5–10 mg/l, whereas breast milk produced at 6 months of lactation only contains 0.3–0.5 mg/l [29]. Since infant formula contains ~4–7 mg of zinc/l, formula-fed infants will receive about the same amount of zinc as breastfed infants during the neonatal period, but by 6 months of age they will consume more than 10 times as much. Although zinc is of particular importance during rapid growth, the prudence of such high intakes of zinc may be questioned. Similarly, the iron concentration of early milk is about 0.4–0.6 mg/l and at 6 months about 0.2 mg/l, whereas most infant formulas contain 4–12 mg of iron/l. The possibility of excessive intakes of these essential nutrients exists, particularly as they are known to compete with each other and other micronutrients for absorptive pathways. Further, in addition to iron, copper is considerably higher in infant formula than in breast milk (about 4 times), which means that the prooxidative potential of formula is much higher than that of breast milk. This may be of concern as even healthy term infants have shown evidence of oxidative stress during early infancy [30]. Since the human term infant is born with significant stores of iron and copper, and these are mobilized during early life, it may be advisable to limit the iron and copper content of formula for young infants. It is apparent that 'individualizing' infant formulas to specific age periods would make it possible to adjust the micronutrient concentrations to levels closer to those in breast milk at any given time during lactation, although they should always be somewhat higher than in breast milk due to their lower bioavailability from formula [31].

Concept

Every day, the mother/caregiver will prepare formula to feed the infant. To date, a single source of formula has been used from the early newborn period to late in infancy. If instead age-specific products were made available, it would be possible to provide the formula-fed infants with nutrient intakes corresponding to their needs at any given age. For example, there may be a 'starter' formula for the first 2 weeks, another one for the next month, one for 2–4 months, one for 4–6 months and one for infants older than 6 months. Not only could the nutrient composition of these formulas be tailored towards the requirements during each period, but there would be a possibility to add bioactive components during appropriate times – these components may be especially important during early life and, with regard to proteins, become digested/inactive in infants of older age. It should not be difficult to convince mothers about the biological 'soundness' of this approach; parents are acutely aware that their infants progress quickly through different developmental stages and will not be surprised that their nutrient needs also change.

References

1 Polberger S, Lönnerdal B: Simple and rapid macronutrient analysis of human milk for individualized fortification: basis for improved nutritional management of very low birth weight infants? J Pediatr Gastroenterol Nutr 1993;17:283–290.
2 Polberger S, Räihä NCR, Juvonen P, et al: Individualized protein fortification of human milk for preterm infants: comparison of ultrafiltered human milk protein and a bovine whey fortifier. J Pediatr Gastroenterol Nutr 1999;29:332–338.
3 Arslanoglu S, Moro GE, Ziegler EE: Adjustable fortification of human milk fed to preterm infants: does it make a difference? J Perinatol 2006;26:614–621.
4 Dewey KG, Heinig MJ, Nommsen LA, et al: Growth of breast-fed and formula-fed infants from 0 to 18 months: the DARLING Study. Pediatrics 1992;89:1035–1041.
5 Harzer G, Haug M, Bindels JG: Biochemistry of maternal milk in early lactation. Hum Nutr Appl Nutr 1986;40A(suppl 1):11–18.
6 Lönnerdal B, Adkins Y: Developmental changes in breast milk protein composition during lactation; in Sanderson IR, Walker WA (eds): Development of the Gastrointestinal Tract. Decker, Hamilton, 2000, pp 227–244.
7 Dewey KG, Finley DA, Lönnerdal B: Breast milk volume and composition during late lactation (7–20 months). J Pediatr Gastroenterol Nutr 1984;3:713–720.
8 Lönnerdal B: Effects of maternal dietary intake on breast milk composition. J Nutr 1986;116: 499–513.
9 Forsum E, Lönnerdal B: Effect of protein intake on protein and nitrogen composition of breast milk. Am J Clin Nutr 1980;33:1809–1813.
10 Lönnerdal B, Forsum E, Hambraeus L: A longitudinal study of the protein, nitrogen and lactose contents of human milk from Swedish well-nourished mothers. Am J Clin Nutr 1976; 29:1127–1133.
11 Dewey KG, Lönnerdal B: Milk and nutrient intake of breastfed infants from 1 to 6 months: relation to growth and fatness. J Pediatr Gastroenterol Nutr 1983;2:497–506.
12 Rudloff S, Lönnerdal B: Solubility and digestibility of milk proteins in infant formulas exposed to different heat treatment. J Pediatr Gastroenterol Nutr 1992;15:25–33.
13 Lönnerdal B, Hernell O: Effects of feeding ultrahigh-temperature (UHT)-treated infant formula with different protein concentrations or powdered formula, as compared with breast-feeding, on plasma amino acids, hematology, and trace element status. Am J Clin Nutr 1998;68:350–356.
14 Kunz C, Lönnerdal B: Re-evaluation of the whey protein/casein ratio of human milk. Acta Paediatr 1987;81:107–112.
15 Lönnerdal B: Nutritional and physiologic significance of human milk proteins. Am J Clin Nutr 2003;77:1537S–1543S.
16 Davidson LA, Lönnerdal B: Persistence of human milk proteins in the breast-fed infant. Acta Paediatr Scand 1987;76:733–740.
17 Kunz C, Rudloff S, Baier W, et al: Oligosaccharides in human milk: structural, functional and metabolic aspects. Annu Rev Nutr 200;20:699–722.
18 Obermeier S, Rudloff S, Pohlentz G, et al: Secretion of ^{13}C-labelled oligosaccharides into human milk and infant's urine after an oral [^{13}C]galactose load. Isotopes Environ Health Stud 1999;35:119–125.
19 Newburg DS, Ruiz-Palacios GM, Morrow AL: Human milk glycans protect infants against enteric pathogens. Annu Rev Nutr 2005;25:37–58.
20 Chaturvedi P, Warren CD, Altaye M, et al: Fucosylated human milk oligosaccharides vary between individuals and over the course of lactation. Glycobiology 2001;11:365–372.
21 Moro G, Minoli I, Mosca M, et al: Dosage-related bifidogenic effects of galacto- and fructooligosaccharides in formula-fed term infants. J Pediatr Gastroenterol Nutr 2002;34:291–295.
22 Kovacs A, Funke S, Marosvölgyi T, et al: Fatty acids in early human milk after preterm and full-term delivery. J Pediatr Gastroenterol Nutr 2005;41:454–459.
23 Fleith M, Clandinin MT: Dietary PUFA for preterm and term infants: review of clinical studies. Crit Rev Food Sci Nutr 2005;45:205–229.
24 Lucia Bergmann R, Bergmann KE, Haschke-Becher E, et al.: Does maternal docosahexaenoic acid supplementation during pregnancy and lactation lower BMI in late infancy? J Perinat Med 2007;35:295–300.

25 Bhattacharya A, Banu J, Rahman M, et al: Biological effects of conjugated linoleic acids in health and disease. J Nutr Biochem 2006;17:789–810.
26 Dewey KG, Lönnerdal B: Infant self-regulation of breast milk intake. Acta Paediatr Scand 1986;75:893–898.
27 Dewey KG, Heinig MJ, Nommsen LA, et al: Breast-fed infants are leaner than formula-fed infants at one year of age: the DARLING study. Am J Clin Nutr 1993;57:140–145.
28 Butte NF: Energy requirements of infants. Publ Health Nutr 2005;8:953–967.
29 Fransson G-B, Lönnerdal B: Zinc, copper, calcium and magnesium in human milk. J Pediatr 1982;101:504–508.
30 Friel JK, Friesen RW, Harding SV, Roberts LJ: Evidence of oxidative stress in full-term healthy infants. Pediatr Res 2004;56:878–882.
31 Lönnerdal B: The effects of milk and milk components on calcium, magnesium and trace element absorption during infancy. Physiol Rev 1997;77:634–699.

Discussion

Dr. Vaarala: Are there differences in the breast milk of mothers living in a high-versus low-hygiene environment? You have done some studies in Peru, and together with Dr. Savilahti we have seen that probiotics may induce an increase in total IgA in serum and feces, and one could think that secretory IgA, for example in breast milk, may be higher in mothers living in a low-hygiene environment because the gut microbiota might stimulate IgA.

Dr. Lönnerdal: It's quite possible but I am not aware of any such studies. What we looked at in Peru was the common belief that women who had infections produced breast milk of inferior quality and therefore should not nurse. We questioned the factual basis for that, and did studies in Peruvian women who had infections during early lactation and looked at the composition of their milk as compared to milk from women who had no infection [1]. We repeated the study in another cohort during mid-lactation when milk production was more established and found no differences in composition [2]. Their pathogen load certainly was very different, and did not affect milk composition, but that does not exclude the possibility you are referring to.

Dr. Björkstén: There is a study from the 1980s comparing milk from Swedish and Pakistani mothers and, if I recall correctly, there were surprisingly small differences in IgA levels between the two rather extreme environments.

Dr. Lönnerdal: I think there was no difference in total secretory IgA but in the specific secretory IgA levels towards certain antigens.

Dr. Björkstén: Yes, because obviously the Swedish and Pakistani mothers had been exposed to different microbes, but the total levels were similar.

Dr. Walker: The advantage of sIgA in breast milk is that it provides antibodies against microorganisms in the maternal environment which is also the infants' environment. As you mentioned, what you see is a difference in the actual type of sIgA compared to total.

Dr. Koletzko: We have actually been discussing the staged approach in Europe for many years but so far have not found a manufacturer willing to do that. Obviously there is not a huge volume that could be used but the concept is very convincing. You pointed out the effect of heat treatment on lowering bioavailability, and you showed the data for protein and copper. Jacques Rigo has also found very similar effects in his studies of nitrogen balance on mineral bioavailability. These heat-treated products are used due to the fear of enterobacter contamination, particularly in newborn and premature infants where obviously the concern about lowering bioavailability would be greatest. Should we be more careful in using heat-treated products and could UHT products play a role? I would assume they would have less of a problem.

Dr. Lönnerdal: Certainly extensive heat treatment would affect protein digestibility and as you indicated this has indirect effects on the bioavailability of several minerals. I think it is a good idea because as far as I know UHT is as efficient with régard to bacteriological quality. I don't know what it would take to change manufacturing into this direction, but we have done clinical studies on that aspect and found much better utilization of amino acids [3]. We therefore may be able to lower the protein level in formula and therefore avoid the high levels of BUN found in formula-fed infants. I think that any heat treatment that would maintain bacterial quality while minimizing heat exposure would be beneficial.

Dr. Haschke: We continuously talk about the microbiota and whether there are differences or not. I would like to mention that we tend to forget the godfather of this idea, Willy Heine from Rostock. He attended several of these workshops in the 1980s showing that the same microbiota can be achieved with a formula in which there is lactalbumin and a low protein and high whey fraction. Unfortunately he was working in the Eastern German environment and was not able to publish in proper journals. Only when he went to Houston did he finally have access to good journals in which he could show his findings. The second comment is from the industrial perspective. At present there is a push situation from science to industry to add lactoferrin and secretory IgA because science shows advantages. On the other hand I would like to point out that there must be some understanding that there is a long development process for this kind of formula because these are ingredients which need to be approved by regulatory agencies, the Food and Drug Administration or European Food Safety Association (EFSA), and that requires long-term clinical trials, even from two centers, on safety and then on efficacy, and then come the regulatory hurdles. Even if a company could be convinced that these ingredients should be in, it will take time. I already had the same reaction when we discussed this one year ago in Vietnam at another workshop. You showed a difference between breastfeeding and formula feeding in terms of intake. Do you really think it is only the formula? There are so many variables: the attitude; the mode of breastfeeding; if the baby cries then it is taken to the breast which only takes few seconds, whereas if the baby starts to cry the mother has to prepare the formula fresh if the rules are followed, she has to get up in the night and go to the kitchen. Has anybody looked at these factors which provide so much inconvenience. If formula-fed infants are fed more often, really on demand, couldn't the same pattern be achieved?

Dr. Lönnerdal: It is a very complex issue and we have also done some studies showing self-regulation by the breastfed infant [4]. Thus, even if the breastfed infant has more milk available it will not take it. We don't know why; it is most likely some neuroendocrine regulation that is occurring. I think that for a formula-fed infant part of it is parental control, part of it may even be easy access. There are preliminary studies showing that when smaller holes in the nipple of the bottle are used, the infant is forced to fight for the content and intake will be reduced.

Dr. Salminen: I just wanted to comment on the idea knowing a little bit about the EFSA side: it really is a long process and we are dealing with the most well-regulated and safeguarded part in our food supply when we talk about infant formula. As I look at the process once you are ready with your scientific discovery, it will probably still take 2 years to get on the ingredient list, to have the scientific opinions of the EFSA panel, and to have the commission approve your ingredients. So we are really talking about a long-term process unless you have something that is immediately lifesaving and could actually go faster.

Dr. Lönnerdal: You are correct and I believe formulas should be tightly regulated. However, we should not give up. It is a long process and we have to set our goals which I think have been fairly modest previously; we need to raise that barrier a little bit higher.

Dr. Bier: I wanted to come back to the stepwise issue. Putting aside the study Dr. Koletzko told us about the other day about the effect on weight, what should be measured to know that this makes any difference at all and how long is it going to take us to find that out? I don't have an immediate end point at which I will know whether that is going to make a difference or not. By enlarge for the formula-fed infants you may be showing us a mean or average intake; for the breastfed infant we take that as a requirement level but really it is not a generous requirement, it is a marginal requirement level. So if we look at populations and there is a child whose protein requirements are on the high end and we start stepping down, what is the public health perspective of that? How do we even know? What do we use to tell us that this has any human beneficial effect?

Dr. Lönnerdal: That's why I think this workshop has been very stimulating. We have to use new approaches to measure outcomes which I did not have time to discuss here. What you are saying may be correct but what happens if you have a breastfed infant who has a high protein requirement and a mother producing a low protein breast milk – what is the consequence for that infant? There have been very few studies on individual infants who were followed by analyzing the diet of that particular infant. This could now be combined with some metabolomic approaches to study how each infant responds metabolically. It has always been thought that the breastfed infant just meets its requirements but not much more. How much evidence do we have for that? I believe that if breastfed infants are that close to meeting their requirements, wouldn't we see a whole lot of breastfed infants having nutritional problems?

Dr. Bier: I guess some people would say we really don't know that answer either. Let's look at this from the other perspective of requirements. If someone came into the nutrition community and said, I am going to make all my nutrition recommendations on the basis of the estimated average requirement for all the other nutrients at age 15, we would have 10,000 nutrition scientists stand up and say, what are you crazy. So here we are saying this in some ways for the newborn. I don't know the answer to this but it just seems to me that there are inconsistencies here, that we have great unknowns about that.

Dr. Hernell: I was actually thinking along the same lines. In Sweden we used to have two and even three formulas during the first 6 months, and the change in breast milk is of course a continuum. So what would you envision if we turned back and again had more formulas; how many would you suggest during the first 6 months?

Dr. Lönnerdal: More than two perhaps. I have talked to many formula manufacturers and it has always been said that the mother is not ready for such an 'educated' message. I don't think that it is true because any mother knows that a newborn baby is not the same as a 1-month-old baby, or as a 3-month-old baby, and it would not be difficult to understand the nutrient requirements and physiological needs do change with age and that you need to change the infant's diet. How many products that are practically possible will be up to the formula industry, but I still think that any step to make them more diversified and more fit to their needs would be a step forward. We actually did a study in Taiwan in which we used a staged approach and in our publications we documented benefits with regard to metabolic responses [5, 6].

Dr. Isolauri: Going back to the discussion on microbes and probiotics we had at the beginning, our early data in diarrhea patients, rotavirus diarrhea patients, and vaccine studies as well as in milk-allergic children showed that the enhancement of IgA as assessed by the Elispot method was also antigen-specific and transient. Interestingly then the experimental data showed that the effect was also related to the formula we were using. So we do not achieve the same effects on immunostimulation in formula-fed children that we see in breastfed babies, and also there are differences in the effects if we give children hydrolyzed protein or unmodified milk protein. Therefore these effects are strain-specific but depend on the host and the food matrix as well. Finally, in your slide two breast milk oligosaccharides are listed: galacto-oligosaccharides and fructo-oligosaccharides. Is it correct, or what is the justification for listing fructo-oligosaccharides as breast milk oligosaccharides?

Dr. Lönnerdal: I think that's a mistake, I did not show that fructo- and galacto-oligosaccharides are in breast milk. Those are the ones being used in formula in an attempt to achieve the prebiotic effect of the human milk oligosaccharides. As far as I know those are not in breast milk.

Dr. Brandtzaeg: I would like to come back to the possibility of adding secretory IgA to the formulas as you mentioned. In my opinion, it can never be achieved with the broad range of antibodies that occur in breast milk, reflecting both the antigen exposure of the mother's mucous membranes in the airways and the gut. There were many attempts to elicit secretory IgA antibodies in cow's milk 20 years ago. Of course that was against a selective antigen used for local immunization, a special bacteria or pathogen. In the end it was deemed to be unethical because of the need for complete Freund's adjuvant with oil and mycobacteria which gave rise to terrible abscesses in the cow's udder. So that was stopped for ethical reasons. Perhaps you could use serum IgG instead of secretory IgA antibodies. But as you mentioned, IgG is easily degraded in the gut lumen. However, perhaps it is not so much of a problem at the beginning, in the first postnatal weeks, so that is one realistic option. But, nevertheless, I think there is a lot of information coming up now that the individualized spectrum antibodies provided by breast milk are needed because there are receptors for IgA on the lymphoid tissue in the gut which will guide the mother's IgA back to the baby's immune system and thus actually introduce the right antigens to the developing immune system to stimulate a homeostatic immune response as part of the tolerance mechanisms. So in this way secretory IgA in breast milk actually is a sort of link between the mother and the developing infant's immune system to direct the immune responses in the gut-associated lymphoid tissue.

Dr. Lönnerdal: I have never believed that any type of produced secretory IgA would have the functions of the breast milk secretory IgA, but I have heard that there are companies producing bovine secretory IgA which they obtained by exposing the cows to a cocktail of pathogens that many human infants are exposed to. I don't know how far they have come, but serious attempts are going on and it may be possible that a small part of the functional secretory IgA in breast milk could be copied by that approach.

Dr. Brandtzaeg: As you mentioned, this disappeared from the literature for ethical reasons.

Dr. Isolauri: This kind of hyper-immune milk is used for instance in intensive care to reduce the risk of clostridium infections.

Dr. Brandtzaeg: But that is mainly based on IgG.

Dr. Venter: Why isn't any eicosapentaenoic acid (EPA) added to infant formulas? They all contain arachidonic acid (AA) and docosahexaenoic acid but there is no EPA.

Dr. Koletzko: In fact the EPA content in formula is limited both in the European legislation and in the guidance provided by the Codex Alimentarus Commission that was adopted this summer. The guidance is given that a formula should not contain high amounts of EPA because EPA is not found in breast milk in appreciable amounts, only in very small amounts, and it is not found in infant tissues. There is some concern that EPA acts as a metabolic competitor with AA, and as Dr. Isolauri raised the other day AA is not only bad but it has important biological functions. Some of the early studies in preterm infants have reported that formula with a high EPA content was associated with reduced infant growth. So unless that is resolved there is caution about adding high amounts of EPA.

Dr. Michaelsen: Dr. Bier asked about what to measure and I would suggest that IGF1 would be interesting to measure, at least at the group level. We have data where we looked at IGF1 during the first year compared to IGF1 at 7 years of age and there is a reverse relation. It seems that there is a programming of the IGF1 axis where breastfed infants have low values while they are breastfed and then higher values later on. There are a few studies suggesting that breastfed infants are taller as adults and somehow this fits to the whole hypothesis of the relation between early growth velocity and later disease. We could not get immediate responses on what it means in the long-term, but I think it is fascinating to look at this programming of IGF1 as well.

Dr. Lönnerdal: I think it is a very good idea. Clinical studies evaluating changes in infant formula composition should look at response factors. IGF1 is certainly one, and if we use proteomic or genomic approaches we could follow a wider array because to date most clinical studies have followed very few parameters. It will be nice when a much wider array of biomarkers can be used in clinical studies.

Dr. Saavedra: This was a great presentation of the multiple things that we obviously need to start thinking about. From a historical perspective we have improved these alternatives to breast milk substitutes principally by a process of trial and error. For example, we found that cow casein caused problems in formula, so it was decreased because even though there is a lot of casein in human milk casein, the cow casein is very different. We knew that we needed to given iron and found that if we gave the same amount of iron in breast milk this led to many anemic babies, so we had to increase the levels. Then we recognized the antigenecity of cow's milk, so we tried to bring it down. In the end, what we are really doing is finding ways to decrease the complications that come from not exclusive breastfeeding. I think a better paradigm would probably be to try to get compositionally 'closer' to breast milk, but rather, we should work on getting functionally closer to breast milk, that is, causing less complications in children who aren't exclusively breastfed. For example, we need to decrease the metabolic and immunologic complications that come from not exclusively breastfeeding, and if we focus on understanding those implications, both the metabolic and immunologic ones which are the bigger ones, then we have something to fix. We then have a reason to go after all these interesting potential ingredients, but not simply adding ingredients because they happen to be in breast milk. We would be adding things like EPA and cholesterol if that was the case (just because 'they are in breast milk'). Does that make sense?

Dr. Lönnerdal: It makes sense but I am not sure I like it. It seems more to be a reactive approach than a proactive approach and to kind of find out when something is wrong we need to fix it. I would like to reemphasize that we cannot use breast milk as a perfect model, but I still think we can use it as a goal for several nutrients, but not all of them.

Dr. Saavedra: The only answer I would have is that until we know what the issues are, it is just going to be very hard to try to copy.

Dr. Gluckman: We know increasingly from experimental work in rats that short periods of changes in nutrition during lactation can have enormous effects on the offspring in the long-term. The issue that does crop up is that of fine tuning the match between nutritional requirements at different stages during what is a very long lactation cycle in relationship to the time of human development and the need of the organism. I don't know how we address that because this is limited to what you clinical people can do in terms of studying human beings and making interpretations. Do you have a view as to which if any of the various animal species is useful for studying these questions? Whether epigenetics or other biomarkers are used to address these questions, animal models could play a large role if there was an animal model that could be found useful.

Dr. Lönnerdal: Excellent question, and I think my response would be that for each individual nutrient or group of nutrients and for each developmental stage there may be a good animal model. For example, we have documented that when it comes to iron we have been able to replicate findings from human infants in rat pups. For example, we have done radioisotope studies in rat pups and found very similar results to those obtained from stable isotope studies in human infants at corresponding developmental stages. I think that animal models, such as piglets or rat pups, can be very valuable, but they need to be validated.

Dr. Gluckman: You focused largely on micronutrients and immune-related substances. There is increasing interest in hormones and other factors in milk. To what extent has it been looked at systematically in human versus other milk? Formula has very low levels of IGF1 and IGF2 and human milk has quite significant levels of IGF1 and IGF2, and there are the issues of leptin and prolactin, particularly in early milk.

Dr. Lönnerdal: It is possible that rodent models may be less valid for studying hormones and growth factors. However, Park et al. [7] have done very interesting studies on IGF1, and IGF-binding proteins in the piglet model and for those the piglet seems to be a valid model. As I stated before, for each group of compounds or nutrients, the appropriateness of the animal model chosen must be taken into consideration.

Dr. Gluckman: I really wasn't asking a question in relation to animal models, I wanted to know to what extent are those of you who are interested in human formula design thinking about the issues of the small bioactive? For example there is literature on IGF1 and IGF2 in terms of gut maturation in particular. The other point I would like to raise is the one about bottle-fed babies drinking more than breastfed babies; this intrigues me because the issue of what creates satiety in an infant is something we do need to understand more about. There is growing comparative literature on the ratio or sources of energy in setting satiety, in other words whether it is from protein or carbohydrates or from lipids. It would be interesting to know whether the ratios of energy sources are different between breastfed and formula-fed infants because it could be anticipated that if there is an altered ratio favoring the non-protein energy sources as a ratio, not as an absolute amount, the food volume intake would tend to be greater.

Dr. Haschke: We know that during the breastfeeding protein is initially high; at the end fat is higher, so this probably answers your question.

References

1 Lönnerdal B, Zavaleta N, Kusunoki L, et al: Effect of postpartum maternal infection on proteins and trace elements in colostrum and early milk. Acta Paediatr 1996;85:537–542.
2 Zavaleta N, Lanata C, Butron B, et al: Effect of acute maternal infection on quantity and composition of breast milk. Am J Clin Nutr 1995;62:559–563.
3 Lönnerdal B, Hernell O: Effects of feeding ultrahigh-temperature (UHT)-treated infant formula with different protein concentrations or powdered formula, as compared with breastfeeding, on plasma amino acids, hematology, and trace element status. Am J Clin Nutr 1998;68:350–356.
4 Dewey KG, Lönnerdal B: Infant self-regulation of breast milk intake. Acta Paediatr Scand 1986;75:893–898.
5 Lönnerdal B, Chen CL: Effects of formula protein level and ratio on infant growth, plasma amino acids and serum trace elements. I. Cow's milk formula. Acta Paediatr Scand 1990;79: 257–265.
6 Lönnerdal B, Chen CL: Effects of formula protein level and ratio on infant growth, plasma amino acids and serum trace elements. II. Follow-up formula. Acta Paediatr Scand 1990;79: 266–273.
7 Park YK, Monaco MM, Donovan SM: Delivery of total parenteral nutrition (TPN) via umbilical catheterization: development of a piglet model to investigate therapies to improve gastrointestinal structure and enzyme activity during TPN. Biol Neonate 1998;73:295–305.

Bier DM, German JB, Lönnerdal B (eds): Personalized Nutrition for the Diverse Needs of Infants and Children.
Nestlé Nutr Workshop Ser Pediatr Program, vol 62, pp 205–222,
Nestec Ltd., Vevey/S. Karger AG, Basel, © 2008.

Human Milk Oligosaccharides: Evolution, Structures and Bioselectivity as Substrates for Intestinal Bacteria

J. Bruce German, Samara L. Freeman, Carlito B. Lebrilla, David A. Mills

Department of Nutrition, University of California, Davis, CA, USA

Abstract

Human milk contains a high concentration of diverse soluble oligosaccharides, carbohydrate polymers formed from a small number of monosaccharides. Novel methods combining liquid chromatography with high resolution mass spectrometry have identified approximately 200 unique oligosaccharides structures varying from 3 to 22 sugars. The increasing complexity of oligosaccharides follows the general pattern of mammalian evolution though the concentration and diversity of these structures in homo sapiens are strikingly. There is also diversity among human mothers in oligosaccharides. Milks from randomly selected mothers contain as few as 23 and as many as 130 different oligosaccharides. The functional implications of this diversity are not known. Despite the role of milk to serve as a sole nutrient source for mammalian infants, the oligosaccharides in milk are not digestible by human infants. This apparent paradox raises questions about the functions of these oligosaccharides and how their diverse molecular structures affect their functions. The nutritional function most attributed to milk oligosaccharides is to serve as prebiotics – a form of indigestible carbohydrate that is selectively fermented by desirable gut microflora. This function was tested by purifying human milk oligosaccharides and providing these as the sole carbon source to various intestinal bacteria. Indeed, the selectively of providing the complex mixture of oligosaccharides pooled from human milk samples is remarkable. Among a variety of Bifidobacteria tested only *Bifidobacteria longum* biovar *infantis* was able to grow extensively on human milk oligosaccharides as sole carbon source. The genomic sequence of this strain revealed approximately 700 genes that are unique to infantis, including a variety of co-regulated glycosidases, relative to other Bifidobacteria, implying a co-evolution of human milk oligosaccharides and the genetic capability of select intestinal bacteria to utilize them. The goal of ongoing research is to assign specific functions to the combined oligosaccharide–bacteria–host interactions that emerged from this evolutionary pressure.

Copyright © 2008 Nestec Ltd., Vevey/S. Karger AG, Basel

Milk and Lactation: Genomics as a Toolset to Reveal Unknown Biological Values of Milk Components

Milk is the only biomaterial that evolved to nourish growing mammals. Survival of mammalian offspring consuming milk as their sole food exerted a strong Darwinian selective pressure on the biochemical and genetic evolution of the lactation process, leading to the appearance of components that promote health and survival. This evolutionary pressure led to the proteins, peptides, complex lipids and oligosaccharides in higher order structures coming together as a complex, multi-component, yet highly organized food – milk. Although most research has focused on the essential nutrients present in milk, interestingly these are typically as essential to the mother as to the infant. Milk research has thus principally revealed the quantities, forms and bioavailability of the essential nutrients for infants. Nonetheless, in addition to the essential nutrients, the evolution of lactation led to a myriad of nonessential factors. Research to date has recognized that these nonessential compounds, structures and configurations act as growth factors, toxin-binding factors, antimicrobial peptides, prebiotics and immune regulatory factors within the mammalian intestine. Importantly, these trophic macromolecules deliver nutritional functions that, though not essential, provide biological advantages within the intestine and throughout the body that contribute to neonatal mammalian survival. The tools of genomics are beginning to provide the means to apply innovative strategies to accelerate our understanding of the functionality of the subsets of genes that are the products of evolutionary pressure on lactation – those expressed in milk [1, 2].

The Biology of Lactation

Mammary epithelial cell biology research has described the various stages of lactation, the physiology of the mammary gland, the physiology and supporting role of non-epithelial tissues, the energetics of lactation, the regulation of genes and proteins expressed during lactation, and the biochemical processes that occur within lactating mammary epithelial cells and the mammary gland. Unfortunately, to date, little research on lactation biology has focused on the primary underlying driving force for this biological process: the nutrition of the infant.

Milk composition, mammary function and the genes associated with lactation vary across mammalian species. These variations in the composition of milk and in the functions of milk across species point toward the adaptation of milk compositions to the environmental niches, reproductive strategies, and nutrients and growth requirements of different mammalian infants. Thus, the diversity of molecules and structures in different milks reflects the diverse functions of milks emerging through mammalian evolution and the mother–infant pair as an intense Darwinian engine. Integrating the various cellular processes of lactation with the nutritional functions of the nonessential molecules and structures produced by lactation will need both the tools of genomics and systems biology and the ingenuity of researchers. Essential nutrient annotation is relatively straightforward, an essential nutrient eliminated from the diet of an infant will produce a deficiency symptom every time, in every infant. However, nonessential components, structures and complexes are presumably beneficial only in a specific situation. Defining the situation is therefore necessary to defining the benefit itself. The development of the mammary gland throughout evolution illustrates the progression and context of the mammary gland to success of the offspring [3].

Infant Nourishment

Nourishing the mammalian neonate is the most obvious role of milk, and the success of mammals attests to the values of milk as an initial food source for the young of these species. The demands on milk as a sole source of nutrition are remarkable. All of the essential macronutrients, water, vitamins, minerals, amino acids and fatty acids, plus the basic structural and energetic intermediates needed to sustain life, must be delivered to the neonate in a highly absorbable form that is appropriate to the species and the stage of development – all at minimal energy cost to the mother. Lactation research has illuminated many of the biological processes needed to mobilize the essential biomolecules from maternal stores and to convert them into dispersed, transportable and bioavailable structures in milk.

Milk also provides myriad benefits to the growth, development and health-supporting processes of the young and mothers beyond the essential nutrients. The nonessential components of milk are not understood as well as those of essential nutrients, but research is now beginning to focus on their roles in the wellbeing of neonates. The research strategies needed to discover these properties are different from those used to discover the properties and roles of essential nutrients. Essential nutrients can be studied with relative ease because their elimination from the diet of animals leads to overt signs of deficiency in each individual. Nonessential nutrients and their functions, however, are only valuable within a particular context, thus investigations of benefits of nonessential nutrients must first recognize the context in which they are valuable.

Functions of Milk

The evolutionary origins of milk proteins and mammary regulation define the key functions of milk and the mammary gland. The evolution of the mammary gland likely involved adaptive recruitment of existing precursor genes through alteration of regulatory sequences to allow expression in primitive mammary glands and, duplication and mutation of structural sequences to acquire new functions from preexisting primitive proteins. The earliest mammary function after provision of nutrition was possibly the passing of protective advantages on to offspring by immunoglobulins, thus aiding selection for survival. This paved the way for the elaboration of myriad protective functions that we are only now beginning to appreciate.

The functions of milk generally can be considered supportive of both mammalian mothers and infants through several mechanisms. Milk provides nourishment of infant offspring; disease defense for the infant; disease defense for the mother; regulation or stimulation of infant development, growth or function; regulation or stimulation of maternal mammary tissue development, growth or function; inoculation, colonization, nourishment, regulation and elimination of infant microflora; and inoculation, colonization, nourishment, regulation and elimination of maternal mammary microflora.

Milk Oligosaccharides

Given the evolution of milk as a product of epithelial secretions nourishing mammalian offspring, the presence of non-digestible oligosaccharides would appear to be paradoxical. The question, why would milk contain indigestible material, has challenged scientists studying milk for decades. The presence and particularly the remarkable abundance of oligosaccharides in human milk as the third largest solid component have led investigators to propose biological, physiological and protective functions to these molecules [4–6]. Certainly, the number and structural diversity of these molecules would allow more than one function. However, to date, the detailed structural basis of these myriad functions is not yet understood. Recently, human milk oligosaccharides (HMOs) have been demonstrated to selectively nourish the growth of highly specific strains of bifidobacteria thus establishing the means to guide the development of a unique gut microbiota in infants fed breast milk [7–9]. Certain oligosaccharides derived from the mammalian epithelial cells of the mother also share common epitopes on the infant's intestinal epithelia known to be receptors for pathogens. The presence of such structures in milk have been hypothesized to have evolved to provide a direct defensive strategy acting as decoys to prevent binding of pathogens to epithelial cells, thereby protecting infants from diseases [10].

Consistent with the potential for multiple nutritional and biological functions, human milk is comprised of a complex mixture of oligosaccharides that differ in size, charge and abundance [11]. HMOs are composed of both neutral and anionic species with building blocks of 5 monosaccharides: D-glucose, D-galactose, N-acetylglucosamine, L-fucose, and N-acetylneuraminic acid. The basic structure of HMOs include a lactose core at the reducing end and are elongated by N-acetyllactosamine units, with greater structural diversity provided by extensive fucosylation and/or sialylation wherein fucose and sialic acid residues are added at the terminal positions [10]. The ability to understand the diversity of biological functions of HMOs has been hindered to date in part because of the lack of detailed structural knowledge of the overall complexity of HMOs in breast milk. At present, about 200 molecular species have been identified in a pooled human milk sample consisting of mostly neutral and fucosylated oligosaccharides [12].

The analytical methods that are capable of separating and characterizing the various sugar compositions and structures of oligosaccharides in human milk include high-performance liquid chromatography (HPLC), high pH anion exchange chromatography (HPAEC), capillary electrophoresis and various mass spectrometry platforms (MS) [13–21]. These methods as currently used are technically cumbersome, incapable of producing large quantities of highly purified isolated molecules and, as a result, there is little information on many of the basic biological properties of this class of molecule. Even with respect to the variation in abundances and structures across the human condition, little information has been developed. As a result the variation in nourishment that is likely to occur between different infants in different breastfeeding situations is also lacking. Combining the lack of basic information on the diversity of HMOs between different lactating humans, on changes in oligosaccharide compositions and abundances during the course of lactation and on the role of genetic, dietary and physiological determinants on the structures and abundances of HMOs it is difficult to predict at present to what extend variations in health outcomes of different breastfed infants is due to variation in the oligosaccharides delivered in their milk.

To establish the various functions associated with the diverse HMO structures the details of variations in compositions and abundances of oligosaccharides among humans and during lactation need to be measured. Characterization of HMO has been accomplished using HPAEC and HPLC in combination with derivatization techniques [4, 21–24]. The identification of HMOs was based on the retention time of commercially available milk oligosaccharide standards and their quantification was relative to the amount of standards. In one study, a decrease in the total concentration of oligosaccharides was observed from the first weeks postpartum to about half the concentration after one year. In the same report, the absolute and relative concentrations of HMOs between individual donors and at different stages of lactation varied significantly [22]. Asakuma et al. [24] analyzed the level of several neutral oligosaccharides in human milk colostrums for 3 consecutive days from 12 Japanese women. The concentrations of 2′-fucosylactose and lactodifucotetraose on day 1 were found to be substantially higher than those on days 2 and 3. On the other hand, the lacto-*N*-tetraose concentration increased from days 1 to 3. These data are compelling that variation in the structures and abundances of the various oligosaccharides in human milk are variable and it now becomes of considerable scientific and practical interest to understand the regulatory basis of these variations (genetics, diet, physiological state of the mother/infant, pathological state of the mother/infant, etc.).

The arrival of HPLC-Chip TOF/MS technology provides the analytical means to take a new strategy to routinely profile oligosaccharides in human milk [9, 11, 12]. This analytical technique employs an integrated microfluidic chip coupled with a high mass accuracy time-of-flight mass analyzer. Using this analytical platform nearly daily profiles of oligosaccharides in human milk samples were determined for different individual human donors (fig. 1). The levels of milk oligosaccharides and their heterogeneity were investigated both within the individual donor and among multiple donors at different stages of lactation. This approach is designed to provide basic knowledge on HMOs in normal humans as the key compositional basis to understanding the relationship between the levels of milk oligosaccharides and the specific functions these biomolecules contribute to maternal and infant health and development.

Analysis of Milk Oligosaccharides

Milk is a highly complex mixture of biomolecules with overlapping physical, chemical and biological properties. To study each class of these molecules at present it is necessary to isolate them in preparative scale. The initial steps of oligosaccharide chemical, structural and functional analysis used physical methods to separate oligosaccharides from the balance of milk components. Thus cells, lipids and proteins were separated from milk serum [8, 11]. In these laboratory scale studies, a combination of the centrifugation and liquid/liquid extraction was effective in removing lipids, proteins, and small molecules and concentrate oligosaccharides from single milk samples or various pooled milks. The oligosaccharides were desalted and concentrated using GCC-SPE to purify and partially fractionate oligosaccharides. Nonporous graphitized carbon cartridge (GCC; a material similar to PGC; Supelco, State College, Pa., USA) proved to be very effective in removing salts, monosaccharides, detergents (SDS and Triton X-100), proteins (including enzymes), and reagents for the release of oligosaccharides from glycoconjugates (such as hydrazine and sodium borohydride).

Once isolated, various analytical goals were established for the oligosaccharide research. The determination of the precise structural assignments for all HMOs was the first priority. Once in place, however, it was important to develop high throughput methods to analyze large numbers of samples to determine the distributions, concentrations and variations in biological samples from human milk to microbial fermentation studies. Finally, highly quantitative methods were necessary to establish which oligosaccharides were consumed by which bacteria during fermentation studies. This required the development of isotopic enrichment protocols to quantitatively compare entire mixtures of oligosaccharides before and after particular treatments.

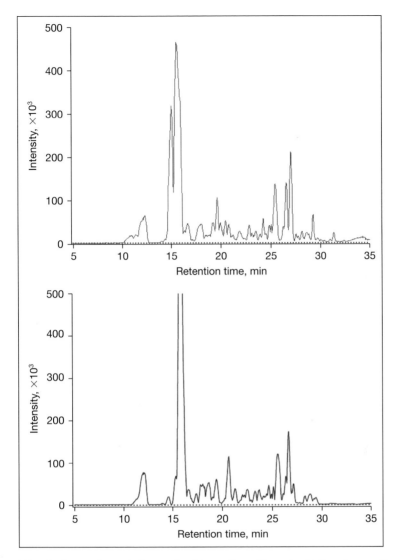

Fig. 1. Comparison of oligosaccharide profiles of breast milk from two mothers on day 6 of lactation. Oligosaccharides analyzed by the Agilent nano-LC chip TOF system.

For structural analyses, the strategy to annotate the human milk glycome was to perform tandem mass spectrometry, specifically infrared multiphoton dissociation, to obtain the sequence and connectivity of each residue and the position of the fucoses and the sialic acids and employ exoglycosidases to differentiate between isomers and determine ambiguous structures [12].

211

For routine analyses of oligosaccharide, samples in high throughput were analyzed using a microfluidic HPLC-Chip/MS technology developed with the active collaboration of Agilent Terchnologies Inc. [11]. The microfluidic HPLC-Chip was made using laser-ablated and laminated biocompatible polyimide film. The chip consists of an integrated sample loading structure, a packed LC separation column, and nanoelectrospray tip. It is hydraulically interfaced with LC pumps and an autosampler through a face-seal rotary valve. A nanoliter pump was used to deliver an LC gradient at 300 nl/min. The chip was interfaced to an o-TOF/MS for online nanoESI. Both the on-chip enrichment column and on-chip LC separation column were packed with porous graphitized carbon media.

For accurate quantitation of oligosaccharides by matrix-assisted laser desorption/ionization-Fourier transform ion cyclotron resonance mass spectrometry (MALDI–FTICR MS), a method using an internal deuterium-labeled standard was developed. In summary, oligosaccharides recovered from the microbial supernatants (100 μl) were reduced by adding 100 μl of 2.0 m sodium borohydride or sodium borodeuteride. Isotopic abundance ratios provided a highly accurate and detailed determination of the precise molecular differences between control and treated mixtures [9].

Infant Microflora

At birth, developing a healthy, protective and metabolically active gut microflora consisting of a wide range of bacteria in various ecological niches along the intestine (termed the infant's microbiome) is considered to be important to the acute health of the infant and the maturation of its intestinal system [25, 26]. Although there are some suggestions that infants are specifically exposed to bacteria prior to birth [27], mammalian infants are generally believed to be born with an intestine that is ostensibly sterile and is hence immediately exposed to various ingested bacteria [28]. Given the likelihood of the infant being challenged by (if not actually perfused in) a large number of aggressive pathogens, and considering the naïve status of both the innate and adaptive immune system of infants, the conditions that lead to and support the bacteria that colonize the infant's intestine have likely been under a very strong Darwinian pressure for survival throughout mammalian and particularly primate evolution. Albeit crude measures of this process have catalogued that breastfed infants are distinctive from adults and non-breastfed infants with an unusual abundance of bacteria generally characterized as bifidobacteria [7]. How Bifidobacteria establish such predominant numbers in breastfed infants and whether their abundance and/or growth properties provide distinct protection to the infant is the subject of intensive ongoing investigations [8, 29]. Several molecules have been proposed as candidates for the putative bifidobacterial growth factors including antimicrobial peptides, antibodies and milk oligosaccharides [5, 30]. Hence it is of considerable interest to know precisely how different bacteria are established in the gut of the newborn infant and in particular to understand what in breast milk leads to the unusual accumulation and persistence of the protective microbiome of breastfed infants. Therefore, a research strategy was developed to ascertain whether the oligosaccharides in human milk when isolated would provide a highly selective growth response in different species of intestinal bacteria.

Selective Microbial Fermentation of Milk Oligosaccharides

The functions of oligosaccharides in stimulating the growth of beneficial bacteria remain poorly understood. If oligosaccharides in milk are to be net beneficial by virtue of their selective stimulation of uniquely protective bacteria, the mechanisms behind this selectivity must be understood. Oligosaccharides purified from human milk were provided as the sole carbon source in a microbial growth assay inoculated with various bacteria. The bioselectivity of these oligosaccharides for specific bacterial growth are remarkable. Growth curves against time for 6 strains of Bifidobacteria are shown in figure 2. While all strains of Bifidobacteria grew well on lactose and several grew successfully on inulin, only *Bifidobacteria longum* biovar *infantis* grew successfully on HMOs as the sole carbon source supporting their growth.

Oligosaccharide Specificity by Different Bacteria

To determine the precise nature of the oligosaccharides that are consumed by different bacteria, the deuterium isotope enrichment technique was used to measure the difference in abundance of each of the different oligosaccharides before and after microbial fermentation. The flow sheet describing this technique is shown in figure 3a, and typical results in figure 3b. By incubating various bacteria with the milk oligosaccharide mixture and quantifying each of the respective mass-based structures, it is possible to build a map of the grazing strategy of different bacteria [31]. Using this approach *B. longum* bv. *longum*, *B. longum* bv. *infantis*, and *B. breve*, used as example bifidobacterial species isolated from the gut in infant and adults, were profiled for their selectivity in fucosylated and neutral HMO consumption oligosaccharides. *B. infantis* preferably consumed oligosaccharides with a degree of polymerization of ≤ 7 (m/z 1389 and below). These are quantitatively the most abundant oligosaccharides in pooled human milk. These data further suggest a direct relationship between what the mammary gland is producing and what the *B. infantis* strain consumes.

The implications of these data are clear. With infants consuming breast milk and digesting and absorbing all biomolecules possible, the abundance of

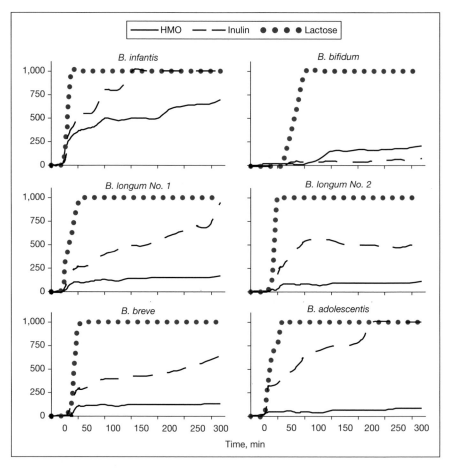

Fig. 2. Growth curves for different strains of bacteria using lactose, inulin and human milk oligosaccharides (HMO) as their sole carbon source. Modified from Ward et al. [8].

the milk oligosaccharides combined with the lack of enzymatic capabilities by the infant to digest them, the major biomolecule class reaching the infant's lower intestine will be the complex oligosaccharides. All bacteria that are attempting to colonize the infant's intestine will be forced to compete based on these oligosaccharides as their major carbon source. This places a prohibitive premium on the genetic capabilities of different bacteria to consume oligosaccharides. It is now the focused objective of this research to identify various strains of bacteria capable of consuming HMOs and to characterize

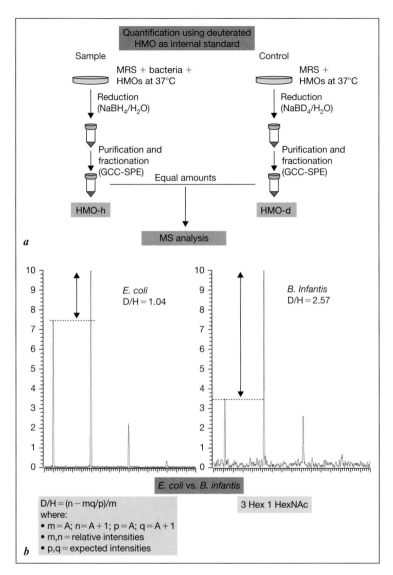

Fig. 3. **a** Flow sheet of the method of glycoprofiling using isotope enrichment and mass ratio quantitation. **b** Typical data comparing *E. coli* and *B. infantis* consumption of specific oligosaccharides.

the genomes of these organisms with sufficient detail to understand the basis of their unique ecological niche (breastfed infants) and the Darwinian advantage that this remarkable product of co-evolution provides to the breastfed infant.

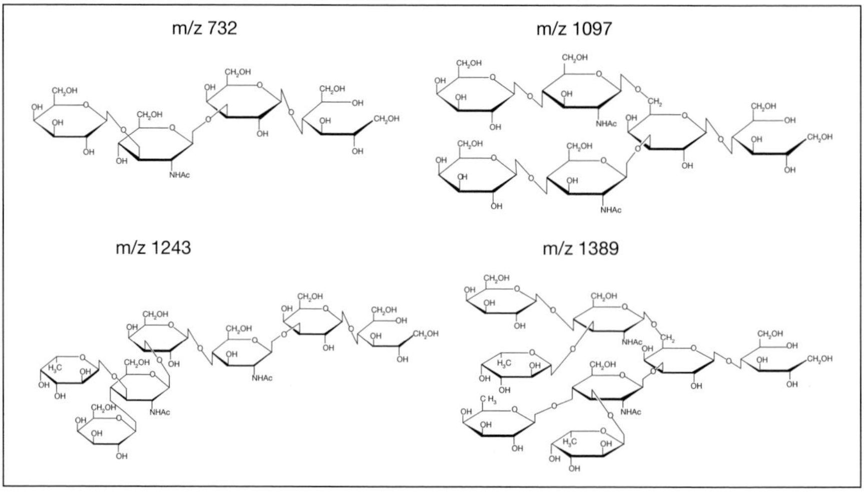

Fig. 4. Structures of human milk oligosaccharides consumed by *Bifidobacteria infantis*.

Personalization of Infants

It is intriguing to speculate on the role of the diverse oligosaccharide products found in human breast milk. Results to date demonstrate clearly that samples of breast milk from different mothers exhibit different concentrations, structures and lactational variation in their oligosaccharides. Do these variations provide infants with an unusual advantage? Do variations in the physiology of the mother or the infant trigger these variations? Would infants in particular environments, growth stages or physiological states take advantage of selective variations in the amounts of oligosaccharides? These are questions that must await future research to be resolved. Nonetheless, the intimate relationship between breast milk, infants and their resident microflora argues compellingly for active research in this area. It should be undertaken quickly to determine how oligosaccharide levels vary in different humans. Once accurate methods are in routine practice around the world, it will be possible to map the composition of HMOs with various health outcomes from diarrhea to allergy.

References

1 German JB, Dillard CJ, Ward RE: Bioactive components in milk. Curr Opin Clin Nutr Metab Care 2002;5:653–658.
2 German JB, Schanbacher FL, Lönnerdal B, et al: International milk genomics consortium. Trends Food Science & Technology 2005;vol 17(12):656–661.
3 Schanbacher FL, Talhouk RS, Murry FA: Biology and origin of bioactive peptides in milk. Livestock Production Science 1997;vol 50(1–2):105–123.
4 Coppa GV, Gabrielli O, Pierani P, et al: Changes in carbohydrate composition in human milk over 4 months of lactation. Pediatrics 1993;91:637–641.
5 Kunz C, Rudloff S, Baier W, et al: Oligosaccharides in human milk: structural, functional, and metabolic aspects. Annu Rev Nutr 2000;20:699–722.
6 Bode L: Recent advances on structure, metabolism, and function of human milk oligosaccharides. J Nutr 2006;136:2127–2130.
7 Harmsen HJM, Wildeboer-Veloo ACM, Raangs GC, et al: Analysis of intestinal flora development in breast-fed and formula-fed infants by using molecular identification and detection methods. J Pediatr Gastroenterol Nutr 2000;30:61–67.
8 Ward RE, Niñonuevo M, Mills DA, et al: In vitro fermentation of breast milk oligosaccharides by *Bifidobacterium infantis* and *Lactobacillus gasseri*. Appl Environ Microbiol 2006;72:4497–4499.
9 Niñonuevo MR, Ward RE, LoCascio RG, et al: Methods for the quantitation of human milk oligosaccharides in bacterial fermentation by mass spectrometry. Anal Biochem 2007;361:15–23.
10 Newburg DS, Ruiz-Palacios GM, Morrow AL: Human milk glycans protect infants against enteric pathogens. Annu Rev Nutr 2005;25:37–58.
11 Niñonuevo M, An H, Yin H, et al: Nanoliquid chromatography-mass spectrometry of oligosaccharides employing graphitized carbon chromatography on microchip with a high-accuracy mass analyzer. Electrophoresis 2005;26:3641–3649.
12 Niñonuevo MR, Park Y, Yin H, et al: A strategy for annotating the human milk glycome. J Agric Food Chem 2006;54:7471–7480.
13 Thurl S, Muller-Werner B, Sawatzki G: Quantification of individual oligosaccharide compounds from human milk using high-pH anion-exchange chromatography. Anal Biochem 1996;235:202–206.
14 Chaturvedi P, Warren CD, Ruiz-Palacios GM, et al: Milk oligosaccharide profiles by reversed-phase HPLC of their perbenzoylated derivatives. Anal Biochem 1997;251:89–97.
15 Charlwood J, Tolson D, Dwek M, Camilleri P: A detailed analysis of neutral and acidic carbohydrates in human milk. Anal Biochem 1999;273:261–277.
16 Nakhla T, Fu DT, Zopf D, et al: Neutral oligosaccharide content of preterm human milk. Br J Nutr 1999;82:361–367.
17 Shen ZJ, Warren CD, Newburg DS: High-performance capillary electrophoresis of sialylated oligosaccharides of human milk. Anal Biochem 2000;279:37–45.
18 Suzuki M, Suzuki A: Structural characterization of fucose-containing oligosaccharides by high-performance liquid chromatography and matrix-assisted laser desorption/ionization time-of-flight mass spectrometry. Biol Chem 2001;382:251–257.
19 Pfenninger A, Karas M, Finke B, Stahl B: Structural analysis of underivatized neutral human milk oligosaccharides in the negative ion mode by nano-electrospray MS(n) (part 1:methodology). J Am Soc Mass Spectrom 2002;13:1331–1340.
20 Pfenninger A, Karas M, Finke B, Stahl B: Structural analysis of underivatized neutral human milk oligosaccharides in the negative ion mode by nano-electrospray MS(n) (part 2:application to isomeric mixtures). J Am Soc Mass Spectrom 2002;13:1341–1348.
21 Sumiyoshi W, Urashima T, Nakamura T, et al: Determination of each neutral oligosaccharide in the milk of Japanese women during the course of lactation. Br J Nutr 2003;89:61–69.
22 Chaturvedi P, Warren CD, Altaye M, et al: Fucosylated human milk oligosaccharides vary between individuals and over the course of lactation. Glycobiology 2001;11:365–372.
23 Musumeci M, Simpore J, D'Agata A, et al: Oligosaccharides in colostrum of Italian and Burkinabe women. J Pediatr Gastroenterol Nutr 2006;43:372–378.
24 Asakuma S, Urashima T, Akahori M, et al: Variation of major neutral oligosaccharides levels in human colostrum. Eur J Clin Nutr 2007 [Epub ahead of print].

25 Kelly D, Conway S, Aminov R: Commensal gut bacteria: mechanisms of immune modulation. Trends Immunol 2005;26:326–333.
26 Forchielli ML, Walker MA: The role of gut-associated lymphoid tissues and mucosal defence. Br J Nutr 2005;93(suppl 1):S41–S48.
27 Perez PF, Doré J, Leclerc M, et al: Bacterial imprinting of the neonatal immune system: lessons from maternal cells? Pediatrics 2007;119:e724–e732.
28 Fanaro S, Chierici R, Guerrini P, Vigi V: Intestinal microflora in early infancy: composition and development. Acta Paediatr Suppl 2003;91:48–55.
29 Palmer C, Bik EM, Digiulio DB, et al: Development of the human infant intestinal microbiota. PLoS Biol 2007;5:e177.
30 Gyorgy P, Norris RF, Rose CS: Bifidus factor. I. A variant of *Lactobacillus bifidus* requiring a special growth factor. Arch Biochem Biophys 1954;48:193–201.
31 LoCascio RG, Ninonuevo MR, Freeman SL, et al: Glycoprofiling of bifidobacterial consumption of human milk oligosaccharides demonstrates strain specific, preferential consumption of small chain glycans secreted in early human lactation. J Agric Food Chem 2007;55: 8914–8919.

Discussion

Dr. Isolauri: You verbalized the historical view that human milk oligosaccharides (HMOs) are good and bifidobacteria are good, and thus we should increase bifidobacteria biota as if the bifidobacterium level were a health benefit per se. We have shown for instance that allergic infants have different bifidobacteria than healthy infants. So it makes a lot of sense that also HMOs have specific effects on different bifidobacteria.

Dr. German: One of the things that has actually been very intriguing is that we had no idea that this was going to be the way things worked out. We were very surprised about the differences in bifidobacteria and frankly the opportunity to now begin to assign these functions. We have started working with a company to deliver DNA chips so we can provide the means, for your program for example, to analyze quantitatively all the bifidobacteria in a very specific way, not by the technique of culture but by identifying each strain, which we think is actually going to be necessary now that it is clear that they are so different.

Dr. Walker: Does the quantitative composition of oligosaccharides substantially change with time?

Dr. German: As mothers, humans are about the most persistent oligosaccharide producers that we have found. Although primates for the most part tend to persist in their oligosaccharide support, rhesus monkeys, for example, are relatively similar to humans, but humans hold onto that production capability. But it is still too early to know exactly what the basis is. At the present time there is no evidence that there is a rapid decline in a specific subset or a specific group, they persist for quite a long time much of the way through lactation.

Dr. Walker: It is my understanding that in the first short period of postpartum life bifidobacteria are very important players but then as other organisms expand they play a lesser role. Does that have to do with other substrates that are available to stimulate colonizing bacteria?

Dr. German: From an ecological point of view it becomes very interesting because basically as long as the oligosaccharides in human breast milk are those things that are coming along, initially the bifidobacteria will in essence proliferate. The strategy of the mother recruiting an entire life form to babysit her infant is ingenious. But you can imagine that the bacteria that are going to begin to succeed in that environment will be the ones that can take that which the bifidobacteria are throwing away, and we see evidence of that already, such as your data that the gut begins itself to nourish. As the gut itself begins to mature successfully, it takes over a very important feeding role, and diversity begins to establish. It could be that not only are the initial bifidobacteria directed through oligosaccharides, but also a subsequent proliferation of species. Although this is a very recent elaboration in evolution, the long oligosaccharides seem to be the ones in similar studies showing binding. How these will in essence be able to provide surrogate binding sites for other bacteria even viruses is not yet known, so the ways with which the milk is regulating the intestinal ecosystem is quite complex. The fact that we are so unique relative to other primates suggests that there have been some things that humans have done in their recent history that unusually threatened infants from a pathogenic perspective, which again may say that unless there is a very threatening pathogenic environment, benefit won't necessarily be seen, and that may be why infant formula that does not contain these things hasn't shown any substantial difference in outcome. We haven't put infants in the sorts of pathogenic environments. It is possible that relatively similar primates don't have the amounts because they are relatively solitary and their infants are not exposed to the sorts of unusual clustered living that humans are.

Dr. Walker: Because oligosaccharides represent such a high percentage of the total content of breast milk, I always think that they are clonically fermented and then short-chain fatty acids were being taken up as an energy source. But from what you said, it seems that there is not so much fermentation going on. What is their use in addition to that; have you thought about that evolutionarily?

Dr. German: We have, and to a certain extent we have to start back at square one now that these molecules can be analyzed in high throughput, and especially to measure the entire ensemble, expose them to bacteria, viruses, etc., and then see what oligosaccharides are selectively taken up. Then we can identify and begin to functionally annotate those molecules. It is going to be a fascinating area of nutrition.

Dr. Bier: The classification of bacteria was at least historically based on relatively crude phenotypic types of things, and here you have given us one, I think these have an n of 1 genome. How stable is this genome in that species across the human population; what are the differences between those adult and infant genomes, and do we know, for example, in the gut ecology of the infant that the functions that aren't present in one bacteria aren't replaced by something else in the ecological system? It seems that we should at least have an n of 2 or 200, or something.

Dr. German: With the Joint Genome Institute (JGI) we have just finished sequencing 8 more. We have picked up some from sources in India, Africa and a couple in the United States, so even within *Bifidobacterium infantis* there are interesting differences within the genome. So there is a certain amount of diversity there, and it is certainly going to be an interesting area. There are other bacteria that look as though they will be able to grow but not as successfully and perhaps not as competitively. But interestingly it may mean that if you are not inoculated with the *B. infantis* you might begin to get some unusual bacteria which may be one of things that we see from cesarean section infants, for example. We are sequencing as fast as the JGI will give us capacity on sequencers, and thankfully we are getting better. We also want to be able to build the tools to be able to take this to human infant samples and begin to document that they are there in numbers and abundance. Also, where they are in human mothers because clearly they are being inoculated. If these bacteria are passed from mother to daughter through generations, a cesarean section in a sterile birth and incubator growth, keeping the infant away from these, could actually break that chain, and therefore at least the daughters should be re-inoculated so that they can keep that legacy going.

Dr. Räihä: Do the oligosaccharides cross the placenta? I am asking this because of the difference between a fetus who is developing to term in utero versus a fetus who is born prematurely and then receives quite a lot of oligosaccharides from the mother.

Dr. German: We are actually now taking the tools to a variety of other biofluids, and certainly the placenta will be studied. At this point we don't know; there are no data, and this must be pursued.

Dr. Gluckman: Do you know anything about maternal health and effects on oligosaccharide profile or maternal nutritional profile? You said each mother produces only roughly 130 over 200 possibilities. What about the 70 that are not produced? Is there a consistent pattern where the high variation is in the long chain?

Dr. German: No, that's interesting, in fact when you say 130 that doesn't mean that all mothers produce 130; there are some mothers who are producing only approximately 35. So there is variation and we don't know the difference. We are now in the process of recruiting samples from all over the world, from India, Gambia, South America, to answer those questions. Because there actually are infants and mothers in much more difficult situations in many respects and greater variation in outcomes, we think we can begin to assign some of those differences to more functional endpoints.

Dr. Gluckman: Is there a core group that is always produced?

Dr. German: The ones I showed are always there. To date we have never found a mother who doesn't produce the core that supports the *B. infantis;* the variation is primarily in the long ones.

Dr. Kunz: There was excellent work from Sweden, the United States, and Finland about 25–30 years ago demonstrating exactly 150 oligosaccharides. Coming back to the placenta, as far as we know these oligosaccharides are produced exclusively in the mammary gland and are based upon lactose. In my opinion there is no reason why they should pass the placenta unless we find other places where they are produced. You mentioned that these oligosaccharides are not digested. That's true but it doesn't mean that they are not absorbed. By using stable isotopes, we have shown in term and preterm infants that a small percentage (1–2%) are excreted in the urine of these infants [1]. Depending on the blood group and the secretory specificity, if an infant receives per suckling 50–150 mg bactoentitrose, which is the core structure, this must be absorbed and nobody knows exactly why. But this amount circulates in the blood and some will be excreted. This means that we have to investigate the systemic effects of milk oligosaccharides as well. I also agree that in animal species there is only a low number of milk oligosaccharides, basically of sialylated components. Each species, goat milk, sheep milk, gorilla and so on, all has an individual pattern. We don't know yet what this means. You showed 6 or 7 structures which are very specific regarding the functions of the bifidobacteria. The amount of oligosaccharides depends very much on the mother's Lewis specificity and secretory status. Meaning that if samples are analyzed, within a few days the Lewis activity, Lewis A or Lewis B activity or the secretory status, is known. Then there are 3 different patterns: the first group has a large amount of oligosaccharides 120–150; in the second group there are perhaps only 100, and the third group, only 10% of the population, is non-secretor and Lewis B and Lewis A negative and only has about 50 or 60. What do these very different patterns of milk oligosaccharides mean?

Dr. German: Actually that was one of the reasons for the underlying enthusiasm for the subject of this meeting and this workshop. There are aspects of diversity within the human condition that when looked at in some initial clinical trials of, for instance, diarrhea outcomes in Mexico City, differences in diarrhea in children can be assigned to secretory status. So we are confident that there is a pot of gold at the end of this but it is going to take a substantial amount of research. What we are going to establish are these encouraging specific bacteria, and then, are they binding to specific pathogens? This is a field that needs very good high throughput tools. It is a very important thing, and while bacterial stimulation has been our focus up until now, I think we are ready to begin to answer that sort of question, but it is going to take large studies. Individualizing outcomes takes a great deal of resources.

Dr. Corthésy: A very provocative presentation, at least for microbiologists. Since milk contains a high amount of lactose and the gut is lined with highly glycosylated proteins, why would bacteria select HMO to grow?

Dr. German: The initial thought would be that the lactose goes to the infant and the infant digests and absorbs that long before the lower intestinal bacteria so what we are basically likely to see is that the intestine is excluding everything but the oligosaccharides because of the infant's role in competing for digestible and absorbable molecules. The hidden oligosaccharides or next phase of glycobiology actually is in all the glycosylated proteins and lipids and I think that is going to make this area at least as complicated. If you look at the proteins and the extent of diversity of glycosylation of proteins and the fragments you get from proteolysis, one would argue that if a protein was only providing amino acids for nutrition, evolution would not select to decorate it and leave it as amino acids to be rapidly absorbed. If proteins were glycosylated by a sort of a backwards evolutionary logic there is a likely function to that and that means that we are also going to be enriching the infant intestine with specific glycosylated peptides for example, and how the different bacteria then compete for that will be another aspect of the ecology. Unfortunately Carlito Lebrilla and his group are still developing the tools for high throughput glycoproteomics, so by next year we should be able to report on those methods, but it is going to change the story as well. We still don't know what lactose does. I think that lactose may actually participate in this mother–infant conflict. We don't talk about this, but the infant has a 100% investment in its mother's milk. However, the mother has only a 50% investment in feeding the infant and so there is a fundamental conflict. The mother wants to wean off that infant and so while stopping breastfeeding is in the interest of the mother, it is not in the interest of the infant. How do you do that? One thought, and it is a very interesting idea, is that lactose is there in part because lactase can then be shut off, and lactose then becomes unpleasant and the breastfeeding experience becomes unpleasant. So looking at evolution and all the aspects of milk, there may be some things in milk that are of benefit to the mother—infant pair that are not actually in the infant's best interest. So when we start looking at the overall picture, it is going to be complicated.

Dr. Berry: As I recall, there are 2 or 3 marine mammals whose breast milk doesn't contain lactose. Have you had a chance to look at some of these more exotic species to see if oligosaccharides are missing?

Dr. German: We haven't been that extensive yet. In terms of our approaches, we have primarily been looking at the primate lineages to see if we could explain when and where they appeared and perhaps then be able to speciate the bacteria associated with that. There are certainly anecdotes of some very interesting animals and what they eat and their oligosaccharides. We have elephant milk because it is supposed to be very rich in milk oligosaccharides as well, but we're early on and in those sorts of analyses.

Dr. Berry: Are you suggesting that lactose is the building block for the oligosaccharides? If there is no lactose, then theoretically oligosaccharides couldn't be made?

Dr. German: There are two questions. One is if lactose can't be made, then the oligosaccharides can't be made, but lactose can actually be made, and just completely decorates all of it. Actually I believe marsupials can produce lactose. So lactose even though we think it is mammalian, it is a little bit earlier than that and defines that decision to become an epithelial secretor of these materials. Interestingly in the early development of kangaroos and similar marsupials, they appear to live basically on lactose and oligosaccharides.

Dr. Netrebenko: In the case of bottle feeding, what kind of oligosaccharides, prebiotics, could be the best source for the growth of *B. infantis*? Are there differences between the protective function of, for example, *B. infantis* and *Bifidobacteria longum*?

Dr. German: To be honest in terms of what you would supply to get the function of the *B. infantis* selection is right now one of the big challenges. What we see from things like inulin, is it supports a pretty discouraging broad range of bacteria and so I am not sure that in the long term we will think of inulin as being an infant-appropriate oligosaccharide source. The great dilemma for any one in the industrialization of this is where you are going to get HMOs. They are unique, and remember if they proliferate in a variety of places then bacteria would have proliferated, those gene sets would have been co-opted presumably by a variety of pathogens and lose selectivity. The heart of glycobiology is this constant competition between the organism decorating itself and pathogens trying to find adherence. Basically when a pathogen finds a way to do that, then disease occurs; the flue epidemics are a classic example where a new viral form is able to bind and get into human cells because of that difference. What we see in the commercial future is first oligosaccharides identical to human milk, but then there is no reason why we couldn't actually enhance this whole dimension to accelerate the evolution of humans to keep ahead of pathogens. The future of this I think is very exciting. Human milk has given us a paradigm but I would not think that industrially we will stop there. One could imagine actually getting much more sophisticated and the future probiotics being very sophisticated and individualized bacteria that are being selected for and evolved industrially to live on oligosaccharides that we are able to make. We will never make them more simple, we will make them more complex.

Dr. Strandvik: The mucous layer in the intestine needs fucose and sialic acid for the synthesis. Might it be that in the newborn and in early life the oligosaccharides are just substrates for the mucus before infants get other feeding?

Dr. German: Absolutely, sialidase may actually be one of the benefits of these bifidobacteria, that they are actually able to take sialic acid off the oligosaccharide and deliver it to the intestinal cells. That is certainly one of the hypotheses we are pursuing, the gene capability is there. I think it is a really good idea and would be one of the possible reasons to explain this co-evolution that bacteria are providing a catalytic activity that in essence doesn't exist in the infant.

Dr. Strandvik: that Would also explain a little about some of the variation because the fucosyltransferases are genetically determined in the human [2]. So that might be one point to explain the variation.

Dr. German: Absolutely and when you think about it from an evolutionary perspective, metabolites can frequently evolve faster, especially in a quantitative sense, than whole gene products. So in essence glycobiology is a great evolutionary machine itself and so you can see a rapid change in oligosaccharide amounts and patterns without massive changes in genes, but in the activities and regulation of the complement of enzymes.

References

1   Rudloff S, Pohlentz G, Diekmann L, et al: Urinary excretion of lactose and oligosaccharides in preterm infants fed human milk or infant formula. Acta Paediatr 1996;85:598–603.
2   Henry SM: Molecular diversity in the biosynthesis of GI tract glycoconjugates. A blood-group-related chart of microorganism receptors. Transfus Clin Biol 2001;8:226–230.

Bier DM, German JB, Lönnerdal B (eds): Personalized Nutrition for the Diverse Needs of Infants and Children.
Nestlé Nutr Workshop Ser Pediatr Program, vol 62, pp 223–237,
Nestec Ltd., Vevey/S. Karger AG, Basel, © 2008.

Opportunities for Improving the Health and Nutrition of the Human Infant by Probiotics

Seppo Salminen[a], Erika Isolauri[b]

[a]Functional Foods Forum, and [b]Department of Pediatrics, University of Turku, Turku, Finland

Abstract

The newborn is first colonized by microbes at birth. The colonizing bacteria originate mainly from the mother's gut, vaginal tract and skin. The origin of the microbiota and its development depend on genetics, mode of delivery, early feeding strategies and the hygienic conditions around the child. The indigenous microbiota of an infant's gastrointestinal tract is modulated through contact and interaction with the microbiota of the parents and the infant's immediate environment. After delivery breastfeeding continues to enhance the original inoculum by specific lactic acid bacteria and bifidobacteria and bacteria from the mother's skin enabling the infant gut microbiota to be dominated by bifidobacteria. These bacteria set the basis for gut microbiotia development and modulation along with breastfeeding and the environmental exposures such as antibiotic administration. Modifying this exposure can take place by probiotic bacteria when breastfeeding is not possible. Thus, incorporating specific probiotics selected for the development of the infant's gut microbiota may form a beneficial possibility for future infant feeding purposes. Many current probiotics have documented strain-specific health-promoting effects, and most of the effects that have been demonstrated in infants and children. The target in infants is to modify the gut microbiota to resemble that of the healthy breastfed infant and to counteract deviations or aberrancies present in infants at risk of specific diseases. Thus, providing specific selected probiotics to the mother to balance the intestinal microbiota during pregnancy and to the infant after birth. As the disturbed succession during early infancy has been linked to the risk of developing infectious, inflammatory and allergic diseases later in life, it is still of great interest to further characterize both the composition and succession of microbiota during infancy. With new methodologies we have been able to identify more specific aberrancies in microbiota prior to or during different disease states.

Introduction

According to current thinking, the newborn is colonized by microbes at birth. The colonizing bacteria originate mainly from the mother's gut, vaginal tract and skin, and bacteria can transfer from the gut to the infant as shown by probiotic intervention studies [1]. The origin of the microbiota and its further development depend on genetics, mode of delivery, early feeding strategies and the hygienic conditions around the child. The indigenous microbiota of an infant's gastrointestinal tract is modulated through contact and interaction with the microbiota of the parents and the infant's immediate environment. Bacteria are present in the environment of the infant prior to and after delivery, and breastfeeding continues to enhance the original inoculum by specific lactic acid bacteria and bifidobacteria enabling the infant's gut microbiota to be dominated by bifidobacteria. These bacteria set the basis for gut microbiotia development and modulation along with breastfeeding and the environmental exposures. Modifying the exposure can take place by probiotic bacteria when breastfeeding is not possible. Thus, incorporating specific probiotics selected for the development of the infant's gut microbiota may form a beneficial possibility for future infant feeding developments.

Many currently used and proposed probiotic bacteria have a scientifically demonstrated effect on human health [2, 3]. Most clinically demonstrated effects have been shown in infants and children. These may take place through a modifying effect on the relatively simple gut microbiota in infants. To improve infant nutrition we have to consider the development of gut microbiota along with the means to influence the process through dietary intervention with specific probiotics. The target in infants is to assist the development and maintenance of gut microbiota to resemble that of the healthy breastfed infant and to counteract deviations or aberrancies present in infants at risk of specific diseases. This forms the basis for healthy individual gut microbiota which promotes the health and wellbeing of the infant. Thus, providing specific selected probiotics to the mother to balance the intestinal microbiota during pregnancy and to the infant after birth will have an influence on the healthy microbiotia development and wellbeing.

Probiotics: The Definition

Probiotics are live microbial food supplements with demonstrated positive effects on host health [2, 3]. This definition indicates that not all lactic acid bacteria or bifidobacteria are probiotic bacteria. The safety and efficacy of each probiotic strain has to be demonstrated in carefully controlled human clinical studies [2, 3]. Scientific reports often refer to probiotic properties without specific documentation in intervention studies. However, even closely related species and strains may have significantly different health properties and thus have to be documented individually. An example is found in *Lactobacillus rhamnosus* studies. When two closely related *L. rhamnosus* strains were assessed in the treatment of rotavirus diarrhea, one was found to be effective and the other had no clinical effect on the duration of rotavirus diarrhea [4]. In other studies, viable *L. rhamnosus* GG (ATCC 53103) was reported effective in alleviating atopic eczema in infants. The same strain in a nonviable form was ineffective and caused side effects when administered to a similar infant population [5, 6].

Probiotics often act by modifying the process of intestinal microbiotia development or by affecting the composition and activity of developed microbiota [3]. In addition to microbiotia effects, probiotics can also act by direct contact with the mucosal cells facilitating cross-talk between the host and microbes [7]. Current probiotics have several demonstrated beneficial effects on infant health. These include the maintenance of healthy intestinal microbiotia development and counteracting deviations observed in gut inflammatory diseases or preceding them [8, 9]. The best studied effects have been demonstrated in the treatment and prevention of rotavirus diarrhea [10–12]. Other studies have been reported on the prevention of antibiotic-associated diarrhea with specific *Lactobacillus* GG [13, 14]. Probiotics have been demonstrated to reduce the risk of necrotizing enterocolitis in preterm neonates and, meta-analyses suggest that this may be the case in infants with less than 33 weeks gestation. Many of the described effects have been verified in meta-analysis studies, but only the most recent ones consider probiotics on a strain-specific basis [15–18].

How Do Probiotics Differ?

Each probiotic strain is a unique bacterium with its own strain-specific properties as already demonstrated when the strain differences were discussed. The unique properties are today best described by assessing the strain properties and some example strains. Genomic information has revealed a lot of new data on the probiotic properties. As an example, *Lactobacillus acidophilus* NCFM is a very acid tolerant strain which, upon entering the stomach, activates its adhesion ability by contact with stomach and bile secretions and adheres to the small intestinal mucosa [19, 20]. *Bifidobacterium longum*, on the other hand, is adapted to the lower part of the intestinal system to utilize breast milk oligosaccharides or intestinal mucus secretion as nutrient [21]. This makes *B. longum* an excellent bacterium in the intestinal tract of a breastfed infant. The strain also has special adhesive systems which may include microfimbriae to facilitate its adhesion to intestinal mucosa and probably also immune effects through this contact [21].

It has been suggested that combining specific probiotics may be useful in counteracting complicated microbiotia deviations. However, combining probiotics has also yielded significantly different clinical effects. An example again is the efficacy of *L. rhamnosus* strain GG (ATCC 53103) which has alleviated symptoms of atopic disease in infants [10]. On the contrary, when the same probiotic was administered in combination with *Bifidobacterium lactis, Propionibacterium freudenreichii* and *L. rhamnosus* LC 705, no clinical effect on symptoms of atopic eczema were observed [22]. In a prevention study, where the combination was administered to mothers prior to delivery and infants after birth, an effect on the prevention of atopic eczema was observed [22].

As all microbes have shuttle differences which may influence clinical outcomes, it is especially important to define the probiotic strains used as well as possible.

Intestinal Microbiota

Gut Microbiota in Neonates

The first colonizing bacteria in the infant gut originate from the mother's gut, vaginal tract and skin. Prior to birth the fetus is considered microbiologically sterile. However, this has been challenged recently by the demonstration of exposure of the fetus to bacteria in the amniotic fluid and through the placenta [23]. Thus it appears that the newborn is exposed to bacteria already prior to birth and the source of the original inoculum may vary. How the microbiota originates depends on genetics, mode of delivery, early feeding strategies, and the hygienic conditions around the child. Recently, it has been suggested that stress and dietary habits during later pregnancy and prior to birth may have a significant impact on the microbiota at the time of delivery thus influencing the quality and quantity of first colonizers of the newborn [24, 25].

Breast Milk

Human milk is generally considered the optimal nutrition for neonates as it contains the required nutrients and some protective compounds needed by the neonate. The diet of the mother has an effect on breast milk composition including the fatty acid composition and this in turn influences the adhesive properties of specific bacterial species and strains of bacteria. Many of the components such as oligosaccharides and fatty acids influence early microbial colonization of the infant gut. There is abundant evidence that breast milk also transmits bacteria to the infant gut [26, 27]. Many pathogens have been shown to arise in breast milk from the mother's skin and more bacteria from the infant's gastrointestinal tract and mouth [26]. However, breast milk also contains a natural bacterial inoculum which has an impact on the developing infant's microbiota [27, 28]. Perez et al. [28] have shown that some bacterial signatures in breast milk are common in the infant's feces and mother's blood samples. In mouse studies translocation from the gut to mammary gland via mesenteric lymph nodes has been described [29, 30].

Transfer of Breast Milk Microbiota

Expressed human milk contains commensal bacteria which are specific to the environment and the mother. Breastfeeding exposes the milk duct to skin bacteria and also intestinal bacteria from the neonate. In normal breast milk the bacterial content depends on contamination with the skin, skin bacteria in general, breastfeeding (feedback from the infant) and contamination with gut bacteria. Additionally there are the bacteria originating from the mother's gut. These bacteria and their combinations accelerate the adjustment of the infant's gut microbiota to adapt to the environment of the mother and child. They are likely to have a significant impact on the succession and establishment of the type of microbiota (fig. 1).

In recent studies it was demonstrated that breast milk contains around 3,000 bacteria/ml and an average of almost 10^3 bifidobacteria/ml [26, 27]. The milk from an individual mother may contain from 1 to 5 different bifidobacterial species. Transfer of the maternal bacteria via breast milk may be a natural means of reinforcing the colonization of the gastrointestinal tract of the neonate. Thus, breast milk forms a unique personalized source of bacteria typical of the particular environment in which the mother and infant reside.

Impact of Breast Milk Microbes on the Health of the Child

The microbial provocation originally obtained from the mother changes over time. Yet it appears that large numbers of bifidobacteria and lactic acid bacteria form an essential supplementary bacterial inoculum to the breastfed infant. Generally, a competitive exclusion effect between breast milk microbes and their impact on gut microbiota is a factor that may shape the succession of microbiota during breastfeeding and weaning. By reinforcing the original inoculum from the mother and by providing breast milk oligosaccharides, the mother acts as a constant source of both probiotic bacteria and prebiotics to the newborn. This supplementation is likely to modify and shape the normal gut microbiota. As several studies have suggested a protective impact of breastfeeding against different intestinal tract-associated diseases, the colonization effects may provide one explaining mechanisms for the observed effects [30, 31] and suggest a basis for the development of healthy gut microbiota.

Succession of Microbial Communities

The step-wise process of indigenous microbiotia establishment begins with facultative anaerobes such as the enterobacteria, coliforms, lactobacilli and

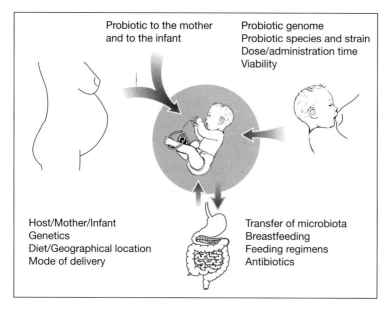

Probiotic to the mother
and to the infant

Probiotic genome
Probiotic species and strain
Dose/administration time
Viability

Host/Mother/Infant
Genetics
Diet/Geographical location
Mode of delivery

Transfer of microbiota
Breastfeeding
Feeding regimens
Antibiotics

Fig. 1. Factors affecting microbial colonization of the mother and the infant with points of intervention with probiotics.

streptococci first colonizing the intestine. These are rapidly succeeded by bifidobacteria and lactic acid bacteria.

The development of infant gut microbiota is usually characterized by the following steps: early colonization at birth with facultative anaerobes depending on the mode of delivery with rapid succession by anaerobic genera such as *Bifidobacterium, Bacteroides, Clostridium* and *Eubacterium.* Molecular methods indicate that lactic acid-producing bacteria may account for less than 1% of the total microbiota while bifidobacteria can range from 60 up to 90% of the total fecal microbiota in breastfed infants. In formula-fed infants the microbiota is more complex, but depends on the composition of formula. The new techniques indicate that the greatest difference in the microbiota of breastfed and formula-fed infant lies both in the bifidobacterial numbers and species composition within the intestinal microbiota, while the lactic acid bacteria composition appears to be rather similar. *Bifidobacterium breve, Bifidobacterium infantis* and *B. longum* are frequently found in fecal samples of breastfed infants, whereas the most common lactobacilli in both breastfed and formula-fed infant feces constitute *L. acidophilus* group microorganisms such as *L. acidophilus, L. gasseri* and *L. johnsonii.* In general, the differences between the breastfed and formula-fed infants have decreased along with the improved composition of infant formulas [32].

Probiotic Effects on Immune Responses

Specific probiotic bacteria are involved and may assist in the development and maintenance of the gut immune homeostasis by either influencing microbiotia composition and metabolic activity or by directly modulating immune responses through gut mucosal signaling pathways. These mechanisms strengthen the epithelial barrier function and may inhibit pathogen adhesion to mucosal surfaces and consequent growth and invasion. Probiotics can interact with the mucosal immune system via the same pathways as commensal bacteria, specifically via interaction with epithelial cells and dendritic cells. Through this interaction there is an influence on both innate and adaptive immune responses. Probiotic effects on immune responses appear to be immune-regulating rather than immune-activating. In vitro and in vivo studies in mice and humans have shown that probiotics may predominantly modulate dendritic cell and T regulatory cell activity rather than T-helper responses per se. For example, *Lactobacillus casei* Shirota strain was shown to increase the Th1 response in an animal model of diabetes but to inhibit Th1 responses in an animal model of allergic disease, suggesting an effect at the T-regulatory cell level [8–10]. As with probiotics in general, each effect is unique to a defined strain and no extrapolation can be made on the properties of closely related strains.

Probiotic Benefits to Infant Nutrition

The best documented benefits of specific probiotics have been demonstrated in the reduction in the risk of gastrointestinal diseases such as necrotizing enterocolitis, rotavirus diarrhea, antibiotic associated side effects, and the treatment and prevention of atopic diseases. Probiotic combinations, apart from *B. lactis* Bb12 and *L. rhamnosus* GG combined, have not been successful in infants. Several intervention studies, especially on atopic diseases, are currently on their way, under evaluation and being published as indicated in a recent review [33].

The practical benefits of specific probiotics and specific probiotic combinations in infant nutrition may lie in the early microbiotia modification.

First, modifying the microbiota of the pregnant mother is important. This approach may provide benefits to the microbiota and the wellbeing of the mother during pregnancy by influencing both the composition of intestinal microbiota and the consequent metabolic activity. Specific bifidobacteria and lactic acid bacteria have been demonstrated to be transferred from the mother to the infant during delivery and during breastfeeding [34]. Thus, the balance of mother's intestinal tract microbiota and vaginal microbiota may influence the outcome in the infant. Microbiota may also predispose infants to later health problems as has been reported for atopic diseases [35] and recently for obesity development [36, 37].

Second, specific probiotic bacteria may be important for providing microbial stimulus to the intestinal microbiota during early infancy to assist in establishing a healthy gut microbiota and the barrier against harmful microbes and detrimental dietary components. Similarly, as the infant receives lactic acid bacteria and bifidobacteria via breast milk during breast-feeding, these are likely to deliver some of the beneficial effects associated with breastfeeding, such as protection against diarrheal diseases, atopic diseases and even obesity. Thus, it may be important to correct potential deviations in infant microbiota and to offer formula-fed infants bacterial stimuli in a form of safe probiotic lactic acid bacteria and bifidobacteria. It could be that the probiotic bacteria-supplemented formulae may better mimic the effects provided by breastfeeding. These aspects have been discussed by the North American and European expert group reports [38, 39].

Conclusions

The most important focus point in probiotic research for infant nutrition is to recognize the individual properties of specific probiotics. Each strain is different and the properties of each strain and the combinations of each strain are unique. Therefore, the scientific documentation behind probiotics always focuses on specific probiotic strains or specific probiotic combinations.

The current scientific contributions to infant health clearly include shortening of the duration of rotavirus diarrhea, reduction in risk of rotavirus diarrhea, reduction in the risk of antibiotic-associated side effects, alleviation of atopic eczema symptoms, and prevention of atopic eczema, and balancing of the deviated infant microbiota.

The healthy human microbiota is metabolically active and acts as a defense mechanisms for our body. Deviations in its composition are related to multiple disease states within the intestine but also beyond the gastrointestinal tract. Components of the human intestinal microbiota or organisms entering the intestine may have both harmful or beneficial effects on human health and clearly the genomic approach on the human infant side and the probiotic side will assist in formulating new approaches to benefit infant health.

The available information focuses mostly on the crucial role of infant microbiota and the first colonization steps to later health. Especially bifidobacteria play a key role in this process. The mother–infant contact has an important impact on initial development. The mother provides the first inoculum at birth, promotes the bifidogenic environment through prebiotic galacto-oligosaccharides in breast milk and introduces environmental bacteria through her skin and other contact with the infant, thus providing the means to promote guidance to the development of individually optimized microbiota under the existing environmental conditions for each infant.

The future target is to further clarify both the sequelae and the succession of microbial communities especially during and after weaning and during the first years of life. Another target is to understand the use of specific probiotics and prebiotics to influence microbiotia development and maintenance as well as dietary management of the reported health-related microbiotia deviations.

Potential Future Approaches

The knowledge on intestinal microbiotia acquisition and intestinal microbiotia development increases rapidly. This facilitates the understanding on the impact of probiotics on intestinal microbiotia composition and metabolic activity. Successful probiotics have two main characteristics: the ability to colonize the infant intestinal tract, influence the microbiota, and its composition and activity effects and immunological properties. These have been the main targets for probiotics. Recent studies have also indicated that intestinal microbiota can act on the host signaling system to have an impact on host health. Such developments enable the thorough understanding of intestinal microbiota and help to identify the right probiotic strains or combinations to counteract or to normalize particular well-characterized microbiotia aberrancies. These will require carefully designed intervention studies to establish the suggested effects and to apply them to practical infant nutrition guidelines and practices.

References

1 Penders J, Thijs C, Vink C, et al: Factors influencing the composition of the intestinal microbiota in early infancy. Pediatrics 2006;118:511–521.
2 Salminen S, Bouley MC, Boutron-Rualt MC, et al: Functional food science and gastrointestinal physiology and function. Br J Nutr 1998;80(suppl 1):S147–S171.
3 WHO 2001. Guidelines for assessing probiotics. http://www.who.int/foodsafety/fs_management/en/probiotic_guidelines.pdf
4 Majamaa H, Isolauri E, Saxelin M, Vesikari T: Lactic acid bacteria in the treatment of acute rotavirus gastroenteritis. J Pediatr Gastroenterol Nutr 1995;20:333–338.
5 Isolauri E, Arvola T, Sutas Y, et al: Probiotics in the management of atopic eczema. Clin Exp Allergy 2000;30:1604–1610.
6 Kirjavainen PV, Salminen SJ, Isolauri E: Probiotic bacteria in the management of atopic disease: underscoring the importance of viability. J Pediatr Gastroenterol Nutr 2003;36:223–227.
7 Di Caro S, Tao H, Grillo A, et al: Effects of *Lactobacillus GG* on genes expression pattern in small bowel mucosa. Dig Liver Dis 2005;37:320–329.
8 Isolauri E, Salminen S, Ouwehand A: Manipulation of the gut microbiota: probiotics. Best Pract Res Clin Gastroenterol 2004;18:299–313.
9 Isolauri E, Salminen S: Probiotics, gut inflammation and barrier function. Gastroenterol Clin North Am 2005;34;437–450.
10 Saavedra JM, Bauman NA, Oung I, et al: Feeding of *Bifidobacterium bifidum* and *Streptococcus thermophilus* to infants in hospital for prevention of diarrhoea and shedding of rotavirus. Lancet 1994;344:1046–1049.

11 Sandhu BK, Isolauri E, Walker-Smith JA, et al: A multicentre study on behalf of the European Society of Paediatric Gastroenterology and Nutrition Working Group on Acute Diarrhoea. Early feeding in childhood gastroenteritis. J Pediatr Gastroenterol Nutr. 1997;24:522–527.

12 Arvola T, Laiho K, Torkkeli S, et al: Prophylactic *Lactobacillus GG* reduces antibiotic-associated diarrhea in children with respiratory infections: a randomized study. Pediatrics 1999;104:e64.

13 Vanderhoof JA, Whitney DB, Antonson DL, et al: *Lactobacillus GG* in the prevention of antibiotic-associated diarrhea in children. J Pediatr 1999;135:564–568.

14 Szajewska H, Ruszczynski M, Radzikowski A: Probiotics in the prevention of antibiotic-associated diarrhea in children: a meta-analysis of randomized controlled trials. J Pediatr 2006;149: 367–372.

15 Johnston BC, Supina AL, Vohra S: Probiotics for pediatric antibiotic-associated diarrhea: a meta-analysis of randomized placebo-controlled trials. CMAJ 2006;175:377–383. Erratum in: CMAJ 2006;175:777.

16 Sazawal S, Hiremath G, Dhingra U, et al: Efficacy of probiotics in prevention of acute diarrhoea: a meta-analysis of masked, randomised, placebo-controlled trials. Lancet Infect Dis 2006;6:374–382.

17 Deshpante G, Rao S, Patole S: Probiotics for prevention of necrotizing enterocolitis in preterm neonates with very low birthweight: a systematic review of randomized controlled trials. Lancet 2007;369:1614–1620.

18 Altermann E, Russell WM, Azcarate-Peril MA, et al: Complete genome sequence of the probiotic lactic acid bacterium *Lactobacillus acidophilus* NCFM. Proc Natl Acad Sci USA 2005;102:3906–3912.

19 Pridmore RD, Berger B, Desiere F, The genome sequence of the probiotic intestinal bacterium Lactobacillus johnsonii NCC 533. Proc Natl Acad Sci USA 2004;101:2512–2517.

20 Schell MA, Karmirantzou M, Snel B: The genome sequence of *Bifidobacterium longum* reflects its adaptation to the human gastrointestinal tract. Proc Natl Acad Sci USA 2002;99:14422–14427.

21 Viljanen M, Savilahti E, Haahtela T, et al: Probiotics in the treatment of atopic eczema/dermatitis syndrome in infants: a double-blind placebo-controlled trial. Allergy 2005;60:494–500.

22 Bakardjiev AI, Theriot JA, Portnoy DA: *Listeria monocytogenes* traffics from maternal organs to the placenta and back. PLoS Pathog 2006;2:e66.

23 Bailey MT, Lubach GR, Coe CL: Prenatal stress alters bacterial colonization of the gut in infant monkeys. J Pediatr Gastroenterol Nutr 2004;38:414–421.

24 Kirjavainen PV, Kalliomaki M, Salminen SJ, Isolauri E: Postnatal effects of obstetrical epidural anesthesia on allergic sensitization. Allergy 2007;62:88–89.

25 Heikkila MP, Saris PE. Inhibition of Staphylococcus aureus by the commensal bacteria of human milk. J Appl Microbiol. 2003;95:471–478

26 Gueimonde M, Laitinen K, Salminen S, Isolauri E: Breast milk: a source of bifidobacteria for infant gut development and maturation? Neonatology 2007;92:64–66.

27 Martin R, Heilig H, Zoetendal E, et al: Cultivation-independent assessment of the bacterial diversity of breast milk among healthy women. Res Microbiol 2007;158:31–37.

28 Perez PF, Dore J, Leclerc M, et al: Bacterial imprinting of the neonatal immune system: lessons from maternal cells? Pediatrics 2007;119:e724–e732.

29 Martin R, Langa S, Reviriego C, et al: The commensal microflora of human milk: new perspectives for food bacteriotherapy and probiotics. Trends Food Sci Technol 2004;15:121–127.

30 Becker AB: Primary prevention of allergy and asthma is possible. Clin Rev Allergy Immunol 2005;28:5–16.

31 Rinne M, Kalliomaki M, Arvilommi H, et al: Effect of probiotics and breastfeeding on the bifidobacterium and lactobacillus/enterococcus microbiota and humoral immune responses. J Pediatr 2005;147:186–191.

32 Collado MC, Jalonen L, Meriluoto J, Salminen S: Protection mechanism of probiotic combination against human pathogens: in vitro adhesion to human intestinal mucus. Asia Pac J Clin Nutr 2006;15:570–575.

33 Prescott SL, Björkstén B: Probiotics for the prevention or treatment of allergic diseases. J Allergy Clin Immunol 2007;120:255–262.

34 Gueimonde M, Sakata S, Kalliomaki M, et al: Effect of maternal consumption of lactobacillus GG on transfer and establishment of fecal bifidobacterial microbiota in neonates. J Pediatr Gastroenterol Nutr 2006;42:166–170.

35 Kalliomäki M, Kirjavainen P, Eerola E, et al: Distinct patterns of neonatal gut microflora in infants developing or not developing atopy. J Allergy Clin Immunol 2001;107:129–134.

36 Collado MC, Kalliomaki M, Salminen S, Isolauri E: Fecal microbiota composition may predict overweight in children. J Pediatr Gastroenterol Nutr 2007;44:e325.

37 Kalliomäki M, Collado MC, Salminen S, Isolauri E: Early differences in fecal microbiota composition in children may predict overweight. Am J Clin Nutr 2008;87:534–538.

38 Michail S, Sylvester F, Fuchs G, Issenman R: Clinical efficacy of probiotics: review of the evidence with focus on children. NASPGHAN Nutrition Report Committee. J Pediatr Gastroenterol Nutr 2006;43:550–557.

39 Agostoni C, Axelsson I, Braegger C, et al: Probiotic bacteria in dietetic products for infants: a commentary by the ESPGHAN Committee on Nutrition. J Pediatr Gastroenterol Nutr 2004; 38:365–374.

Discussion

Dr. Björkstén: Thank you for this elegant presentation and I agree basically with everything you said. However, I would like to suggest that perhaps we should have an alternative approach. One may question the evidence for strain specificity. I think that the traditional reductionist approach of one molecule or one specific bacteria may not be an optimal approach. The internal ecology is as complex as the ecology of a jungle. Going for one specific strain would of course be wonderful for the industry.

Dr. Salminen: To a certain extent I would agree and I was actually not promoting a single strain approach at all. I was rather demonstrating that especially in the infant gut microbiota, when we try to modulate it, we have to be primarily safe rather than sorry. Therefore we have to select the safest alternatives, and I am quite convinced that these alternatives won't work for you and me. With such a complex environment, only in early childhood do we have the luxury of a simple microbiota which can be influenced in a simple way. That is exactly the reason why most of the studies showing clinical efficacy to probiotics are actually from infants.

Dr. Björkstén: I agree with this. I think at this stage it is alright to include various strains of lactobacilli in the meta-analyses, provided that the studies were done properly. It may be that differences in the outcome of various studies are more a consequence of different environments than of different strains. You quoted Dr. Prescott's and my recent review summarizing the allergy-prevention studies [1]. Three of them were positive and one negative. Although there were different strains, the major difference between the studies may actually be that in the negative study, treatment only started after birth, while in the three positive studies treatment started in the pregnant mothers.

Dr. Salminen: That is certainly one explanation, but I still question and I have asked the producers several times to provide information on the strain that was used in the negative study, because it would be very interesting for the scientific community to understand what the properties are in a particular strain that might have influenced the outcome. So far I have not had an answer from the producer concerning the strain or the preclinical and safety studies on it.

Dr. Hernell: 25 years ago Dr. Björkstén and myself were involved in writing guidelines for milk banks in Sweden and there was always concern about the bacterial contamination of breast milk – that was before the hygiene hypothesis. When the bacterial count in the breast milk was too high, we recommended that the mothers clean their breasts and nipples and the amount of bacteria dropped very significantly. Have you checked what happens with the bifidobacteria in the milk if the mother cleans her breast?

Dr. Salminen: We of course tried to have sampling procedures as clean as possible; if the sampling procedures were not clean we would have had much higher concentrations.

For instance, there is a study from Spain that almost suggested that breast milk like yogurt has 10^7 CFU/ml and I am sure that part of those bacteria were really from the sampling procedures and from the skin. For us having perhaps 10^2 to 10^3 CFU/ml, I think this is realistic and we significantly reduced contamination by doing that. The important thing that should also be discussed is that when we think about personalized nutrition, breast milk is really personal in the way that the bacteria are also adjusted to the environment of the mother. It is meant for that particular baby living in that particular environment, it is not meant for somebody living in New York City or somebody living in Japan, but that particular surrounding; that is what makes it virtually impossible to personalize the bacterial content unless the approach is to use a safe bacterium, a specific member of the healthy intestinal gut microbiota, in infants who remain healthy for years to come.

Dr. Prescott: I have more of an answer than a question. The strain that we used is also known as LAFTI-10. It was used by Clancy et al. [2] who recently published a paper on it. It is produced by DSM Foods in Australia. The company that provided it to me asked us to use a different trade name, so I hope that helps.

Dr. Salminen: That certainly helps but it also returns us to our discussion yesterday that the basic principle in all studies would be to use the International Culture Collection numbers so that we would know what type of bacteria there is.

Dr. Prescott: Absolutely, and as I previously indicated we commenced this study in the 1990s before any of the other studies had been published. It was very difficult to know which strain to choose in any of these studies, and our choice was limited by what was available at the time. There was also very little information in the area at the time, so I am sure you agree.

Dr. Savilahti: You started by remembering our mothers as the source of gastrointestinal microflora, and then you said that some lactobacilli come from vegetable sources. How large a proportion of gastrointestinal flora originates from nonhuman sources, from the soil, from drinking water, from the feces of other animals? It is known that children who grow up on farms have fewer allergies, which is thought to be because they inhale lipopolysaccharides but they actually also eat feces from the cattle, and we know that if there are a lot of cats and dogs, allergy is reduced. Do these other sources permanently change our microbiota?

Dr. Salminen: I don't think it is important whether they permanently change; what happens in early childhood is. For instance we haven't seen the probiotics that are used today to permanently colonize anybody, but it is important how the success of the microbiota is facilitated during early life, and certainly the success is different if you live in a different environment. Several speakers have pointed out that there are differences between countries and certainly if we live in the US, Europe, Australia, Japan, most of our food technologists have always been taught to kill all the bacteria in our food supply. We have worked together with Indonesian researchers, and there is a totally different environment. There are the natural lactic acid bacteria, bifidobacteria from all environmental sources, from the food supply, from water, from the hygienic conditions, the exposure is totally different. So basically we are trying to reverse what food technology has done to us, trying to introduce some of the friendlier bacteria back, the ones that we have always wiped out during the last 50–60 years.

Dr. Savilahti: Are these bacteria human specific or are they specific for other species?

Dr. Salminen: Bacteria are very difficult. I know that the early definition of probiotics actually said that we should have bacteria of human origin, but what is of human origin? Does it mean that any bacteria we have eaten and stays for a while in our intestinal content, or something that is only adhering to our mucosa that we never see in the fecal samples? I think it is easier to define what you have, especially in infants; you have a healthy gut microbiota defined in such a way that those children remain healthy for years to come, and you look at the composition and the types of safe bacteria there that you can take. We have all sorts of passersby that cause transient diarrhea in adults and children; we have viruses that cause transient diarrhea, change the metabolic profile and activity of our intestinal microbiota, so it is quite difficult to say whether something is really of human origin or whether it is specific to humans. We then also have to understand the adaptability of bacteria. There was a wonderful article on *Bacteroides fragilis* in *Science* 2 years ago [3] and, just by its position in the gastrointestinal tract, a single strain can take at least 12 different phenotypes that act totally differently, and it depends on the stimuli provided by the intestinal mucosa, by the interaction with the intestinal mucosa, and the same bacteria which we analyze in the feces is one form but it could be 12 different forms in the upper intestinal tract. So bacteria are very adaptable, and whether they are really specific or not to one mammalian species I wonder. We did a study with Dr. Arthur Ouwehand in our laboratory where we compared the species specificity, looking at opossums from Australia, crocodiles, cats, cows, humans, and actually there was no real species specificity [4]. Adhering bacteria adhered; if you want to displace a pathogen you can do it in an opossum or a crocodile as well as you do it in a human. So the idea is to select the ones that are really members of what is healthy and normal to your species.

Dr. Isolauri: I want to summarize what we mean by identifying the strain and identifying the population. Our studies [5, 6] are frequently compared with that of Brouwer et al. [7]. In our studies [5, 6] at weaning breastfed infants were given extensively hydrolyzed formula with or without probiotics, then after that treatment period they were challenged and then only those who had cow's milk allergy fulfilled the study criteria. The opposite was done in the Netherlands study [7], in which formula-fed infants of the same age were given extensively hydrolyzed formula, and then an open challenge was made with cow's milk which was negative. So even though the patient population was infants, some were allergic, some were not, some had gut involvement, and others didn't, but then they had different microbiota to begin with. So it is also very important to chose the food matrix and the target population.

Dr. Klassen-Wigger: Thank you for your presentation that nicely summarized the current evidence on the efficacy of probiotic strains that can be of interest for an infant population. However, some of the strains that you were referring to are D-lactate producers and as such current regulation does not allow their use in infant nutrition. Do you think that the scientific community is trying to pave the way for changing this legislation or at least trying to get a bit more evidence about this?

Dr. Salminen: I think that is a very good and complicated question. If I look at it from the point of view of the regulatory authorities, for instance the European Food Safety Authority (EFSA), safety is of primary importance, and that is why there are hurdles that actually do prevent many of the new products from becoming available on the market. If I recall correctly, this matter of lactic acid product safety was studied for one of the strains beforehand, but it still doesn't exclude the fact that, especially in German-speaking countries, the regulation is very strict. So that is another point, harmonizing the regulations even within the countries of the European Union is happening only little by little. Going back to safety, there is also the EFSA safety assessment procedure. We currently have the qualitative presumption of safety document which is available on the EFSA website (http://www.efsa.europa.eu/EFSA/efsa_locale-1178620753812_1178667590178.htm). I actually recommend all of you to have a look before you go into a clinical intervention study. If you go to the EFSA website, search for QPS, you will find a number of documents that actually list the safety studies and safety assessment of different types of probiotic products in Europe. Again in the US it is a totally different ball game of course, and as far as I understand there is no such list on the FDA net basis at the moment. But EFSA is really focusing on that, not only in the human area but also in the animal probiotics area, and there are very strict criteria for the safety assessment, which will probably make it even harder for some of these products to find their way to the consumers, or lengthen the time at least. But on the other hand, as I said, it is better to be safe when you deal with bacteria.

Dr. Björkstén: We have actually looked at D-lactic acid production by one of the probiotic *Lactobacillus* strains and also looked at the evidence behind the caution for D-lactic acid-producing bacteria. The studies were merely suggestions from the 1960s rather than studies and there is no novel documentation. It just shows how the bureaucracy hangs around for ever. So I don't think that it is an issue. We have always said that the mother is the source of the bacteria and that is obviously true for some strains in vaginally delivered babies. Dr. Hernell referred to studies that were done when we were younger. Dr. Gothefors in our team showed for *Escherichia coli* that it was equally common that the baby got the strain from outside and subsequently colonized the mother. This was under somewhat other hygienic conditions 35 years ago in Sweden than we have today. So it may be more complicated than only blaming the mother.

Dr. Salminen: I always say that you can't blame your mother; you can only thank your mother for what you have got. She has certainly done her best and under the circumstances given what can be given. It is a process and not only the mother; what has happened before defines it. We actually have a couple of papers in which we describe this mother–infant transfer of microbiota, and it must be taken into account that it is not always possible for the mother to understand or have an impact on what she is giving her offspring [8–10].

Dr. Walker: I want to come back to what Dr. Isolauri mentioned several times, that is the matrix in the succession of bacteria. Could you comment on that?

Dr. Salminen: I think the genomic information that I showed very simple examples of is actually quite important. For instance, let's think about health foods; quite often we take these capsules that pass all these triggers which are important for at least those 3 sample model strains. It should also be carefully considered whether the bacteria in a food matrix thrive on that particular matrix or whether they are given in a dormant state. I think this is as important as the strain itself.

Dr. Koletzko: Allow me to come back to the question of D-lactic acid and the comment that Dr. Björkstén made. I fully agree that in most infants and children it is probably a nonissue, but I would be careful with concluding that it is not a safety concern. We have been measuring D-lactic acid for a number of years now and have regularly seen cases of D-lactic acidosis in children with short bowel syndrome. The symptomatology is exactly as that which veterinarians describe as the drunken cow's syndrome. It is a neurological disturbance which most people probably would not associate with D-lactic acid until they have actually measured it and seen it. It is easy to treat short bowel syndrome either with dietary changes or antibiotics. But I think it needs to be looked at before we conclude that it is a nonissue in infants.

Dr. Björkstén: May I just comment on that very briefly? I didn't say that it's a non-issue in short bowel syndrome, I said that it is a nonissue with regard to the use of probiotic bacteria.

Dr. Koletzko: I agree that it is probably a nonissue in most cases, but I think we should have some data before we draw that conclusion.

Dr. Salminen: I can only say that it has been extensively considered by several authority working groups, and I don't think there is a big change for the time being. It is still being considered and I quite agree that the early studies were not well done. We also went to those to look where the ban, so to say, originates, but there are also some worries regarding the information which makes people cautious.

Dr. Haschke: Just to contribute to the more recent data, there is a study by Claude Bachman, presently under review, looking at a huge cohort with regard to D-lactic acid excretion when those kinds of bacteria where added to a starter formula. I can only say that in a double-blind study there was no higher excretion as compared to controls.

Dr. Isolauri: Just a brief comment on the mother–infant transfer of bacteria. Even though the child's first inoculum frequently comes from the mother, it is not passive. This means that the child does not directly get those bifidobacteria which the mother carries.

References

1 Prescott SL, Björkstén B: Probiotics for the prevention or treatment of allergic diseases. J Allergy Clin Immunol 2007;120:255–262.
2 Clancy RL, Gleeson M, Cox A, et al: Reversal in fatigued athletes of a defect in interferon gamma secretion after administration of *Lactobacillus acidophilus.* Br J Sports Med 2006;40:351–354.
3 Coyne MJ, Reinap B, Lee MM, Comstock LE: Human symbionts use a host-like pathway for surface fucosylation. Science 2005;307:1778–1781.
4 Rinkinen M, Westermarck E, Salminen S, Ouwehand AC: Absence of host specificity for in vitro adhesion of probiotic lactic acid bacteria to intestinal mucus. Vet Microbiol 2003;97: 55–61.
5 Majamaa H, Isolauri E: Probiotics: a novel approach in the management of food allergy. J Allergy Clin Immunol 1997;99:179–185.
6 Isolauri E, Arvola T, Sütas Y, et al: Probiotics in the management of atopic eczema. Clin Exp Allergy 2000;30:1604–1610.
7 Brouwer ML, Wolt-Plompen SA, Dubois AE, et al: No effects of probiotics on atopic dermatitis in infancy: a randomized placebo-controlled trial. Clin Exp Allergy 2006;36:899–906.
8 Grönlund MM, Gueimonde M, Laitinen K, et al: Maternal breast-milk and intestinal bifidobacteria guide the compositional development of the Bifidobacterium microbiota in infants at risk of allergic disease. Clin Exp Allergy 2007;37:1764–1772.
9 Gueimonde M, Laitinen K, Salminen S, Isolauri E: Breast milk: a source of bifidobacteria for infant gut development and maturation? Neonatology 2007;92:64–66.
10 Gueimonde M, Kalliomäki M, Isolauri E, Salminen S: Probiotic intervention in neonates – will permanent colonization ensue? J Pediatr Gastroenterol Nutr 2006;42:604–606.

Bier DM, German JB, Lönnerdal B (eds): Personalized Nutrition for the Diverse Needs of Infants and Children.
Nestlé Nutr Workshop Ser Pediatr Program, vol 62, pp 239–252,
Nestec Ltd., Vevey/S. Karger AG, Basel, © 2008.

Do We Need Personalized Recommendations for Infants at Risk of Developing Disease?

Olle Hernell, Christina West

Department of Clinical Sciences, Pediatrics, Umeå University, Umeå, Sweden

Abstract

Current nutrition recommendations, directed towards populations, are based on estimated average nutrient requirements for a target population and intend to meet the needs of most individuals within that population. They also aim at preventing common diseases such as obesity, diabetes and cardiovascular disease. For infants with specific genetic polymorphisms, e.g. some inborn errors of metabolism, adherence to current recommendations will cause disease symptoms and they need personalized nutrition recommendations. Some other monogenic polymorphisms, e.g. adult hypolactasia, are common but with varying prevalence between ethnic groups and within populations. Ages at onset as well as the degree of the resulting lactose intolerance also vary, making population-based as well as personalized recommendations difficult. The tolerable intake is best set by each individual based on symptoms. For polygenetic diseases such as celiac disease, type-1 diabetes and allergic disease, current knowledge is insufficient to suggest personalized recommendations aiming at primary prevention for all high-risk infants, although it may be justified to provide such recommendations on an individual level should the parents ask for them. New technologies such as nutrigenetics and nutrigenomics are promising tools with which current nutrition recommendations can possibly be refined and the potential of individualized nutrition be explored. It seems likely that in the future it will be possible to offer more subgroups within a population personalized recommendations.

Copyright © 2008 Nestec Ltd., Vevey/S. Karger AG, Basel

Introduction

Historically, the main objective of nutrition recommendations was to prevent deficiency disorders. Today nutrition recommendations have shifted their main focus from prevention of deficiency disorders to maintaining good health and preventing major chronic diseases, e.g. coronary heart disease (CHD), obesity, diabetes, cancer and osteoporosis. Our recent understanding that early nutrition may impact on morbidity in these diseases in adult life [1] has turned nutrient recommendations for pregnant women and infants into an even more challenging task. So far, dietary recommendations target populations, or subgroups of populations, e.g. infants, children, pregnant and lactating women and elderly, but not individuals. Below we discuss whether there is a need to make nutrition recommendations more personalized, in particular for infants with an increased risk of certain diseases, and if we have sufficient scientific basis for such a change.

Nutrient Requirements and Dietary Recommendations

Nutrient recommendations are based on scientific knowledge taking into account food habits and health conditions within the target population. Generally, observational and experimental studies are the basis for decisions on nutrient requirements, for associations of diet and health, and for food-based recommendations. The requirement for a nutrient in a population can be described as a cumulated dose-response relationship. In the Nordic Nutrition Recommendations [2] as well as in the European Union Scientific Committee for Food Recommendations [3], the average requirement denotes the intake of a nutrient that represents the average requirement for a group of individuals. This corresponds to the estimated average intake recommendations used in the UK [4] and USA [5]. Studies using biochemical indicators on 'status' after feeding diets with different amounts of a nutrient exceeding what is required to elicit clinical deficiency symptoms are often used to define the average requirements of a population. Nutrient balance studies and/or factorial methods are also used to assess average requirements and make decisions on recommendations, particularly for minerals. Hence, current nutrient recommendations are not for individuals, but variations in requirements between individuals of the same age and sex are taken care of by adding a margin of safety, e.g. +2 SD to the calculated average requirement. The reference intake in the Nordic Nutrition Recommendations [2], the reference nutrient intake in the European Union [3], recommended daily allowance in the USA [4] and population reference intake in the UK [5] refer to the amount of a nutrient that, based on current knowledge, can meet the known requirement and maintain good nutritional status among practically all healthy individuals in the target population.

Geographic Differences in Nutrition-Related Disease Patterns

Epidemiological studies have shown striking differences between populations and countries in the prevalence of many diseases. For instance, there is a strong association between the incidence of CHD and the level of serum cholesterol in a population as well as between the death rate from CHD and the median serum cholesterol concentration, which also mirrors the correlation between CHD deaths and the percentage of fat derived from saturated fatty acids. It is now generally accepted that diet plays a role in the etiology of many multifactorial diseases such as cancer, CHD and diabetes [6]. Hence, besides the basic requirements to maintain body stores and functions, most dietary recommendations are also based on correlations, or at least associations between nutrient intakes and food composition on the one hand and the risk of developing various diseases on the other [2]. Thus, the importance of considering not only recommended intakes based on the average requirement and a safety margin but also maximum intakes or upper limits has caught increasingly more attention [7]. This has generally been adopted for the energy-yielding nutrients, i.e. fat, fatty acids and carbohydrate, but also for some other nutrients. Several controlled intervention studies have shown that a diet in agreement with, for instance, the Nordic Nutrition Recommendations [2], i.e. fat constituting around 30% of the energy (E%) of which no more than 10 E% should be saturated fatty acids (from 2 years of age), rich in dietary fiber, an adequate amount of n-3 fatty acids, and frequent consumption of fruit, vegetables, whole grain products, and regular consumption of fish and regular physical activity, can reduce the risk of or, alternatively, have a beneficial influence on several risk factors for overweight, diabetes and CHD including serum lipids, blood pressure and insulin resistance. The age from which the same recommendations should be applied for children as for adults is however controversial [8]. Although, these recommendations aim at reducing the risk of contracting common diseases on the population level, they do not take into account all possible individual risk factors such as extreme susceptibility due to genetic polymorphisms or to the feeding pattern in infancy.

Nutrigenetics and Nutrigenomics

Genetic variation is known to affect food tolerances among human subpopulations. There are many examples on how nutrients are directly involved in gene regulation, which may have both short- and long-term consequences, as well as on how genetic variation caused by single nucleotide polymorphisms (SNPs) within a gene may affect digestion, absorption, excretion, storage or transport of a nutrient, which in turn may contribute to variation in the requirement for that nutrient and also the risk of disease symptoms. One example is the Ala222Val polymorphism in the methylene tetrahydrofolate reductase gene, which substantially alters folate metabolism increasing the risk of neural tube defects and cardiovascular disease but possibly decreasing the risk of colon cancer [9]. This illustrates that merely increasing the reference intake for the whole population to cover the requirement for folate for this phenotype may at the same time have negative health consequences for the target population. This is important to take into account when decisions on general supplementation programs are made, but also when considering personalized recommendations. All potential consequences need to be known before recommendations are given. Other known polymorphisms, for instance in apolipoprotein E can explain why some individuals respond differently than others to dietary modifications, e.g. aiming at normalizing elevated plasma cholesterol levels [6, 10]. Seemingly healthy individuals have different SNPs of a particular gene. In fact such polymorphisms are normal and only a minority of them causes disease, or may cause symptoms only when a nutrient is consumed in excess [9].

In the area of gene–diet interactions, nutrigenetics and nutrigenomics are two emerging concepts. The former addresses the importance of genotype (mainly SNPs) on the risk of nutritionally related disease. It has developed from the assumption that certain genetic polymorphisms measurably alter nutritional deficiency. Genetic polymorphisms are identified and studied to see if they modulate the relationships between nutritional exposure and risk. The aim of nutrigenetics is thus to generate recommendations on an individual basis regarding the risk and benefit of specific dietary components.

Nutrigenomics addresses the inverse relationship. It focuses on the effect of food-borne components on gene transcription, proteomics and metabolomics, and involves the characterization of gene products and the physiological function and interaction of these products, promoting an increased understanding of how nutrition influences metabolic pathways and homeostatic control. The premise in this case is that diet influences disease through mechanisms regulating gene expression. Nutritional genomics aims to identify the genetic variation that accounts for individual reactions to dietary components. It is obvious that nutrigenomics is much more difficult to use in nutritional research than nutrigenetics [10, 11]. The question is whether such individual differences impact on dietary recommendations to the extent that they become individualized for each genetic makeup. In this context it should however be noted that if the data used to set the reference intake (recommended daily allowance) and upper limits are based on a diverse population, these should encompass most of the genetic variation in that population.

Some Examples from Monogenic Disorders

Phenylketonuria

Phenylketonuria (PKU) is a classical autosomal recessive inherited deficiency of the enzyme phenylalanine hydroxylase, resulting in a lost or reduced capacity to convert phenylalanine to tyrosine, a substantial increase in phenylalanine in serum, and severe mental retardation unless dietary phenylalanine is restricted [12]. The prevalence varies between populations but in Caucasians 1 infant per 12,000 born is diagnosed with PKU. Large numbers of SNPs within the gene have been described. Because of the severity of the disease and the profound preventive effect of early dietary treatment, many countries now screen all newborn infants for raised levels of phenylalanine (the Guthrie test). Patients diagnosed with PKU are subject to personalized dietary recommendations, illustrating that for a few genotypes this already exists. So far neonatal screening is carried out for a few monogenic diseases but, with technical developments in recent years, the possibility of screening for many more inherited metabolic diseases has emerged [13].

Familial Hypercholesterolemia

Familial hypercholesterolemia (FH) is a co-dominant inherited disorder characterized by very high concentrations of low-density lipoprotein cholesterol (LDL-C) and a severely increased risk of premature CHD. The clinical phenotype and, hence, premature death from CHD is much more pronounced for homozygotes than for heterozygotes. While homozygous individuals are rare (1 per million), the heterozygous condition, typically referred to as FH, is relatively common (1 per 300 to 1 per 500 in most countries). The underlying reason is a mutation in the LDL-receptor gene [14] with severely reduced clearance of LDL particles from the circulation. More than 800 different mutations have been identified and, as for PKU, the phenotypic expression varies considerably. Obviously, some mutations result in more severe clinical phenotypes than others depending on what exact function of the protein is affected. However, also individuals who share the same SNP in the LDL-receptor gene may differ substantially in clinical presentation of the disease. It seems that additional factors influence the clinical course of FH, e.g. modifying genes. Several factors, including various lipases and apolipoproteins, e.g. apolipoprotein E polymorphisms, seem to have such a modifying effect on LDL-C for several common polymorphisms of FH [10]. Another modifier is of course diet, which is used in the treatment of hypercholesterolemia. It is interesting to note that while FH is a much more prevalent disease than PKU, and it is well established that the atherosclerotic process starts early in life and that FH results in severe risk for premature morbidity and mortality [14], there is no general screening for FH and most countries do not recommend general pre-symptomatic diagnosis and early preventive dietary intervention [15]. In fact, most countries do not screen children of parents diagnosed with FH due to early CHD, which may seem doubtful from an ethical point of view.

Adult Hypolactasia

Geographic variation in disease patterns results from both dietary and genetic differences. An example on how genetic variation may affect food tolerance is adult hypolactasia, a normal condition among mammals including man, encompassing around 70% of the world's population. After weaning there is a gradual reduction in the activity of the lactase-phlorizin hydrolase enzyme, which hydrolyzes lactose to absorbable glucose and galactose. Lactase persistence can be regarded as a mutant phenotype (autosomal dominant trait), which arose 5,000–10,000 years ago coinciding with the domestication of cattle. 95% of people of Asian origin carry the adult hypolactasia genotype, compared to 80% of African-Americans and less than 5% of Caucasians of northern European and Scandinavian descent [16]. Recently Ennath et al. [17] ascribed adult hypolactasia in caucasians to one major mutation (C13910T) located approximately 14 kb upstream from the LCT locus, the gene coding for lactase-phlorizin hydrolase. Interestingly, different mutations seem to have appeared around the same time among Africans and Caucasians [18]. The sensitivity to lactose differs considerably between individuals with the same genetic polymorphism, and symptoms may appear already in early childhood in Asian populations while they rarely occur before teenage or adolescence in Finns [16]. Therefore, it must be pointed out that while adult hypolactasia is a laboratory diagnosis, lactose intolerance is a clinical diagnosis. Thus confirming that the adult hypolactasia genotype is not sufficient for personalized dietary recommendations. The capacity to digest lactose varies between individuals, with age and a number of other factors, again illustrating that gene–diet interactions are indeed complex. The tolerable intake is best decided on by each individual based on symptoms.

Some Examples from Polygenic Disorders

Celiac Disease

Celiac disease (CD) is a chronic inflammatory disease of the small intestine, affecting genetically susceptible individuals. Virtually all CD patients express the HLA-DQ2 and/or HLA-DQ8 alleles. Other as yet not identified genes account for at least half of the genetic risk. CD is caused by failure to establish and/or maintain tolerance to dietary prolamins in wheat, barley and rye, and particularly to wheat gliadin. Active disease is associated with an intestinal lesion, typically showing villous atrophy, crypt hyperplasia, and increased numbers of lymphocytes within both the epithelium and the lamina propria [19]. Clinical and histological improvements are seen upon withdrawal of wheat, barley, and rye from the diet, which is the only current treatment of CD. Most likely each separate genetic risk factor is fairly frequent in the general population, suggesting that a combination of some of these genes and their interaction with the environment induce CD, making it a chronic disease of multifactorial etiology.

In the mid 1980s, Sweden experienced a unique epidemic of symptomatic CD in children below 2 years of age. The incidence reached levels higher than ever reported at that time. It decreased as quickly as it had increased to the level seen before the epidemic [20]. The most plausible cause of the epidemic was a variation over time of some causal factors affecting a large fraction of the Swedish infant population as only children below 2 years of age were affected. Changes in infant feeding practices were suspected to be the culprit. In a case-referent study we could indeed demonstrate that early infant feeding practices contributed to the epidemic. If gluten is introduced slowly while the mother is still breastfeeding, the risk for the child to contract CD before 2 years of age is reduced (odds ratio (OR) 0.59; 95% confidence interval (CI) 0.42–0.83) [21] compared to if gluten is introduced after breast feeding has been discontinued. The longer the mother continues to breastfeed after gluten has been introduced into the diet, the greater the protective effect seems to be. Moreover, the amount of gluten given during the first 2 weeks after the first exposure also was found to be an independent risk factor. Based on the distribution of flour consumption of the referents we found that consuming large amounts (corresponding to the upper third of the distribution) as compared to small or medium amounts (lower and middle third of the distribution) increased the risk (adjusted OR 1.5, 95% CI 1.1–2.1) [21]. These observations led to new national recommendations on gluten introduction in 1997, i.e. to change the age at introduction from 6 months to between 4 and 6 months as for other complementary foods, and to introduce small amounts of gluten gradually, preferentially while the mother is still breastfeeding. The new recommendations coincided with the observed rapid decline at the end of the epidemic [20], suggesting that primary prevention of CD may be possible by dietary recommendations. However, Sweden as most other European countries has adopted the WHO recommendation on exclusive breastfeeding for 6 months, i.e. again to postpone gluten introduction to 6 months of age, a change that preceded the abrupt increase in the epidemic in 1983 [20]. Thus, these two recommendations may be in conflict unless mothers continue to breastfeed beyond 6 months of age. Would it therefore be justified to adopt personalized dietary recommendations to reduce the risk for children below 2 years of age to contract CD? One possibility would be to test infants with first-degree relatives who have CD for the HLA-DQ2 and DQ8 haplotype. Should they carry one of them, their parents could be advised to introduce gluten between 4 and 6 months and encourage the mothers to continue breastfeeding well beyond the introduction. However, it is not yet known if cohorts born after as compared to during the epidemic carry less life-time risk of contracting CD. An ongoing Swedish screening study will answer if primary prevention by dietary guidelines is at all possible [22].

Type-1 Diabetes

There are indications that the pathogenic process leading to type-1 diabetes (T1D) starts very early in life and during childhood the incidence has shifted towards lower age in many countries. As for CD the early feeding pattern may modulate the risk of developing T1D in genetically susceptible individuals. Moreover, patients with T1D are at increased risk of developing CD. Not only are breastfed infants at less risk than formula-fed infants of developing

T1D but also the timing of the introduction of both gluten-containing solids and cow's milk as well as the amount of cow's milk consumed at 1 year of age have been suggested to affect the risk. It is possible that introduction before 3 months confers a greater risk than between 4 and 6 months of age [23, 24]. However, exactly how weaning habits affect the risk for T1D is still not clear. The ongoing Trial to Reduce IDDM in Genetically at Risk, which tests the hypothesis that weaning to an extensively hydrolyzed infant formula will decrease the incidence of T1D, as demonstrated in animal models, will hopefully solve the question on the role of cow's milk protein in the pathogenesis. Until then and until more is known about which genes besides HLA are crucial, it seems premature to give personalized advice for high-risk infants besides encouraging breastfeeding; although besides the introduction of milk as a potential risk factor, it seems that the same strategy suggested for CD could also be applied to the prevention of T1D.

Allergic Diseases

The prevalence of allergy and asthma is increasing and approximately 20% of the world population suffers from IgE-mediated allergic diseases. Individuals with a family history of atopy have an increased risk of developing IgE sensitization and typical symptoms of eczema, allergic asthma, allergic rhinitis and/or allergic conjunctivitis. Immune programming starts early in life and several approaches to prevent IgE sensitization have been implemented over the years. However, there are no reliable genetic and immunologic markers to identify an infant at risk, which complicates primary prevention of IgE sensitization. A positive family history is the most reliable predictor of allergy in infants [25]. Dietary measures in the prevention of allergy have included avoidance of dietary antigens during pregnancy and breastfeeding with no evidence of long-term prevention of allergy. Rather, such a diet could be harmful by adversely affecting maternal as well as fetal nutrition [26]. Studies exploring the effects of breastfeeding in the prevention of allergy have produced conflicting results, and an obvious shortcoming is the lack of randomized studies for ethical reasons. However, in a Cochrane review, exclusive breastfeeding for 6 vs. 3–4 months did not significantly reduce the risk of allergic disease [27]. The Section of Pediatrics of the European Academy of Allergy and Clinical Immunology recommends breastfeeding combined with avoidance of solid foods and cow's milk for the first 4–6 months of life in the prevention of allergic disease in high-risk infants. When breastfeeding is not possible, feeding of a hypoallergenic formula is recommended [28]. However, it is recognized that studies underlying these recommendations have methodological shortcomings [28, 29], and elimination diets in the long-term prevention of allergy have been inconclusive.

The decline in microbial exposure during early childhood is one of the most probable reasons for the increasing incidence of allergic disease in the Western world. Both epidemiological studies and gnotobiotic animal models have been supportive of such a hypothesis [30]. Gut microbiota is a major stimulus of the immune system and is suggested to act by inducing T-cell immune regulation. This has driven the idea of using probiotics, mainly bifidobacteria and lacto-bacilli, for the treatment and prevention of allergic disease. Today, dietary preventive strategies are moving from allergen avoidance towards controlled dietary antigen exposure and stimulation of the gut microbiota via pre- or probiotics. Some studies have demonstrated a positive effect of probiotics in the treatment and prevention of eczema while other studies do not support these findings, and no clear preventive effect has been demonstrated on sensitization or any allergic disease other than eczema [for review see, 30].

Prebiotics, non-digestible fermentable oligosaccharides stimulating the growth and/or activity of a limited number of bacteria in the colon, can influence gut microbial composition and activity. Including prebiotics in the infant diet in the prevention of allergy is a promising approach, but so far data from clinical studies are limited. Data on pre- and probiotics in the treatment and prevention of eczema are still preliminary and inconclusive, and at this stage it is too early to recommend such treatment for all infants at risk. However, if parents still wish to try probiotic supplements in addition to standard treatment of eczema, personalized recommendations could be considered provided well-documented probiotic strains are used.

Conclusion

In conclusion, current nutrition recommendations are directed towards populations and are based on estimated nutrient requirements for these populations. Hence, these recommendations should cover most of the existing genotypes within a population. For certain infants with specific genetic polymorphisms, e.g. some inborn errors of metabolism, adherence to current nutrition recommendations or food-based recommendations will cause disease symptoms and they already need personalized nutrition recommendations. It can be foreseen that modern nutrigenetics will allow more diagnoses to be included in this group within a near future. Other SNPs, e.g. adult hypolactasia causing lactose intolerance, vary considerably between ethnic groups and within populations. Age at onset and sensitivity also vary making population-based as well as personalized recommendations difficult. For polygenetic diseases such as CD, T1D and allergic disease, current knowledge is too limited to suggest personalized recommendations for all high-risk infants, although it may be justified to provide such recommendations should the parents ask for them. With refined methodology and a growing understanding of nutrigenomics, our capacity to identify larger groups of the population who would benefit from personalized nutrition- and food-based recommendations will increase. However, who will pay the cost and who will have the competence to make these recommendations?

References

1 Lucas A: Programming by early nutrition in man. Ciba Found Symp 1991;156:38–50.
2 Nordic Nutrition Recommendations 2004, ed 4. Copenhagen, Nordic Council of Ministers, 2004.
3 Commission of the European Communities: Nutrient and Energy Intakes for the European Community. Reports of the Scientific Committee for Food, 31st series. Luxembourg, Office for Official Publications of the European Communities, 1993.
4 Committee on Medical Aspects of Food Policy: Dietary Reference Values for Food Energy and Nutrients for the United Kingdom. Report on Health and Social Subjects. London, HMSO, 1991.
5 Food and Nutrition Board: Dietary Reference Intakes for Energy, Carbohydrate, Fiber, Fat, Fatty Acids, Cholesterol, Protein, and Amino Acids (Macronutrients). Washington, National Academic Press, 2002.
6 Gibney MJ, Gibney ER: Diet genes and disease: implications for nutrition policy. Proc Nutr Soc 2004;63:491–500.
7 Aggett PJ, Bresson J, Haschke F, et al: Recommended dietary allowances (RDAs), recommended dietary intakes (RDIs), recommended nutrient intakes (RNIs), and population reference intakes (PRIs) are not 'recommended intakes'. J Pediatr Gastroenterol Nutr 1997;25: 236–241.
8 Öhlund I, Hörnell A, Lind T, Hernell O: Dietary fat in infancy should be more focused on quality than on quantity. Eur J Clin Nutr 2007; [Epub ahead of print].
9 Stover PJ: Influence of human genetic variation on nutritional requirements. Am J Clin Nutr 2006;83(suppl):436S–442S.
10 Corella C, Ordovas JM: Single nucleotide polymorphisms that influence lipid metabolism: interaction with dietary factors. Annu Rev Nutr 2005:341–390.
11 Arab L: Individualized nutritional recommendations: do we have the measurements needed to assess risk and make dietary recommendations. Proc Nutr Soc 2004;63:167–172.
12 Waters PJ: How PAH gene mutations cause hyperphenylalaninemia and why mechanisms matters: insights from in vitro expression. Hum Mutat 2003;21:357–369.
13 Therrell BL, Adams J: Newborn screening in North America. J Inherit Metab Dis 2007;30: 447–465.
14 Rodenburg J, Vissers MN, Wiegman A, et al: Statin treatment in children with familial hypercholesterolemia. The younger the better. Circulation 2007;116;664–668.
15 Haney EM, Huffman LH, Bougatsos C, et al: Screening and treatment for lipid disorders in children and adolescents: systematic evidence review for the US Preventive Services Task Force. Pediatrics 2007;120:e189–e214.
16 Heyman MB, Committee on Nutrition: Lactose intolerance in infants, children and adolescents. Pediatrics 2006;118:1279–1286.
17 Ennath NS, Sahi T, Savilahti E, et al: Identification of a variant associated with adult-type hypolactasia. Nat Genet 2002;30:233–237.
18 Tishkoff SA, Reed FA, Ranciaro A. et al: Convergent adaptation of human lactase persistence in Africa and Europe. Nat Genet 2007;39:31–40.
19 Forsberg G, Hernell O, Hammarström S, Hammarström ML: Concomitant increase in IL-10 and pro-inflammatory cytokines in intraepithelial lymphocyte subsets in celiac disease. Int Immunol 2007;19:993–1001.
20 Ivarsson A, Persson LÅ, Nyström L, et al: Epidemic of coeliac disease in Swedish children. Acta Paediatr 2000;89:165–171.
21 Ivarsson A, Hernell O, Stenlund H, Persson LA: Breast-feeding protects against celiac disease. Am J Clin Nutr 2002;75:914–921.
22 Ivarsson A, Myléus A, Wall S: Towards preventing celiac disease – an epidemiological approach; in Fasano A, Troncone R, Branski D (eds): Pediatric and Adolescent Medicine. Front Celiac Dis. Basel, Karger, 2008, vol 12, in press.
23 Wahlberg J, Vaarala O, Ludvigsson J; ABIS-Study Group: Dietary risk factors for the emergence of type 1 diabetes-related autoantibodies in 2 year-old Swedish children. Br J Nutr 2006;95:603–608.
24 Ziegler A-G, Schmid S, Huber D, et al: Early infant feeding and risk of developing type 1 diabetes-associated autoantibodies. JAMA 2003;290:1721–1728.

25 WHO/NMH/MNC/CRA/03.2: Prevention of Allergy and Allergic Asthma. 2002.
26 Kramer MS, Kakuma R: Maternal dietary antigen avoidance during pregnancy or lactation, or both, for preventing or treating atopic disease in the child. Cochrane Database Syst Rev 2006;3:CD000133.
27 Kramer MS, Kakuma R: Optimal duration of exclusive breastfeeding. Cochrane Database Syst Rev 2002;1:CD003517.
28 Muraro A, Dreborg S, Halken S, et al: Dietary prevention of allergic diseases in infants and small children. Part III. Critical review of published peer-reviewed observational and interventional studies and final recommendations. Pediatr Allergy Immunol 2004;15:291–307.
29 Brand PLP, Vlieg-Boerstra BJ, Dubois AEJ: Dietary prevention of allergic disease in children: Are current recommendations really based on good evidence? Pediatr Allergy Immunol 2007; 18:475–479.
30 Prescott SL, Björkstén B: Probiotics for the prevention or treatment of allergic diseases. J Allergy Clin Immunol 2007;120:255–262.

Discussion

Dr. Vaarala: In diabetes research we have seen that there are high-risk and moderate-risk genotypes. Nowadays there is a very high incidence of diabetes in Sweden and Finland, and the proportion of patients carrying the so-called moderate-risk genotype is increasing all the time, therefore the environmental pressure for type-1 diabetes is increasing so that even with a low genetic risk the diabetic phenotype develops. When the incidence of celiac disease was increasing in Sweden, did you find that there were more patients with the DQ8 genotype which is usually quite rare in patients with celiac disease?

Dr. Hernell: I can't answer that because we didn't do genotyping, but I think that it is a very interesting question. However, based on our studies recently I don't think that this is the explanation. There are also other aspects of this epidemic. Our best estimate is that an unfavorable gluten introduction accounted for at most 50% of the increase during the epidemic, which means that there is still 50% to be explained. One factor that also seems to have contributed is if a child had more than 3 infections during the first 6 months, that is actually before the introduction of gluten, compared to fewer infections. Thus, it seems as if infections actually have something to do with the epidemic and indeed recently rotavirus has been implicated as a trigger. It could also be as simple as if you have more infections you probably have an increased gut permeability which results in an increased risk of an untoward reaction when gluten is introduced.

Dr. Szajewska: In addition to what you said, it may be interesting for the audience that there is a randomized control trial financed by the European Union in which we are trying to find out whether or not it is possible to induce tolerance to gluten in genetically predisposed children by introducing small amounts of gluten during breastfeeding between the ages of 4 and 6 months (www.preventcd.com). I know that there are slightly different recommendations compared to other parts of Europe when it comes to the introduction of gluten in Sweden. Can you please comment? My understanding is that gluten is introduced in small amounts and gradually and, as I already asked some time ago, what is a small amount? You said you didn't know, but perhaps you know now.

Dr. Hernell: No, I don't know what it is because in the study we had to define it one way or the other. What we did was actually to calculate at 7 months of age the intake of gluten in cases and controls. We used the controls, the reference group, and graded their intake into the upper one third, the middle one third and the lower one third, and then we took the upper one third of that intake and defined that as a large amount. That was the best we could do. If you want me to give you an exact amount in grams per day, I can't do that.

Dr. Brandtzaeg: Regarding these Swedish experiments; when you have the epidemiology ready and it turns out that you have only delayed the presentation of celiac disease, would that be an advantage or not? There has been a heated discussion on this aspect. Even with the EU project, early induction of tolerance may turn out to be broken later, so this is really an uncertain long-term investigation.

Dr. Hernell: It is, and I don't think there is a simple answer to that question. Probably it was quite naïve to say that if a child is going to have celiac disease it is better to get the diagnosis early and be correctly treated. However, now it seems that celiac disease is a spectrum and we see more and more cases that are diagnosed at an older age and many of them have only vague symptoms and not the typical subtotal villus atrophy. Perhaps they only have an increased number of intraepithelial lymphocytes in the mucosa. Do these children benefit from the treatment to the same extent as infants with severe malabsorption? We really don't know. Moreover, a gluten-free diet is said to reduce the risk of other associated diseases like diabetes, but again I think we don't really know if the preventive effect is the same for all celiacs. There is also the question of transient disease and I think in Finland they have found that it is not uncommon with an increase in transglutaminase antibodies during late infancy that spontaneously normalizes with time. So what does this actually mean? Is it part of developing oral tolerance in those individuals? We really do not know.

Dr. Salminen: The last slide nicely summarizes future opportunities. It is really trying to use modern technology, you see on the top that the diaper is full so you need to do something. On the first line it gives you the urine analysis, the hydration level of the baby and tells you to add vitamin C. In the stool analysis I am still worried about the extra serving of cereals and the figs indicating that the bowel movements are regular, but at least I like the approach to combine high technology with very simple individual recommendations on what to do next.

Dr. Lau: I agree with some of your concerns regarding providing personal recommendations on nutrition requirements, but on the other hand some of the obstacles that you listed are not insurmountable. For example it is true that at the current stage some should probably not be used for routine profiling and then followed by recommendations. We are at a stage where discoveries are being made, and these discoveries can be translated to something even more simple that can be given to the general public and not necessarily using very high profiling as the final step. As far as having a lot of genotype subgroups, it is true that the more homogenous the groupings you can define, the more likely you will be able to actually find the gene step associated with certain types of phenotypes. But that is the reason why these studies need to be done as an international consortium where you would be able to acquire that type of study population. As far as the cost of genotyping, it is expensive but on the other hand there are now resources available that are willing to pay for such studies. For example, the Wellcome Trust actually has an open competition for people to propose studies, and as long as the sample size is large enough to power it, they are willing to take it into consideration and actually underwrite the cost of the genotyping. So there are ways to get around some of these obstacles, including the one that says that nutritional effects may take a long time to manifest. It is very similar to what we are doing in oncology as well, we cannot wait for the tumors to progress before we say this doesn't work. So the effort is to try to find surrogate markers that can correlate with these long-term effects such that you can actually carry out your study in a more realistic timeframe. Plus if you can find the surrogate markers in the blood or plasma that would make it even more feasible because it won't involve any invasive procedure to sample the patient. Yes, these are real concerns but perhaps there are creative ways of getting around these concerns that I hope the community will be willing to take on.

Dr. Hernell: I completely agree with you that we will use these tools, no doubt about that, and they will become simpler and, hopefully, be integrated in the recommendations in the future. But I wanted to point out the problem of extrapolating a future perspective from experiences in specific pharmacological treatments of defined malignant diseases within oncology. I think that when it comes to nutrition the situation is far more complex. When we consider nutrition and particularly individualized nutrition recommendations for healthy populations, the question is whether it is worth doing gene chips on such individuals to start to try to define an optimal diet. My understanding is that it depends on what we actually mean with personalized nutrition recommendations. Does personalized mean strictly individual or does it mean dividing current recommendations into more subpopulations of healthy individuals? As I mentioned, presently we can't even agree on whether we should increase the intake of folic acid for a subpopulation of healthy individuals (pre-pregnant and pregnant women) or for the entire population, so I think we are quite far from individualizing recommendations.

Dr. Walker: I do think there is a role for personalized nutrition in the context of intrauterine nutrition, but I rather disagree with you on the folic acid story. It is a tragedy to have a child with a neural tube defect (NTD), and if we know that 25% of the population has a SNP that requires more folic acid, then I think that is a reason to raise the dose. The same thing has been shown in choline and vitamin D is also in question. So I think these are areas where malnutrition or undernutrition have a profound impact on the patient. I think we really need to concentrate on that and look at genomics, but also move those recommendations along.

Dr. Hernell: I agree with you to some extent but, looking at folic acid fortification, I don't think we have enough information. Every infant born with a NTD is a tragedy and of course we should do everything we can to reduce the risk. However, we must bear in mind the possible risk of increasing the number of cancer cases in the entire population. How many infants born with NTDs could be spared by fortification in a country like Sweden, given that women today are screened and when NTD is diagnosed there is a parental choice to have an abortion? It has been estimated that the figure would be 5–10 cases/year. This needs to be balanced against the incidence of colon cancer in the population. If that incidence increases just a few percent, this would concern many more individuals.

Dr. Walker: But in that instance you could increase folic acid during the pregnancy and then you could reduce it thereafter. I don't think a single increase in folic acid during pregnancy is going to enhance the likelihood of colon cancer that much. So I think in this particular situation 5 cases is 5 cases too many and I think you really need to look at it.

Dr. Hernell: The problem, when I was discussing the Swedish or the European cases, is the question of increasing the intake for the whole population by fortifying flour. But if the recommendation is to increase folic acid intake for women before they become pregnant and then reduce the intake to normal after the first trimester or after pregnancy, that is fine. But the problem is that there is a substantial fraction of those you want to reach who will not be reached by such an approach. So it is very complicated.

Dr. Bier: I wasn't actually planning to talk about folic acid with my comment but I think it is precisely the example that illustrates the benefits of personalized nutrition for the reasons you stated. I think it is clear that we don't have the tools yet to be able to fully deal with personalizing nutrition and I don't think anybody wants too personal nutrition. The case of folic acid is I think the precise reason why impersonalized nutrition is problematic because you are making recommendations for an entire popula-tion. In a sense you treat many thousands of people to find one you need to treat. As one of the people who was in the committee that voted to fortify grain products in the United States for folic acid I can spend a lot of time talking about that. I think if we had, for example, the ability to determine who was going to be personalized that would actually be an advantage in this case. Now we have all of our nutrition recom-mendations that treat the great fraction of the population that doesn't need to be treated.

Dr. Hernell: I completely agree with you; if we had that information we would not have had this discussion.

Bier DM, German JB, Lönnerdal B (eds): Personalized Nutrition for the Diverse Needs of Infants and Children.
Nestlé Nutr Workshop Ser Pediatr Program, vol 62, pp 253–256,
Nestec Ltd., Vevey/S. Karger AG, Basel, © 2008.

Concluding Remarks

This is again to reiterate that these last 3 days have been extremely exciting; this has been one of the most interdisciplinary and collegial meetings I have ever attended. On behalf of the organizers I am delighted with the outcome, and it is quite a challenge to try and summarize it all. Let me go through some of the concepts that we have come up with.

If we are going to take a broad overview of this, if we are going to imagine that we are going to personalize diets for infants and children, we first have to ask the questions: do we really know how children differ; are there meanings for these differences; whatever the consequences of these differences are, are they genuinely the sort of long-term outcomes that one would imagine to be genuinely worthwhile? If there are differences, are we in a position to accurately assess those, are there technologies to distinguish individuals, and then finally, can we act predictably, do we know enough nutrition to genuinely change folate?

At the meeting we tried to look at these perspectives. How do children differ? There were several presentations in which the genetic basis of variation and population is described. *Bert Koletzko* gave a very clear indication that very specific polymorphisms in the gene responsible for desaturating polyunsaturated fatty acids have a meaningful consequence on the level of those products and on their functional role in manipulating a variety of lipid-signaling systems, so some of the variations in people are clearly due to explicit identifiable genetic polymorphisms. But we also found that the environment has an important role. *Seppo Salminen* and several people illustrated, for example, that if a child is born by cesarean section the chances of it being environmentally inoculated with the appropriate bacteria are much less, and so in addition to genetics the infant's environment alone can have a meaningful long-term processing effect on phenotype and outcome. We also heard from various people, notably *Peter Gluckman* at the beginning of the conference, that the environment at a specific window of time, particularly in the infant and childhood period, can imprint that individual to lifelong changes in their

253

ability to manage the environment in which they find themselves. *Peter Gluckman* emphasized that our modern environment is not something that the Darwinian process really had in mind, so we have to be aware that early imprinting can have an effect and that is another extra-genetic effect on our differences. Finally, each of us has different microflora which is established early in life and remains quite persistent through to old age, a very important aspect.

We heard from *Ingegerd Adlerberth* how variability can be established, again not depending on genetics. If we look at the consequences, we could now spend another 3 days on this. There were very illuminating talks on the role of variations in humans on things like immunology and immune outcomes, their ability to resist disease, on allergy and the differences between people both in genetics and imprinting on the microflora, on the development and subsequent severity of allergy. I don't think we any of us were prepared for just how devastatingly *Dennis Bier* would describe the obesity epidemic. Very scary numbers in United States, and I think the rest of the world is desperately hoping that the United States has gone this way on their own but to their horror they are beginning to realize that it is not the case and clearly obesity is a diet-cost phenomenon. On the hills of the obesity epidemic there is an epidemic of metabolic diabetes and the predispositions to diabetes established earlier in life are becoming particularly discouraging. The fact that mothers who are overweight and considerably more predisposed to gestational diabetes pass along that predisposition for diabetes to their infants before they are born, is again an example of a non-genetic but a particularly discouraging aspect of the individual variation that we are forcing upon in the children.

Ching Lau talked about cancer and the variations that he is seeing in the ability to predict how patients respond to treatment. Again these differences are important and the variations due to various aspects of genetics and imprinting are the consequences. We spent actually some very interesting time on the way this should be assessed. It is very clear from all these presentations that the basic idea is to take the genetic genotype and use it as a means to distinguish, to differentiate, the population, will not happen. The complexity of genotyping is just too great for prediction, and we have seen various other ways that our genotype can vary from genetics. The fact that we are different is clear; the fact these differences are important to our lifelong health is also clear, but we also realize that we cannot use genotyping as a simple means to predict lifelong health. We have to use much more innovative and comprehensive assessment technologies to see those differences.

Hans Hofstraat talked about molecular imaging and how far along the industrialization process this has come, bringing the practice to technologies for disease. He was very enthusiastic about the opportunities to be able to bring these routes of technologies and their accuracy in position to the level that we would need to be able to understand the phenotypic variation in terms of diet and health. Genotyping was discussed, and it is clear that these technologies are coming along very successfully.

Jason Chieh talked about the nutrigenomic concept and that there are some very important things that genotyping actually can tell you. Selected genotypic analysis for, as *Dennis Bier* pointed out, susceptibility to methylation and improvement of neural tube defects by folate represents a very obvious opportunity. It is not that we would ignore genotyping, we just can't use it as a sole basis.

Rob Waterland talked about methylation and in fact not only is he able to understand mechanistically the effect of the environment on DNA methylation, he showed that it is increasingly possible to measure this to actually assess in individuals what their early history of life did to their methylation on their own individual DNA, an astonishing advance in methodology. Expression profiling is already being brought to practice in diagnostics for cancer; it is clear that this is a very attractive assessment technology for a variety of health aspects ultimately including nutrition.

Gerry Berry talked about the potential of metabolic profiling using practical examples for a variety of diseases such as PKU. *Piero Rinaldo* also talked about the fact that blood spot analyses, which seems to be a very simple basic technology, are going to be a platform that will serve many of the things that we imagine, and which exist today. Ironically many of the issues that are limiting it are not scientific at all, they are related to the politics of moving forward. And we saw in the meeting that there is a great deal of ongoing debate on how much faster we can move this.

Can we act on these differences, this is sort of the good news in the bad news. This is where nutrition as a science should be delivering the actionable science on which we base the future of diet recommendations for individuals and we have to be honest, this is an area where we need some significant work. *Bo Lönnerdal* talked about proteins and the ability to understand, for example, simple variations in the amount of protein to be delivered even as simply as the phase of infant formula, early infancy, different protein level than later, a very straightforward and as you pointed out a very actionable and potentially important improvement.

Oligosaccharides, *Seppo Salminen* talked about probiotics, the ability to deliver bacteria. This is such a fascinating and growing field that there is little question that in the next few years we will see very individualized probiotics as a concept for particular individuals at risk, etc. *Bert Koletzko* again talked about lipids, the ability to recognize people who need a different lipid profile and then the ability to deliver them. Finally *Bo Lönnerdal* talked about micronutrients and treatment with for example iron, that some individuals in a population are significantly enriched, that their health is improved by the exact same amount of iron added to their diet, but that another group in that population could suffer deleterious consequences. So even something so simple, which we think of as being so straightforward, as iron supplementation genuinely and in certain populations needs an individualized approach. So what do we need to do? It is pretty clear that we need to push methodologies that are associated with getting quantitatively accurate end points in association with diet and health, but this is an important limitation, there is no question. The trials that should be done need to incorporate the kind of methods and mechanisms capable of seeing the texture of the population. If large trials are being conducted we need to know not just how the average mean population responds, but also how the population on an individual level responds. We also have to recognize the importance of accuracy and specificity of ingredients; simply measuring probiotics without knowing for example the genome, oligosaccharides, is not enough. Feeding simple polymers and not knowing what their actual structures and functions are, we need to be much better there.

Finally the industry, it would be very good to see the industry explore methods and to actually begin to consider how to deliver personalized foods to the population. What is the business model that will make this a success? If it costs more money than it delivers, it is not going to work. We have to continue to support multidisciplinary research. *Ching Lau* showed us that capabilities are available; we want to bring those together and that is going to require recruiting scientists from the many disciplines that nutrition has.

We have moved very much forward in our oligosaccharide program; we would never have thought about milk and nutrition before. We brought *Carlito Lebrilla* and *David Mills,* who had not thought about the microbiology of oligosaccharides, a world class analytical chemist and a world class microbiologist together, and they are now working on a very well-defined program. I think *Dennis Bier's* picture of all those walking sticks racing around Finland is proof positive that we clearly need more workshops in the northern countries. On behalf of the organizers, I am delighted that you could come and we will see you hopefully at another workshop.

D.M. Bier, J.B. German, B. Lönnerdal

Subject Index

Subject Index